INJURY CONTROL

In the twentieth century, evidence-based injury prevention and control strategies have contributed to a substantial decline in the number of deaths associated with injury. However, researchers in the field of injury prevention have often gathered their study methods from other disciplines; it can be difficult for injury investigators to locate all of the research tools that can be applied to problems related to injury.

Injury Control: A Guide to Research and Program Evaluation addresses the growing need for a comprehensive source of knowledge on all research designs available for injury control and research. Included in this accessible guidebook is information about choices in study design, details about study execution, and discussion of specific tools such as injury severity scales, program evaluations and systematic reviews. Epidemiologists, health service investigators, trauma surgeons and emergency medicine physicians will find this a useful source for understanding, reviewing, and conducting research related to injuries.

Dr. Frederick P. Rivara is Director of the Harborview Injury Prevention and Research Center and founding President of the International Society of Child and Adolescent Injury Prevention. He is also the head of the Division of General Pediatrics at the University of Washington and has conducted research on injury epidemiology and control for more than two decades.

Dr. Peter Cummings joined the Department of Epidemiology at the University of Washington in 1993 after 21 years in clinical medicine, including 10 years in emergency medicine. His research and publications are related to injuries, emergency medicine, and research methods.

Dr. Thomas D. Koepsell is Professor and former Chair of the Department of Epidemiology at the University of Washington. He has conducted research on the etiology and prevention of injuries and non-communicable diseases for over two decades and is the author of over 200 scientific papers and book chapters.

Dr. David C. Grossman is Co-Director of the Harborview Injury Prevention and Research Center and Associate Professor of Pediatrics at the University of Washington in Seattle. His main research interests are in childhood injuries, firearm injury, suicide, motor vehicle occupant injury, and injuries to rural and Native American populations.

Dr. Ronald V. Maier is Surgeon-in-Chief and Director of Surgical Critical Care at Harborview Medical Center and Director of the Northwest Regional Trauma Center in Seattle, Washington. He is a Fellow of the American Association for the Advancement of Science and an active researcher in the field of injury control.

INJURY CONTROL

A Guide to Research and Program Evaluation

Edited by

Frederick P. Rivara
*Harborview Injury
Prevention and
Research Center
Seattle, Washington*

Peter Cummings
*Harborview Injury
Prevention and
Research Center
Seattle, Washington*

Thomas D. Koepsell
*Harborview Injury
Prevention and
Research Center
Seattle, Washington*

David C. Grossman
*Harborview Injury
Prevention and
Research Center
Seattle, Washington*

Ronald V. Maier
*Harborview Injury
Prevention and
Research Center
Seattle, Washington*

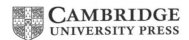
CAMBRIDGE
UNIVERSITY PRESS

PUBLISHED BY THE PRESS SYNDICATE OF
THE UNIVERSITY OF CAMBRIDGE
The Pitt Building, Trumpington Street, Cambridge, United Kingdom

CAMBRIDGE UNIVERSITY PRESS
The Edinburgh Building, Cambridge CB2 2RU, UK
40 West 20th Street, New York, NY 10011-4211, USA
10 Stamford Road, Oaklaigh, Melbourne 3166, Australia
Ruiz de Alarcón 13, 28014 Madrid, Spain
Dock House, The Waterfront, Cape Town 8001, South Africa

http://www.cambridge.org

First published 2001

Printed in the United States of America

Typeface 10$\frac{1}{2}$/13 Times   System 3b2 6.03d [KW]

A catalog record for this book is available from the British Library

Library of Congress Cataloging-in-Publication Data

Injury control: research and program evaluation/edited by Frederick P. Rivara . . . [et al.]
    p. cm.
    Includes bibliographical references.
    1. Accidents–Prevention–Research. 2. Wounds and injuries–Prevention–Research I.
Rivara, Frederick P.

RA772.A25 I55 2000
617.1–dc21   00-027894

ISBN 0 521 66152 8 hardback

Every effort has been made in preparing this book to provide accurate and up-to-date information
that is in accord with accepted standards and practice at the time of publication. Nevertheless, the
authors, editors, and publisher can make no warranties that the information contained herein is
totally free from error, not least because clinical standards are constantly changing through research
and regulation. The authors, editors, and publisher therefore disclaim all liability for direct or
consequential damages resulting from the use of material contained in this book. Readers are
strongly advised to pay careful attention to information provided by the manufacturer of any drugs
or equipment that they plan to use.

Contents

Contributor list

J. Michael Bowling
Injury Prevention and Research
  Center
University of North Carolina,
  Chapel Hill
Chapel Hill, NC

Frances Bunn
Department of Epidemiology and
  Public Health
Institute of Child Health
London UK

Peter Cummings
Harborview Injury Prevention &
  Research Center
Department of Epidemiology
University of Washington
Seattle, WA

Carolyn G. DiGuiseppi
Department of Epidemiology and
  Public Health
Institute of Child Health
London UK

Lois A. Fingerhut
Office of Analysis
Epidemiology and Health Promotion
National Center for Health Statistics
Hyattsville, MD

John Graham
Harvard Center for Risk Analysis
Harvard School of Public Health
Harvard University
Boston, MA

David C. Grossman
Harborview Injury Prevention &
  Research Center
Department of Pediatrics
University of Washington
Seattle, WA

Elizabeth McLoughlin
Trauma Foundation
San Francisco General Hospital
San Francisco, CA

Charles Mock
Harborview Injury Prevention and
  Research Center
Department of Surgery
University of Washington
Seattle, WA

Beth A. Mueller
Harborview Injury Prevention &
  Research Center
Department of Epidemiology
University of Washington
Seattle, WA

Robyn Norton
Institute for International Health
    Research and Development
Crows Nest, AUSTRALIA

Grant O'Keefe
Department of Surgery
The University of Texas
Southwestern Medical Center
Dallas, TX

Lorna Rhodes
Department of Anthropology
University of Washington
Seattle, WA

Michael Rhodes
Professor of Surgery
Thomas Jefferson University
Wilmington, DE

Ralph W. Hingson
Boston University School of Public
    Health
Department of Social & Behavioral
    Sciences
Boston, MA

Jonathan Howland
Boston University School of Public
    Health
Department of Social & Behavioral
    Sciences
Boston, MA

Gregory J. Jurkovich
Harborview Injury Prevention and
    Research Center
Department of Surgery
University of Washington
Seattle, WA

Thomas D. Koepsell
Harborview Injury Prevention &
    Research Center

Department of Epidemiology
University of Washington
Seattle, WA

Jess F. Kraus
Southern California Injury
    Prevention and Research Center
University of California, Los Angeles
School of Public Health
Los Angeles, CA

Ellen MacKenzie
Center for Injury Research and
    Policy
The Johns Hopkins University
School of Hygiene and Public Health
Baltimore, MD

Ronald V. Maier
Harborview Injury Prevention and
    Research Center
Department of Surgery
University of Washington
Seattle, WA

Frederick P. Rivara
Harborview Injury Prevention &
    Research Center
Department of Pediatrics
University of Washington
Seattle, WA

Ian Roberts
Child Monitoring Unit
Institute of Child Health
London UK

Carol W. Runyan
Injury Prevention and Research
    Center
University of North Carolina, Chapel
    Hill
Chapel Hill, NC

Jeffrey J. Sacks
Centers for Disease Control and
    Prevention
Atlanta, GA

Maria Segui-Gomez*
Center for Injury Research and
    Policy
The Johns Hopkins University
School of Hygiene and
    Public Health
Baltimore, MD

Ian G. Stiell
Ottawa Civic Hospital
Loeb Research Institute
Clinical Epidemiology Unit
Ottawa,
Ontario,
CANADA

Helen McGough
Human Subjects Division
University of Washington
Seattle, WA

Robert S. Thompson
Center for Health Studies
Group Health Cooperative of Puget
    Sound
Seattle, WA

Marsha Wolf
Harborview Injury Prevention &
Research Center
Department of Epidemiology
University of Washington
Seattle, WA

*Dr. Segui-Gomez co-wrote the chapter for this book while she was at the Harvard Injury Control and Research Center, Boston, MA.

1

An Overview of Injury Research

Frederick P. Rivara

Accomplishments of Injury Research and Control

During the twentieth century, deaths from infectious diseases have declined dramatically around the world, particularly in industrialized countries. The initial decline occurred due to improved sanitation and public health; more recently it has been due to antibiotics, vaccines, and an increasing emphasis on prevention. Deaths among humankind from injuries have also declined substantially, as shown in Figure 1.1, although the decrease is far less than that for infectious diseases (Baker et al., 1992).

This decline in injury deaths over the last century occurred due to three distinct factors. The first, and in some ways the most important in industrialized countries, has been a general reduction in the exposure to injury hazards as a byproduct of changes in occupations, safer transportation, better housing, and heating, and many other factors that accompanied industrialization. Some hazards such as horses have been replaced by others such as motor vehicles; however, far fewer people are involved in underground mining, smelting of steel, farming, logging, and other dangerous occupations today than there were 100, 50, or even 20 years ago. Building codes have made our homes safer; improvements in highway design and airplane technology have made our travel safer. Equivalent changes in the general environment and the basic application of public health have accounted for far more reduction in infectious disease morbidity and mortality than have antibiotics.

The second factor accounting for the change in injury mortality is more recent: reduction in the risk of dying once injured due to improved medical and surgical care. Much of this improvement in trauma care originated on the battlefield and subsequently moved into the civilian population. The time interval from injury to definitive medical care has decreased dramatically over the course of the century: 12–18 hours in World War I, 6–12 hours in World War II, 2–4 hours in the Korean War, and 1.1 hours in the Vietnam War (Trunkey, 1983). The introduction of early and aggressive fluid therapy, transfusions, antibiotics, new surgical techniques, better instruments for monitoring, and more effective organ support resulted in surgical care making an increasing difference in outcome. Both factors are probably reflected in the declining mortality rate among casualties: 14% in the United States Civil War (1861–65), 8% in World War I (1914–18), 4.5% in World War II (1941–45), 2.5% in the Korean War (1950–53), and 3.6% in the Vietnam War (1965–72)

1

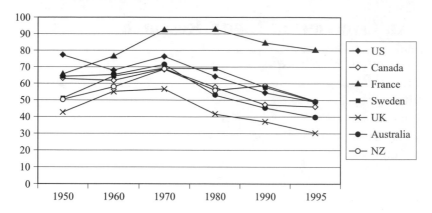

Figure 1.1 Trends in injury mortality for selected countries of the world, 1900–95. Data from Linder and Grove, 1943; Grove and Hetzel, 1968; US Bureau of Census, 1997; UN, 1998.

(Trunkey and Ochsner, 1996). The decline in mortality among those with abdominal war wounds is even more dramatic: 87% in the Civil War, 67% in World War I, and 9% in the Vietnam War. However, further declines in mortality at major trauma centers at the beginning of the twenty-first century will require major breakthroughs in the treatment of traumatic brain injury and multiple organ failure, the most common acute and subacute causes of death among trauma patients.

The third reason for the reduction in injury mortality has been the increasing use of injury control strategies that are based on scientific evidence of their effectiveness. The reduction in traffic mortality per 100 million miles driven is due to the development of safer motor vehicles and roads, and the use of safety equipment such as air bags, seat belts, motorcycle, and bicycle helmets. These advances were based on studies outlining risk factors for injury, and research demonstrating effectiveness of these interventions. Injury prevention strategies have long existed; however, only relatively recently have these interventions been based on firm scientific evidence and rigorous evaluation. It is this evidence-based approach to advances in injury control that holds the most promise in further reducing the impact of injury on our society. The goal of this book is to promote the use of research in the field of injury control and to further advance injury research methods.

History of Injury Research

In many ways, injury research and injury prevention extend back a number of millennia and precede the development of medicine in even its most primitive form. The origins of injury research lie in the age old pursuit of warfare and the desire of leaders to afford at least a modicum of protection to their men, so they could fight on and win their objective. The use of shields in the Trojan War, the use of helmets by the Romans (Simpson, 1996), the development of body armor during the Middle Ages, and the use of military machines, such as those designed by Leonardo da'Vinci for the Duke of Milan are examples of efforts to reduce the risk of injury to a very vulnerable population.

However, the application of the scientific method to injury control did not occur with any regularity until the last 30 years, far later than the use of the scientific method to reduce the burden of disease from infectious agents, for example. The most important reason for this delay in the use of science to control injuries, and one which persists to some degree even today, is the sense of fatalism towards trauma. Injuries are still called accidents, implying a sense of randomness and unpredictability. Trauma is also commonly ascribed to be an act of God, or due to fate. Many blame the injury and its consequences on the victim, and imply they are just rewards for careless or illegal behavior. Few educated people in the last half of the twentieth century would ascribe serious infections as being random events or punishment by God (although human immunodeficiency virus has been evoked as an exception), and hence viewed as non-preventable. Yet, these attitudes have long persisted for injuries both among the public and among professionals (Committee on Injury Prevention and Control, 1999), and have hindered the development of injury control research.

One of the most important milestones in the development of injury research was the publication of *Accident Research: Methods and Approaches* by Haddon et al. in 1964. These authors sought to advance the field of injury (accident) research by compiling together in one place important injury research contributions, and more importantly, to assess the quality of the research, point out pitfalls, and suggest methods to study the injury problem. By bringing together research on injuries from a wide variety of sources and disciplines, their book established the basic principles of the injury field, and is clearly the progenitor of this current volume. Some of the tenets of injury research espoused in their remarkable volume include:

- *Injury as energy transfer*

J. J. Gibson (1961) was an experimental psychologist who recognized in 1961 that injury is due to the transfer of physical energy, either mechanical, thermal, radiant, chemical, or electrical, to the host in an amount which exceeds the threshold for tissue damage. It provided the basis for beginning to view the injury event as separate from the damage to the body, and stimulated others to understand both the limits of tolerance to energy transfer and ways in which this transfer could be mitigated. Many if not most of our injury prevention strategies, such as helmets, air bags, seat belts, and lowered tap water temperature are based on this premise.

- *Biomechanics of injury*

The field of biomechanics is based on understanding the limits of tissue tolerance to energy transfer and designing systems to meet these tolerances. The experiments by John Stapp on himself in a rocket sled in 1957 (Stapp, 1957), the study of survival in falls from as much as 150 feet by DeHaven in 1942 (DeHaven, 1942) and of plane and car crashes in 1952 (DeHaven 1952), the use of barrier tests in 1956 by Severy and Mathewson (1956) to analyze the forces in motor vehicle crashes, and B. J. Campbell's work in 1963 (Campbell, 1963) analyzing the effect of padded dashboards, form the basis of the modern science of injury biomechanics.

• *Use of epidemiology to study injuries*
In 1948, Gordon (Gordon, 1948) outlined the use of the epidemiologic framework to study injuries. He emphasized the interaction of multiple causes, including the agent, host, and environment (encompassing the biologic, physical, and socio-economic environment) in the etiology of injury. In recent years, much attention has been paid to the public health model of injury control. This was in fact laid out by Gordon more than 50 years ago:

> "If home accidents are primarily a public health problem, then that problem is reasonably to be approached in the manner and through the technics that have proved useful for other mass disease problems. This includes first an epidemiologic analysis of the particular situation, an establishment of causes, the development of specific preventive measures directed toward those causes, and finally a periodic evaluation of accomplishment from the program instituted." (Haddon et al., 1964, p. 18)

• *Use of case–control studies to determine injury etiology*
The case–control design has become a cornerstone of modern epidemiology and has been used extensively over the last decade in the injury field. As discussed in chapter 11, the case-control study design has been crucial for examining risk factors for relatively uncommon events, which includes most injuries. One of the first case–control studies in injury control was a study by Haddon et al. (1961) of fatally injured pedestrians in Manhattan. An even earlier case–control study, not featured in this anthology, was a study by Holcomb (1938) examining the risk of motor vehicle crashes related to alcohol.

• *Broadening the framework of injury research to include psychology, sociology, and the social sciences*
Reflecting the diverse background of the three authors, the anthology broadened the base of injury research to include psychology, sociology, and behavioral sciences. They recognized the importance of certain behavior in causing injury, but were among the first to debunk the theory of accident proneness, originally postulated to explain recurrent injury to workers in a British munitions factory (again, the connection between early injury research and warfare) (Greenwood and Woods, 1919). These authors recognized that effective countermeasures for injuries caused primarily by human behavior may in fact be passive measures involving changes to the product or environment rather than attempts to alter behavior.

The contributions collected in *Accident Research: Methods and Approaches* are very clearly the catalyst for the subsequent development of injury research and a second generation of investigators dedicated to the field. Two years after its publication, the National Research Council (1966) published a report, *Accidental Death and Disability: The Neglected Disease of Modern Society*. This focused in particular on trauma care, especially emergency medical services, and trauma research. It emphasized the lack of recognition of injury as a major public health problem, and consequently the poor funding for research in this area. As a result of this report, National Institute of Health funds for the study of the acute care of trauma victims expanded, especially shock and its resuscitation, and the development of trained emergency medical technicians and properly equipped ambulances was made a priority.

That same year, the National Highway Traffic Safety Administration (originally called the National Highway Safety Bureau) was created. Headed by William Haddon, Jr, the foremost injury investigator in the world, the agency sought to improve the safety of vehicles by basing design standards on firm science. Haddon's accomplishment was to take a field which as he said, "has been in its purest sense prescientific" (Haddon, 1967, p. 10) and base it on knowledge and scientific inquiry, while convincing the public this was the right thing to do. As a direct result of his efforts, injury control research has become the most well developed in the automotive field.

Perhaps the most important milestone in injury research during the last two decades was the publication in 1985 of another National Research Council report, *Injury in America* (Committee on Trauma Research, 1985). This report established injury research as a distinct scientific field, which nevertheless incorporated research from a wide variety of disciplines and emphasized an interdisciplinary approach to the problem. *Injury in America* recommended a major investment in injury research and the establishment of a center, based at the Centers for Disease Control and Prevention, which would coordinate a national injury research program. The National Center for Injury Prevention and Control was established, five centers of excellence in the form of Injury Control Research Centers were funded, implementation programs were initiated in state health departments, and research support for individual investigators was made available. The emphasis was on interdisciplinary approaches to injury control.

The publication of *Injury in America* resulted in a remarkable acceleration of injury research not only in the United States, but around the world. The infusion of new money into the field attracted skilled investigators and new trainees. The focus on interdisciplinary research led to the expansion of injury control to intentional injuries, especially those due to firearms. Other injury prevention programs had existed in other parts of the world, in particular the Child Accident Prevention Trust started by Hugh Jackson in the United Kingdom, and the Joint Committee for the Prevention of Childhood Accidents in Sweden led by Ragnar Berfenstam. However, these programs had mostly focused on program implementation, and did not conduct research on acute care or rehabilitation of trauma patients. In the last 15 years, injury research programs have developed in other parts of the world, including New Zealand, Australia, Canada, the United Kingdom, France, India, and elsewhere.

The volume of injury research has expanded almost geometrically in the last 15 years since the publication of *Injury in America*, from approximately 2000 articles per year on trauma, accidents, and injury prevention before 1985 to nearly 5000 articles per year in the last 8 years. Funding has also increased, although it is still far less than for other diseases such as cancer and heart disease with far fewer

	Host	Agent	Physical environment	Social-cultural environment
Pre-event phase				
Event phase				
Post-event phase				

Figure 1.2 Haddon matrix.

potential years of life lost before age 65 and markedly less burden of disability than injuries.

Framework (Models) for Injury Research

The approach to injury research in this volume reflects the approach of the editors and of the Harborview Injury Prevention and Research Center – research should be interdisciplinary and be based on the scientific method. Some of the research methods discussed in this volume are based directly on tools of epidemiology, such as case–control studies. Others are based on social science such as survey designs. Many methods are used across disciplines such as cohort or longitudinal observational study designs and randomized controlled trials for intervention studies.

Much of injury research in the last two decades has occurred in the public health arena and has used the epidemiological model first proposed for injury research by Gordon in 1948. This model includes the host, the agent of injury (energy transfer), the vector for this energy transfer, and the environment (Robertson, 1998). Haddon added another dimension to this model by separating out the factors which pre-dispose an injury producing event to occur from the actual event itself in which energy is transferred to the host in an amount to cause damage. Haddon also added the post-event phase, encompassing transport, emergency care, and reha-bilitation, which affect survival and ultimate outcome once the energy transfer has occurred. Combining these phases of injury with the public health model, he created the now familiar Haddon matrix for the study of injury etiology and prevention (Figure 1.2).

Other disciplines have also made important contributions. The field of auto-motive medicine and motor vehicle design is based on the science of biomechanics, which uses the principles of physics and mechanics to examine the response of the body to mechanical energy transfer (Committee on Trauma Research, 1985; Committee on Injury Prevention and Control, 1999). It establishes the levels of injury tolerance for different tissues in the body, and examines how the energy transfer can be attenuated to decrease or eliminate injury. It also can be used to test the efficacy of interventions involving product design. The field of biomechanics has been most well developed for bony injury (Nahum and Melvin, 1993), but has also played important parts in understanding the pathophysiology of visceral and brain injuries.

Research into violence-related injury has been predominantly conducted by criminologists, psychologists, and sociologists. More recently, violence has come to be viewed as a public health problem as well, and has attracted the interest of more traditional public health investigators. As with other types of injury problems, a variety of disciplines, all based on the scientific method, can contribute to a better understanding of the causes of both intentional and unintentional injuries, their prevention, and control. Psychology and anthropology bring to the injury field an expertise in the study of human factors which increase the risk of injury, as well as the impact of injury on the cognitive, emotional, and mental well being of the individual. Psychology has helped us to understand how people perceive risk and how this influences behavior (Committee on Injury Prevention and Control, 1999). This has been a major contribution to our understanding of how to improve the effectiveness of intervention strategies.

Sociology covers a very wide range of phenomena around the conduct of individuals in relationship to others. It postulates that human actions are limited or determined by the environment. Sociology uses qualitative research techniques as well as quantitative data analysis in both experimental and observational studies. These quantitative research techniques are no different than those used by psychology or epidemiology.

Thus, the framework of injury research as espoused by Haddon can be seen to be inclusive of contributions from a wide variety of disciplines. Epidemiology contributes the basic dimension of host–agent–environment. Psychology and sociology provide us with theoretical models and tools for better understanding the host and environment contributions, respectively. Biomechanics provides us with tools to examine the event phase of injuries, both in injury causation and injury prevention. Medicine and nursing provide the postacute care of the injured patients as well as interventions to reduce risk factors in the host for injury occurrence. All of these disciplines are necessary for the control of injuries.

The Future of Injury Research

At the beginning of the twenty-first century, science is dominated by the Human Genome Project, molecular biology, technology transfer, and information technology. Injury research must incorporate these scientific advances as it searches for etiologic mechanisms of injury, tests new interventions, especially those based on new technology and laboratory discoveries, and examines the impact of interventions on patient outcomes. Figure 1.3 outlines how the different facets of injury research are integrated with one another as well as linked to the advances in biomechanics, molecular biology, and community intervention research.

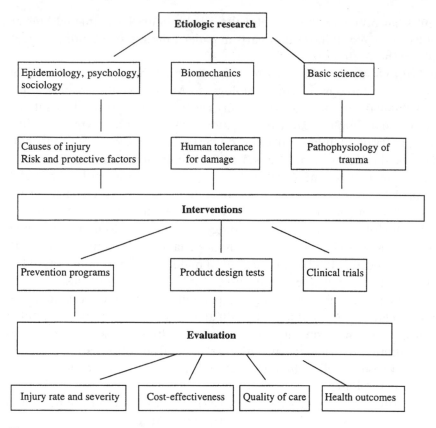

Figure 1.3 Model of injury research.

Etiologic Research

The goal of etiologic studies is to identify cause, defined as "an antecedent event, condition, or characteristic for the occurrence of the [injury] at the moment it occurred, given that other conditions are fixed." (Rothman and Greenland, 1998, p. 8). In other words, if a cause is absent, the injury would not have occurred at that particular time.

The proximate "cause" of injury is transfer of energy to a person at levels which exceed the threshold for tissue damage. Injuries occur frequently in a population, although more serious injury that results in substantial damage and physician care, hospitalization or death is relatively uncommon. Etiologic studies of injuries are concerned with understanding those factors that increase the risk for such injuries or the factors that protect against injury. These factors include the standard epidemiologic dimensions of host, agent, and environment. Risk and protective factors can also be approached from a social science context, and include behavior of the injured individual and of those in the environment, including family and community.

Etiologic research interacts with the laboratory based sciences. Biomechanics contributes to an understanding of the forces acting on an individual and the responses of organs and tissues to these forces. Etiologic hypotheses developed from examination of case series of patients or analysis of large data sets can be tested in the laboratory under controlled experimental conditions. Alternatively, hypotheses derived from laboratory experiments can be tested on a wider population or field basis.

Etiologic research can be carried down to the molecular level to understand how injuries occur and how variations in the host will affect the tolerance and variable response to injury. The Human Genome Project will allow us to understand reasons for individual variations in risk of an injury event, variations in response to energy transfer, and variations in the pathophysiologic cascade of trauma in the organism.

Etiologic research should not be an isolated exercise enumerating a list of risk or protective factors for a particular injury problem. The focus should be ultimately, and always, on better understanding the factors leading to injury in order to intervene with effective prevention strategies. Thus, particular attention should be placed on factors which are mutable. Some have argued that attention to unchangeable risk factors such as age, gender, and socioeconomic status is appropriate because it will allow intervention programs to be better targeted. This is sometimes true, although some of these risk factors are relatively nonspecific (e.g., male gender) and do not allow programs to be appropriately narrowly targeted.

Etiologic studies will usually take the form of cohort or case–control observational studies. These studies compare injured and uninjured individuals to determine host, agent and environment factors which affect the risk of injury. Case series can sometimes provide such information if a powerful association exists. Experimental studies such as randomized controlled trials are usually designed to test the effect of a specific intervention, but will often shed important light on the effect of risk factors on injury occurrence as well. Experimental trials are the tools of the basic sciences and biomechanics in unraveling the human response to energy transfer and trauma.

Design of Prevention Programs

Over the last few decades, a science of prevention has evolved and has resulted in intervention programs, including those for the prevention of injuries, being potentially much more effective. This science is theory driven and rests on a firm foundation of qualitative and quantitative research. Whether it be the Health Belief Model (Becker and Mainman, 1975), the Social Learning Model (Bandura, 1995), the PRECEDE Model (Green and Kreuter, 1991), or the Haddon Matrix described previously (see section on accomplishments of injury research and control) nearly all theory driven interventions provide the opportunity and background for multiple points to intervene in the web of injury causation. Many injury prevention programs have largely ignored the large body of literature on health promotion and disease prevention. Future intervention programs must be science based if increasingly more difficult problems are to be addressed.

Evaluation of Prevention Programs

A key use of research is to evaluate the impact of prevention programs on the rate and/or severity of injury. The injury field has not suffered from a lack of intervention programs, and for nearly all injury problems a variety of interventions have been developed and implemented. However, what has been lacking is rigorous research evaluating the effectiveness of these interventions in reducing injuries, or even the effect on more proximate outcome measures such as changes in risk or protective behavior. The number of rigorous evaluations which have been done is surprisingly small. In a recent review of child injury prevention measures (Rivara et al., 1997), over 50,000 citations were searched for intervention programs; less than 100 rigorous evaluation studies were found. Interventions in some areas of the injury field have been better examined than in other areas. For example, motor vehicle occupant injuries are the most common cause of fatal injury in most developed countries. The impact on injuries of a variety of intervention programs have been examined, especially issues related to occupant protection and driving while intoxicated. Yet, even here there is a dearth of rigorous evaluations (Rivara and MacKenzie, 1999).

Evaluation of intervention programs in medicine and public health has become more rigorous in recent years. The efforts of such groups as the Cochrane Collaboration, the York Center for Dissemination in the United Kingdom, and the U.S. Preventive Services Task Force to examine the effectiveness of clinical and public health interventions across the field of medicine have established controlled trials, especially randomized controlled trials, as the benchmark for program evaluation.

Evaluation of Clinical Interventions for Acute Care and Rehabilitation of Injured Patients

Injury control also includes basic, translational, and clinical trials in acute care and rehabilitation research. For those individuals who have been injured, the goal is to intervene in such a way as to prevent death and to return the person to their pre-injury level of functioning as much as possible. Injury control encompasses this broader mandate and includes the care of the acutely injured patient followed by rehabilitation, as well as primary prevention.

In the last few years, there has been an increasing emphasis on the practice of evidenced-based medicine – basing clinical decisions on scientific evidence of effectiveness (Sackett et al., 1991). For therapeutic interventions, the sine qua non of effectiveness is the randomized controlled trial. This applies not only to drug treatment, but to other interventions such as the use of hypothermia for the treatment of traumatic brain injury (Marion et al., 1997), and cognitive therapy for the rehabilitation of patients with traumatic brain injury (Institute of Medicine, 1997). It can even be applied to direct surgical care; perhaps the most well known example of this was the randomized controlled trial of internal mammary artery ligation for the treatment of angina; this study included thoracotomy without ligation of the arteries in the control patients (Benson and McCallie, 1979).

Rigorous evaluation in acute care and rehabilitation extends beyond therapeutic interventions. It also encompasses evaluation of diagnostic tests and monitoring devices, such as the use of radiography and pulmonary artery catheters in the care of trauma patients, and the evaluation of systems of care such as trauma centers, emergency medical services, training programs, and trauma systems.

In the twenty-first century, one of the key challenges for injury research will be to apply the knowledge that has been gained from the laboratory and test it in a rigorous fashion in patients. This translational research must be done in a rapid but rigorous fashion, using the tools discussed in this volume, in order to bring about further decreases in trauma mortality and morbidity.

There is also a large gap in the dissemination of information. Numerous studies have shown that effective interventions become the standard of care long after they have been shown to be effective (Sackett et al., 1991). The use of meta-analyses and large trials, the publication of systematic reviews, the development of clinical prediction rules, and the dissemination of clinical practice guidelines are designed to decrease the time from innovation to practice change. This has only recently begun to occur in the trauma field (Bullock et al., 1996).

Determination of Injury Outcome

For many years, the outcome of injury control strategies was measured by injury mortality. As with the rest of medicine, there is a need to measure outcomes of interventions in far more sophisticated and sensitive ways (Ware, 1995; Wilson and Cleary, 1995). The impact of different prevention strategies and treatment modalities needs to be assessed by examination of changes in the rate and severity of injuries, the functional outcome of patients in a variety of domains, the impact on family function, the quality of care delivered, and the cost–benefit of different treatment options.

The focus on outcomes from trauma and the effect of different intervention programs will require more sophisticated outcome tools than have been used in injury research to date. These tools must be sensitive to cognitive impairment, as one of the greatest sources of morbidity is that from traumatic brain injury. In addition, they must be easy to administer in the course of normal patient care. Such tools are being developed for general medical problems; they must be tested and adapted for trauma.

Comparisons of outcomes among groups of patients will also require adjustment for variations in injury severity. Injury investigators have led health care in case mix severity adjustment; few other health care problems currently have as good measures of severity. However, the measures we have are still imperfect and must be refined to be more accurate. In addition, they have to date focused nearly exclusively on prediction of mortality; the current need is on prediction of disability.

The focus in health care over the last decade has been on controlling the ever increasing costs of health care. Injury control is no exception. Research is needed to examine the costs of injuries, and the cost-effectiveness and benefit of interventions, both primary interventions such as air bags and helmets as well as acute care and rehabilitation programs such as cognitive therapy for traumatic brain injury. This information will be increasingly important if we are to translate effective interventions into practice.

Conclusions

At the beginning of the twenty-first century, one of humankind's oldest problems – injuries – continues to account for an enormous loss of life and disability in the world. Many of the easy and obvious solutions have been implemented, with a corresponding reduction in injury morbidity and mortality. Further reduction in injury will depend on increasingly more sophisticated research. It is our hope that this volume will help to stimulate such efforts.

References

Baker SP, O'Neill B, Ginsburg MJ, Li G (1992) Injury Fact Book. New York: Oxford University Press.

Bandura A (1995) Self-efficacy in changing societies. New York: Cambridge University Press.

Becker MH, Mainman LA (1975) Sociobehavioral determinants of compliance with health and medical care recommendations. Med Care 13:10–21.

Benson H, McCallie DP, Jr (1979) Angina pectoris and the placebo effect. N Engl J Med 300:1424–9.

Bullock R, Chestnut RM, Clifton G et al. (1996) Guidelines for the management of severe head injury. J Neurotrauma 13:1–734.

Campbell BJ (1963) A study of injuries related to padding on instrument panels. Automotive Crash Injury Research, CAL Report No. VJ-1823-R2, August 1, 1963. Reprinted in: Haddon WJ, Suchman E, Klein D (1964) Accident Research: Methods and Approaches, pp. 696–705. New York: Association for the Aid of Crippled Children.

Committee on Injury Prevention and Control, Division of Health Promotion and Disease Prevention, Institute of Medicine. (1999) Reducing the Burden of Injury: Advancing Prevention and Treatment. Washington, DC: National Academy Press.

Committee on Trauma Research, Commission on Life Sciences, National Research Council and Institute of Medicine. (1985) Injury in America: A Continuing Public Health Problem. Washington, DC: National Academy Press.

DeHaven H (1942) Mechanical analysis of survival in falls from heights of fifty to one hundred and fifty feet. War Medicine 2:586–96. Reprinted in: Haddon WJ, Suchman E, Klein D (1964) Accident Research: Methods and Approaches, pp. 539–46. New York: Association for the Aid of Crippled Children.

(1952) Accident survival – airplane and passenger automobile. Annual Meeting of the Society of Automotive Engineers, January. Reprinted in: Haddon WJ, Suchman E, Klein D (1964) Accident Research: Methods and Approaches, pp. 562–8. New York: Association for the Aid of Crippled Children.

Gibson JJ (1961) The contribution of experimental psychology to the formulation of the problem of safety – a brief for basic research. In: Behavioral Approaches to Accident Research, pp. 77–89. New York: Association for the Aid of Crippled Children.

Reprinted in: Haddon WJ, Suchman E, Klein D (1964) Accident Research: Methods and Approaches, pp. 296–303. New York: Association for the Aid of Crippled Children.

Gordon JE (1948) The epidemiology of accidents. Am J Public Health 39:504–515. Reprinted in: Haddon WJ, Suchman E, Klein D (1964) Accident Research: Methods and Approaches, pp. 18–27. Association for the Aid of Crippled Children.

Green L, Kreuter M (1991) Application of PRECEDE/PROCEED in Community Settings. Health Promotion Planning: an Educational and Environmental Approach. Mountain View, CA: Mayfield.

Greenwood M, Woods HM (1919) The incidence of industrial accidents upon individuals with special reference to multiple accidents. Medical Research Committee, Industrial Fatigue Research Board (Great Britain), Report No. 4. Reprinted in: Haddon WJ, Suchman E, Klein D (1964) Accident Research: Methods and Approaches, pp. 390–6. Association for the Aid of Crippled Children.

Grove RD, Hetzel A (1968) Vital Statistics Rates in the US, 1940–1960. Washington, DC: US Department of Health, Education and Welfare.

Haddon W Jr (1967) Informal remarks. In: Selzer ML, Gikas PW, Huelke DF (eds), The Prevention of Highway Injury. Ann Arbor, MI: Highway Safety Research Institute, University of Michigan, pp. 9–17.

Haddon W Jr, Vailen P, McCarroll JR, Umberger CJ (1961) A controlled investigation of the characteristics of adult pedestrians fatally injured by motor vehicles in Manhattan. J Chronic Dis 14:655–78. Reprinted in: Haddon WJ, Suchman E, Klein D (1964) Accident Research: Methods and Approaches, pp. 232–50. Association for the Aid of Crippled Children.

Haddon WJ, Suchman E, Klein D (1964) Accident Research: Methods and Approaches. Association for Crippled Children.

Holcomb RL (1938) Alcohol in relation to traffic accidents. JAMA 111:1076–85.

Institute of Medicine (1997) Enabling America: Assessing the Role of Rehabilitation Science and Engineering. Washington, DC: National Academy Press.

Linder FE, Grove RD (1943) Vital Statistics Rates in the US, 1900–1940. Washington, DC: US Department of Commerce.

Marion DW, Penrod LE, Kelsey SF, Obrist WD, Kochanek PM, Palmer AM, Wisniewski SR, DeKosky ST (1997) Treatment of traumatic brain injury with moderate hypothermia. N Engl J Med 336:540–6.

National Research Council (1966) Accidental Death and Disability: The Neglected Disease of Modern Society. Washington, DC: National Academy Press.

Nahum AM, Melvin JW (1993) Accidental Injury: Biomechanics and Prevention. New York: Springer-Verlag.

Rivara FP, Thompson DC, Beahler C, Zavitkosky A, Patterson M (1997) Child Injury Prevention. www.hiprc.org/childinjury.

Rivara FP, MacKenzie EJ (eds) (1999) Systematic Reviews of Motor Vehicle Injury Prevention Strategies. Am J Prev Med Supplement, January.

Robertson LS (1998) Injury Epidemiology: Research and Control Strategies. New York: Oxford University Press.

Rosenstock IM (1974) The health belief model and preventive health behavior. Health Education Monogr 2:354–86.

Rothman KJ, Greenland S (eds) (1998) Modern Epidemiology, 2nd edn. Philadelphia: Lippincott-Raven.

Sackett DL, Haynes RB, Guyatt GH, Tugwell P (1991) Clinical Epidemiology. A Basic Science for Clinical Medicine, 2nd edn. Toronto: Little, Brown and Company.

Severy DM, Mathewson JH (1956) Automobile-barrier impacts, Series II. Clinical Orthopaedics 8:275–300. Reprinted in: Haddon WJ, Suchman E, Klein D (1964) Accident Research: Methods and Approaches, pp. 584–95. Association for the Aid of Crippled Children.

Simpson D (1996) Helmets in surgical history. Aust NZ J Surg 66:314–24.

Stapp J (1957) Human tolerance to deceleration. Am J Surgery 93:734–40. Reprinted in: Haddon WJ, Suchman E, Klein D (1964) Accident Research: Methods and Approaches, pp. 554–61. Association for the Aid of Crippled Children.

Trunkey DD (1983) Trauma. Sci Am 249:28–35.

Trunkey DD, Ochsner MG (1996) Management of battle casualties. In: Feliciano DV, Moore EE, Mattox KL (eds), Trauma, 3rd edn, pp. 1023–35. Stamford, CT: Appleton and Lange.

United Nations (1998) Demographic Yearbook, 1996. New York: United Nations.

US Bureau of the Census (1997) Statistical Abstracts of the US, 1997. 117th Edition. Washington, DC: Department of Commerce.

Ware JE (1995) The status of health assessment, 1994. Annu Rev Public Health 16:327–54.

Wilson IB, Cleary PD (1995) Linking clinical variables with health-related quality of life: A conceptual model of patient outcomes. JAMA 273:59–65.

2

Classifying and Counting Injury

Lois A. Fingerhut and Elizabeth McLoughlin

A disease classification is a system of categories to which morbid entities are assigned according to established criteria [World Health Organization (WHO), 1993]. It is used to organize information so as to permit easy storage, retrieval, and analysis of data. The WHO quotes William Farr in 1856 saying "Classification is a method of generalization. Several classifications may, therefore, be used with advantage; and the physician, the pathologist, or the jurist, each from his own point of view, may legitimately classify the diseases and the causes of death in the way that he thinks best adapted to facilitate his inquiries, and to yield general results." (WHO, 1993, p. 73). An injury classification scheme should allow for the capture of information about the nature of the injury, the body region affected, the external cause, intentionality, and circumstances, such as location, activities, and products involved.

This chapter focuses on how injuries are classified and counted, primarily in health data systems, and how the data can be presented and used in research.

Classifying Injury

Injury in the International Classification of Disease (ICD), and the Clinical Modification of the International Classification of Disease (ICD CM)

The ICD, a product of WHO, is the most widely used classification scheme for coding deaths and morbid conditions. It is designed to promote international comparability in the collection, processing, classification, and presentation of mortality and morbidity statistics. The ICD provides the essential guidelines for the coding and classification of cause-of-death and morbidity data.

Most countries use the ICD for coding mortality and morbidity data. However, for morbidity data, the United States developed a clinical modification (ICD CM) to code information from medical records and health surveys [Department of Health and Human Services (DSHS), 1998]. The ICD CM has also been used in other countries, including but not limited to the Netherlands, Israel, Australia, New Zealand, and parts of Spain and Canada. The ICD has undergone periodic revisions. For the 10th revision, Australia has developed its own clinical modification, ICD-10 AM, which New Zealand now also uses. Denmark is using ICD-10 without modification for morbidity coding.

The timing of transition from ICD-9 to ICD-10 has differed by country. ICD-10 was first implemented in 1994 in Denmark, the Czech Republic, and in several other countries. ICD-10 was implemented for mortality coding in the U.S. in 1999; ICD-10 CM will likely be implemented in 2001 or 2002. The WHO maintains a web page indicating the ICD-10 implementation plans for all member countries (see http://www.who.int/hst/icd-10/implemen.htm).

Between 1999 and 2001, the United States and some other countries will code mortality data with ICD-10 and morbidity data with ICD-9 CM. Thus, not only is it important to understand the key differences between ICD and ICD CM, but also between ICD-9 and ICD-10 (Table 2.1) (L'Hours, 1995). The use of two very different classifications poses challenges for data users and data providers for developing data handling and analytic strategies to permit accurate comparisons across mortality and morbidity data and trend analysis across this period.

The National Center for Health Statistics (NCHS) serves as the WHO Collaborating Center for the Classification of Diseases for North America and is responsible for coordination of all official disease classification activities in the United States and Canada relating to the ICD and its use, interpretation, and periodic revision.

Revision Processes for ICD and ICD CM

Until now the ICD has not been updated between revisions. However, a mechanism has been established to provide ICD-10 codes for new diseases where necessary (see http://www.who.int/hst/icd-10/update.htm). The process for updating ICD is independent of the process used in the United States to update ICD-CM annually, which is the joint responsibility of the NCHS and the Health Care Financing Administration (see http://www.cdc.gov/nchswww/about/otheract/icd9/icd9hp2.htm).

Rules and Guidelines for Injury Mortality and Morbidity Coding and Classification

Basic rules and guidelines for mortality coding and classification are found within the ICD volumes (WHO, 1977, 1992, 1993). Adaptations of these for use in the United States can be found in the Instruction Manuals published by NCHS (NCHS, 1998a, b). Similarly, ICD CM coding guidelines for nonfatal injuries are documented in detail (DHHS, 1998).

Coding guidelines differ for mortality and morbidity data. For mortality, the underlying cause of death is the event that initiated the chain of events leading to death; for morbidity, the first-listed external cause-of-injury code is that related to the most serious injury diagnosis. For example, if a person falls down a flight of stairs and sustains a fatal arterial laceration from shards of a broken glass door at the bottom of the stairs, the underlying cause of death would be a fall. If the same person were to survive and be discharged from a hospital, the first-listed or principal diagnosis would likely be the laceration and the associated external cause would be

Table 2.1 Differences between ICD-9 and ICD-10 for injury codes

	ICD-9	ICD-10
Relationship of external cause codes to full classification	Supplemental chapter to the full classification	Integrated into classification, Ch. XX
Labeling	For diagnoses: no letter label For external causes: E	For diagnoses: S and T (Ch. XIX) For external causes: V, W, X, Y (Ch. XX)
Code structure	3-digit numeric code (after E) with 4th digit for specificity	4-digit alphanumeric code
Period in effect	Mortality: 1979–98 Morbidity: 1979–2001	Mortality: 1999– Morbidity: 2001–

Diagnosis codes – primary difference is in structure

Order of diagnosis codes	Nature of injury by body region	Body region by nature of injury. S codes: Injuries to a single body region; T codes: Injuries to multiple or unspecified body regions, poisoning, and certain other consequences of external causes

External cause codes – primary differences are in amount of detail

Poisoning	Extensive detail for "accidental" poisoning, less for self-inflicted, assaultive, and undetermined intent	Considerably less detailed and fewer codes
Firearms	Separate codes to identify rifle, shotgun and larger firearms	Rifle, shotgun, and larger firearms recombined into one code
Transportation	(E810.0–E825.9) first 3 digits capture type of event and 4th digit identifies activity of victim: driver, pedestrian, cyclist, etc.	"V", then identifies mode of transport (vehicle, pedestrain, bicycle, etc.); then identifies circumstances of event (collision, non-collision, etc.), then identifies activity of victim (driver, passenger) and traffic–nontraffic. Many more codes than in previous revision.
Homicide/assault	Very few interpersonal abuse codes	More detailed codes for abuse, neglect, abandonment, identity of perpetrator.
Place of occurrence	Only used with selected unintentional injury codes	Used with external cause codes W00–Y34 (All except "V" codes for transportation)
Activity of victim	No codes	Optional codes for use with all external cause codes

cut/pierce. Consequently, if a researcher is describing the magnitude of, for example, the falls problem in a population by combining mortality and morbidity data, there may be an overall undercount of falls if many serious nonfatal falls are coded as cut/pierce injuries.

Documenting Intent and Mechanism for External Cause of Injury Coding

External cause of injury codes (E-codes) in the ICD capture the circumstances of an injury along two dimensions: intent (unintentional, self-inflicted, assault, undetermined, legal intervention), and mechanism (e.g., fall, drowning, gunshot, fire, motor vehicle collision). In the structure of the ICD, the intent of injury death takes precedence over the mechanism. That is, a coder must first determine intent (e.g., self-inflicted), and then assign the proper mechanism (e.g., fall/jump). Thus, official death rates have been tabulated and presented by intent (e.g., suicide) rather than by mechanism (e.g., fall). However, data users and providers are paying increasing attention to the mechanisms of injury, because evaluation research indicates that passive protection through modification of consumer products and environments is most effective in reducing injury, regardless of intent. However, the intent of injury also can be important when determining effective interventions that involve changes in human behavior (McLoughlin et al., 1997).

Intent:

Determination and documentation of intent (also referred to as "manner of death") for both mortality and morbidity data is problematic. Numerous studies point out the difficulties medical examiners have in assigning intent (Moyer et al., 1989; Young and Pollock, 1993; Hanzlick and Goodin, 1997). Medical examiners (at least in the United States) do not evaluate intent in their investigations in the way that the legal system does; thus medical examiners seem to prefer the word accident compared with unintentional (personal communication from Randy Hanzlick, CDC). The quality and amount of detail on the circumstances of the injury depends largely on the efforts and policies adhered to by medical examiners and coroners, and their access to information from police sources and family informants. Policies are known to vary from jurisdiction to jurisdiction, and the level of reporting detail ... "is left entirely to the judgement, ingenuity, and energy of the certifier" (Rosenberg and Kochanek, 1995).

Problems with documenting intent are not unique to the United States. In France, for example, death certificates are apt to record a cause as an unspecified accident because of confidentiality rules prohibiting more specific data from medicolegal investigations (separate from the reporting of vital statistics) (Smith et al., 1995; Tursz, 1995). In England, the process of certifying an external cause of death involves a legal verdict in almost every case (Rooney, 1996).

Health-care providers also have difficulty ascertaining intent while taking a history about the circumstances causing a patient's injury. Time pressures, treatment responsibilities, severity of injury, and patients' willingness to discuss motives all affect the determination and documentation of intent in the medical record. In most coding systems for nonfatal injuries, the injury is assumed to be unintentional unless noted otherwise. In fact, it was not until 1996 that the guidelines for morbidity coding in the United States included codes for undetermined intent.

Mechanism:

Greater specificity within coding schemes makes it possible to capture important details for subsequent analysis, but it places greater burden for documentation upon the history taker. There is often insufficient detail on the death certificate or medical record to assign a specific external cause code. For example, a coder cannot assign a specific code without knowing whether a person was the driver or a passenger in a motor vehicle collision. Training tools for history takers, including pull-down menus within computerized software prompts, are being developed to assure that essential details are documented on death certificates and medical records.

Injury-related Diagnoses Currently Outside Standard "Injury Codes"

Certain diagnoses that many would classify as injuries or injury-related are currently located in sections of the ICD and ICD CM outside the traditional range of injury diagnosis or external cause codes. These include musculoskeletal conditions related to the knee and the back, certain conditions of the eye such as traumatic cataracts, certain respiratory conditions, and conditions related to drug or alcohol use or dependence (Smith et al., 1991; Fingerhut and Warner, 1997; Donna Pickett, personal communication, 1999).

Researchers continue to refine the definitions of injury within the ICD. For example, a recent analysis of poisoning mortality suggests that ICD-9 code 305, for the nondependent abuse of drug, be included in the definition of poisoning (Fingerhut and Cox, 1998). Including deaths for nondependent abuse increased the annual number of poisoning deaths in the United States in 1995 by 14%. Similarly, in an analysis of drug-related mortality in England and Wales, the authors noted that the coroner's exact words are crucial in determining how drug-related deaths were coded. They concluded that "when quantifying deaths from acute poisoning, it is important to take account of deaths classified under drug dependence and non-dependent abuse." (Christophersen et al., 1998). Using data from a sample of United States emergency departments in 1995–96, the addition of ICD 305 to the traditional external cause codes for poisoning increased the number of visits attributed to poisoning by about 35% (unpublished data from the United States NHAMCS). Impetus for these refinements comes in part from a greater focus on the mechanism of injury, greater availability of external-cause-of-injury-coded morbidity data, a re-examination of acute versus repetitive injury and the complexities of poisoning and drug addiction as manifested in acute episodes versus long-term use (see ICEHS, 1998).

Limitations of the Coding System Regarding Utility for Prevention

The ICD was not designed for prevention purposes. However, because it is available in vital statistics and health system data, it is used for that purpose. Researchers must be aware of the limitations described above for coding intent.

In addition, preventive interventions are often tailored for specific locations or activities. The ICD-9 CM E-codes do include a place code (e.g., street, public building, home, farm). However, because this code must be secondary to a primary E-code, guidelines state that it is never to be used on medical record forms that permit only one E-code. Further, neither the ICD-9 nor the ICD-9 CM identifies injuries as related to major activities such as sports, work, or agriculture. Intimate partner violence could not be identified because ICD-9 does not contain codes to identify the perpetrator in fatal assaults. Essentially, ICD-9 did not include any way to address the concept of what the person was doing at the time of the injury. One important improvement in ICD-10 is activity codes, although much work needs to be done to make them useful for prevention. While ICD-10 does include codes for violence against women and the identity of the perpetrator, no coding scheme can overcome a lack of documentation in an official record or an unwillingness of respondents in population-based surveys to admit to abusive behavior.

Other Injury Classifications

In addition to the ICD, there are other classification schemes that are unique to a specific survey or surveillance system. Information in Table 2.2 should be used as a guide to some of these classifications. Following are detailed examples of another United States classification, an international classification, as well as a proposed classification.

Occupational Injury and Illness Classification System (OIICS):

The Bureau of Labor Statistics (BLS) developed the OIICS to provide a set of procedures for selecting and recording facts relating to an occupational injury or illness. This coding scheme is used for both the Census of Fatal Occupational Injuries and the Survey of Occupational Injuries and Illnesses. Included in OIICS are nature of injury or illness, part of body affected, source (identifies the object or substance that directly inflicted the injury or illness), event, or exposure (describes the manner in which the injury or illness was inflicted by the source), and the secondary source. Each of these five classification structures has four levels of detail from the very general division level to two, three, and four digits of specificity. Such a hierarchical arrangement allows for the classification system to be flexible for the data user. Rules of selection, code descriptions, indices and edit criteria can all be found in the OIICS manual (that can be obtained on-line). Data come from administrative records such as employer logs, and workers' compensation reports (see http://www.bls.gov/oshoiics.htm). The OIICS was designed to be "as compatible as possible with ICD-9 CM" (Toscano et al., 1996). In practice, however, it is not possible to translate OIICS codes directly to ICD-9, or vice versa, making it difficult to compare analyses of data coded by the differing schemes.

NOMESCO

The NOMESCO (Nordic Medico-Statistical Committee) classification was developed to collect information on events resulting in injuries that are treated in emergency departments; its first edition was published in 1984 and the most recent in 1997. The classification has a multiaxial, modular, and hierarchical structure facilitating data collection at different levels of detail. The basic axes of classification include place of occurrence, type of activity, and injury mechanism. There are modules for transportation, occupation, sports, violence, and self-harm, and a product module. NOMESCO is used in some Nordic countries, the Baltic countries, and Greece. The WHO collaborating center in Sweden is responsible for its maintenance and revision (NOMESCO, 1996; Frimodt-Møller, 1998, personal communication). However, NOMESCO's fundamental drawback for use in the United States for national data systems is that it is not compatible with ICD.

ICECI

The International Classification of External Causes of Injury (ICECI) is being developed under the auspices of the WHO by an international working group to remedy some of the shortcomings of the ICD for injury prevention (see section on ICD disadvantages). ICECI, like NOMESCO, is being designed to capture data in emergency departments, but unlike NOMESCO, will be supplementary to the external cause of injury data coded with ICD-10. It will capture more detailed information than ICD-10 about place, activity, product involvement, and intent (including victim–perpetrator relationship). In addition, the ICECI would provide more detail compared with ICD-10 about sports injuries and injuries due to violence (WHO Working Group, 1998).

Counting Injury

Definitions

In order to count injuries, fatal or nonfatal, the researcher must understand the inclusion and exclusion criteria associated with various data bases, or with a particular study design. For example, in the United States vital statistics system, a motor vehicle traffic death is defined without regard to any time interval from crash to death while NHTSA's Fatality and Analysis Reporting System (FARS) includes only those deaths occurring within 30 days of the crash. Similarly, in the recommended definition of an unintentional injury, deaths coded to adverse effects and medical complications are excluded (McLoughlin et al., 1997) while in routine publications of vital statistics, these deaths are included. These can make a large difference in international comparisons of death rates, for example, between Israel and the United States (Barell, 1996).

Counting Fatal Injuries

The primary source for determining the number of deaths in a country in a year is vital statistics.

Underlying Cause versus Contributing Cause:

The underlying cause of death is often the only information reported on a regular basis in vital statistics. For a death resulting from an injury, the underlying cause is

Table 2.2 Classifications (other than the ICD and ICD-CM) used in the coding of injury-related data

Classification	Domain/ownership	Used for/in	Injury diagnosis	External cause	Additional dimension(s)	ICD compatible	References
US based							
OIICS – Occupational Injury and Illness Classification System	Bureau of Labor Statistics	Census of Fatal Occupational Injury (CFOI) Survey of Occupational Injuries and Illnesses (SOII)	Yes	Yes		ICD-9 CM	Toscano et al., 1996 & www.bls.gov/oshoiics.htm
STANGA 2050	NATO	Medical records	Yes	Yes	Sports, battle wounds	Diagnosis codes not external codes	Amoroso et al., 1997 and Smith et al., 2000
Red Cross Wound Classification	Intl Comm of the Red Cross	War surgery	Yes	No		No	Coupland, 1997
CCHPR – Clinical Classifications For Health Policy	DHHS, AHCPR	Medical records (inpatient)	Yes	No		Yes	Elixhauser & McCarthy 1996 and see www.ahcpr.gov/ data/cchpr.htm
Spinal Cord Injury	American Spinal Injury Association	Spinal cord injury assessment	Yes	No		No	www.asia-spinalinjury.org/ publications/index.html
Non-US based							
ICECI (under development)	WHO Working Group on Injury Surveillance	Emergency department injury monitoring	[a]	[a]	[a]	[a]	Consumer Safety Institute, Amsterdam, Netherlands

System	Organization	Type			Coverage		Reference
NOMESCO	Nordic Medico-Statistical Committee	Emergency department injury monitoring	No	Yes	Products, activity, industry	No	NOMESCO, 1996
CHIRPP – Canadian Hospitals Injury Reporting and Prevention Program	Health Canada: Laboratory Centre for Disease Control	Emergency department injury monitoring	Yes	Yes	Activity, safety devices, products	No	Mackenzie and Pless, 1999 www.hc-sc.gc.ca/hpb/icdc/brch/injury.html
EHLASS – European Home and Leisure Accident Surveillance System	Council of Ministers, European Community	Emergency department injury monitoring	Yes	Yes	Product, activity	No	Mulder and Rogmans, 1991
US-based systems with unique injury classification							
NEISS – National Electronic Injury Surveillance System	Consumer Product Safety Commission	Emergency department injury monitoring	Yes	Limited	Only product-related	No	CPSC, 1998
GES – General Estimates System	National Highway Traffic Safety Administration	Traffic-related injury	No	Limited	Only traffic-related crashes	No	NHTSA, 1998 www.nhtsa.dot.gov/people/ncsa/nass_ges.html
FARS – Fatality Analysis Reporting System	National Highway Traffic Safety Administration	Traffic-related injury	No	No	Only fatalities in traffic-related crashes	No	NHTSA, 1998 www.nhtsa.dot.gov/people/ncsa/fars.html

[a] The ICECI is under development.

the external cause rather than the injury diagnosis; for example, a death would be coded to a motor vehicle crash rather than a torn aorta. Information on the injury diagnoses comes from other entries on the death certificate and these are referred to as the contributing causes of death. For analysis, these contributing causes are available on multiple cause-of-death data tapes. For deaths where there is the coexistence of disease and injury, which is common among the elderly, the choice of one as the underlying cause can be dependent on the discretion of the certifier (Hanzlick, 1997).

The linkage between the external cause of death and the injury diagnoses can be important for prevention research. For example, when evaluating motorcycle helmet laws, researchers may need to know which deaths were caused by motorcycle crashes, helmet use by those involved in the crashes, and which of these deaths were caused by fatal head injuries, because helmets protect only the head. Helmet use, not captured by ICD codes, is documented in the United States in the FARS system. (See Table 2.2).

Official Rank/Leading Cause of Death:

Jurisdictions publish official lists of their leading causes of death, using categories based on WHO's recommended tabulation (WHO, 1992). In the United States, ICD-9 used the List of 72 Selected Causes of Death and in ICD-10, the comparable list includes 113 selected causes (NCHS, 1998b). The ICD-10 list for injury deaths follows the traditional emphasis on intent, by including suicide, homicide, and several detailed categories of unintentional injury (WHO, 1992). The problem with these categories is that they ignore the mechanism-specific contributions of, for example, firearms, poisoning, and suffocation. These three mechanisms accounted for 35% of all fatal injury in Australia in 1993–95 and for 42% of all fatal injury in the United States in 1996 (Bordeaux and Harrison, 1996; and unpublished data from NCHS).

Utility of Other Databases:

Specific information about the circumstances of injury deaths is sometimes more complete in data bases other than vital statistics. For example, in the United States circumstances of motor vehicle traffic deaths can be found in Department of Transportation data (FARS), of work-related deaths in Department of Labor data (Census of Fatal Occupational Injury), of deaths resulting from violent crime in Department of Justice data (National Incident-Based Reporting System). For an examination of all U.S. Federal injury-related data bases, see Annest et al. (1996).

Counting Nonfatal Injuries

National estimates of nonfatal injuries are often based on health-care system data (samples of hospital discharges, of emergency room visits) or population-based surveys.

Health Care Systems:

Medical record systems provide information on health-care utilization; that is, who used what services for what medical condition. They are more useful for estimating service utilization (hospital admissions, visits to emergency departments, ambulatory care clinics, or physicians' offices) for a certain medical condition, rather than how many people in a population suffer from that condition. Thus, data users must be aware that trends can reflect changes in systems of care (e.g., the trend away from hospital admission toward ambulatory care for some injuries or insurance practices, which can be a deterrent to seeking medical care) or in record-keeping. For example, these issues have had an impact on the interpretation of burn data. A comparison of the national hospital discharge survey data with that collected by the American Burn Association reveals a sharp decline in burn admissions to hospitals without burn units, which is in contrast with a smaller but steady increase in burn center admissions (Brigham and McLoughlin, 1996). System data can either be based on complete counts or on a sample.

There are some inherent difficulties of using medical records to count injured people. Some data systems include multiple treatments for the same injury in the same facility (e.g., readmissions to hospital), and treatment of one person in more than one department or facility (emergency department and inpatient in same facility or transfer from one hospital to another) (see also Robertson, 1998). A unique patient identifier on medical records could help reduce this "double counting," but concerns about privacy and confidentiality have blocked the adoption of unique identifiers in many jurisdictions. In addition to a patient identifier, however, the date of injury must be included to determine incidence. New Zealand's hospital discharge data has both the identifier and the date of injury (Langley, 1999, personal communication). In England, there is the added complication that one stay in a hospital can be split into several completed consultant episodes; that is, you could be admitted as an emergency under the orthopedic surgeons, but transferred the next day to neurosurgeons and this would be two episodes (Cleone Rooney, Office of National Statistics, 1999, personal communication). Lacking identifiers, treatment episodes rather than people can be counted, or adjustments for overestimation of people injured can be made based upon knowledge derived from other data bases where transfers and readmissions can be identified (see Rice et al., 1989, pp. 30, 31).

Surveys:

Population-based surveys permit estimates of persons injured, because it is the person, rather than the medical system, who reports. Either the injured person or a proxy reporting for the injured person reports on the injury episode, the condition causing the injury, and any product involved in the injury. The relevant measure for prevention purposes is the incidence of injury.

Recall bias presents a challenge to researchers. There is the risk of differential recall depending on the severity of the injury; the longer the time between when the injury happened and when the survey was conducted, the greater the likelihood of not remembering the event (Harel et al., 1994). However, with shorter recall periods, larger samples are needed for estimates of injuries, particularly those that are less common.

In addition, respondents may be more likely to report injuries that occurred prior to the interval of interest. There are substantial differences in the recall periods, the number of screening questions, and periodicity in the national health surveys of 23 countries (NCHS, 1994). In the United States, the National Health Interview Survey (NHIS) is the primary tool for estimating less severe injuries. Because the number of conditions based on the standard 2-week recall period yielded too few injuries for detailed analyses, the 1997 survey used a 3-month recall period (NCHS, 1998). Because the survey asks when the injury happened, analysts have some ability to estimate recall bias.

The severity of nonfatal injury ranges from life-threatening to barely perceptible. It is impossible to measure the total number of minor injuries occurring in a population, due in large part to personal reactions to injury and health-care practices. An injury severe enough for one person to visit an emergency department may, to another person, be nothing more than a painful inconvenience, which might not be recalled in a survey. A child whose parent can readily transport him/her for medical treatment may become an injury statistic, while the child whose parent cannot take off work or who lives in an area without a health-care facility is not included in the estimates (Fingerhut and Warner, 1997).

Use of External Cause of Injury Codes for Non Fatal Injury

In the United States, the absence of routine external cause of injury coding on health system and survey data has hampered researchers' ability to define the injury problem in ways that could facilitate prevention efforts (see Rice et al., 1989; and Fingerhut and Warner, 1997). However, during the 1990s there has been a remarkable increase in the availability of nonfatal data with external cause of injury coding. The U.S. National Hospital Ambulatory Medical Care Survey (NHAMCS) has had external cause of injury coding since 1992, and the U.S. NHIS has since 1997. A 1998 survey found that 36 states routinely collect some level of external cause coding in statewide hospital discharge systems; 23 states require external cause coding in these systems and nine states require external cause coding in their hospital emergency department systems (ICEHS, 1998).

Presentation of Data

Recommended Framework for Presenting External Cause of Injury Data

A standard framework for the presentation of ICD-9 external cause of injury data was developed in 1997 (McLoughlin et al., 1997). The framework permits data users to examine injuries by both intent and mechanism; this helps identify high-risk groups for particular injuries, and facilitates prevention planning and evaluation. It also facilitates comparisons of injury data across countries, studies, jurisdictions, and populations.

There are five columns of intent categories (Table 2.3) and 18 rows for mechanism, selected to accommodate the most frequent categories of fatal and nonfatal

Table 2.3 Deaths due to injury, 1996

Mechanism/cause	Intent/manner of death					
	Unintentional	Suicide	Homicide	Undetermined	Other	All
Motor vehicle traffic	42,522	87	na	11	na	42,620
Firearm	1134	18,166	14,037	413	290	34,040
Poisoning	9510	5080	67	2028	na	16,685
Fall	11,292	645	27	74	na	12,038
Suffocation	4320	5330	762	86	na	10,498
Drowning	3959	361	69	242	na	4631
Fire/hot objects	3845	171	231	106	na	4353
Cut/pierce	97	435	2619	9	1	3161
Struck by/against	903	na	364	na	8	1275
Machinery	926	na	na	na	na	926
Pedal cycle, other	114	na	na	na	na	114
Pedestrian, other	926	na	na	na	na	926
Transportation, other	2119	1	na	na	na	2120
Natural/environmental	1550	10	na	12	na	1572
Overexertion	22	na	na	na	na	22
Other, specified	1564	334	281	18	33	2230
Other, not elsewhere classified	105	201	942	149	17	1414
Not specified	6868	82	1235	315	1	8501
All mechanisms	91,776	30,903	20,634	3463	350	147,126
Adverse effects						3172
All external causes of injury						150,298

Note: E-codes for all categories can be found in McLoughlin et al., 1997. na, not applicable; no E-codes exist for these cells.
Source: National Center for Health Statistics, data from the National Vital Statistics system.

injury. All E-codes of the ICD-9 and ICD-9 CM were assigned to only one cell, thus making all cells in the matrix mutually exclusive. Presenting numbers of deaths in each category of the matrix provides useful information about the mechanism and intent. In addition, by aggregating across categories, data can be summarized by using the marginal totals to describe injury deaths by either mechanism or intent categories (e.g., all deaths caused by poisoning or suicide). The injury matrix excludes those E-codes that pertain to abnormal reactions and complications of medical care and to adverse effects of the therapeutic use of drugs. The framework has been adopted by the NCHS for tabulation in its forthcoming annual vital statistics reports and in reports of the NHAMCS, and it is being adopted by a number of states and local jurisdictions for standard reporting of injury-related data. International analyses of mortality associated with drowning, firearms and poisoning have been done using this framework (Smith et al., 1995; Langley and Smeijers, 1997; Fingerhut et al., 1998)

In early 1999, work had just begun on the development of a framework based on ICD-10 external cause of injury codes, those labeled V-W-X-Y. Unlike the single framework for ICD-9 and ICD-9 CM E-codes, it is likely that ICD-10 and ICD-10 CM will be different enough to warrant separate frameworks.

Proposed Framework for Presentation of Injury Diagnosis Codes

Codes for injury diagnoses include both the nature of the injury (i.e., an open wound) and the anatomic site (i.e., lower limb). To date, no standard exists for the presentation or categorization of injury diagnosis data. For example, there has been no consensus about what a head injury is, or if it differs from a brain injury, or which codes are included in which definition. Under the guidance of the International Collaborative Effort (ICE) on Injury Statistics, work was begun in 1998 to develop a matrix to classify injuries by both their anatomic site and the nature of the injury. All ICD codes in the range 800–999 to be included, and a compatible matrix using ICD-10 CM codes will be developed.

Conclusions

The injury field has made significant progress in classifying and counting injury in the 1990s. But each advance brings its own challenges. One is quality assurance; accurate classifying and counting demands high-quality data. Improvement in the documentation of the circumstances of the injury-causing event is essential for external-cause coding. Methods to monitor the completeness and validity of external-cause coded hospital discharge and emergency department data, which have been developed by some jurisdictions, could usefully be shared with all. The availability of injury morbidity data with external-cause coding opens enormous opportunity for analysis and comparisons across states and countries; valid comparisons must take into account country-and-state-specific differences in data collection and coding guidelines. The challenges posed by the transitions from ICD-9 and ICD-9 CM to ICD-10 and ICD-10 CM are formidable, yet manageable through a continued and coordinated effort by the injury field. Accurate, reliable, and valid injury data contribute significantly to our ability to prevent the pain and burden of injury.

References

Amoroso PJ, Swartz WG, Hoin FA, Yore MM (1997) Total Army Injury and Health Outcomes Database: Description and Capabilities. Technical Note 97-2. Natick, MA: US Army Research Institute of Environmental Medicine.

Annest JL, Conn JM, James SP (1996) Inventory of federal data systems in the United States for injury surveillance, research and prevention activities. Atlanta, GA: Centers for Disease Control and Prevention, National Center for Injury Prevention and Control.

Barell V (1996) Injury data definitions – the need for standards. In: Proceedings of the International Collaborative Effort on Injury Statistics, Vol. II. DHHS Pub no (PHS) 96-1252, pp. 16:1–14. Hyattsville, MD: National Center for Health Statistics.

Bordeaux S, Harrison JE (1996) Injury mortality Australia 1995. Australian Injury Prevention Bulletin 13, September 1996. Adelaide: Australian Institute of Health and Welfare National Injury Surveillance Unit.

Brigham PA, McLoughlin E (1996) Burn incidence and medical care use in the United States: Estimates, trends and data sources. J Burn Care Rehab 17:95–107.

Christophersen O, Rooney C, Kelly S (1998) Drug-related mortality: methods and trends. Office for National Statistics. Population Trends 93:1–9.

Consumer Product Safety Commission (1998) NEISS Coding Manual.

Coupland RM (1997) The Red Cross Wound Classification. Geneva, Switzerland: International Committee of the Red Cross Publications.

Department of Health and Human Services (1998) International Classification of Diseases, Ninth Revision, Clinical Modifications, 6th edition. DHHS Pub no (PHS) 98-1260. Washington DC: DHHS, CDC and Health Care Financing Administration.

Elixhauser A, McCarthy E (1996) Clinical Classifications for Health Policy Research, Version 2: Hospital Inpatient Statistics. HCUP-3 Research Note 1, 180. DHHS Pub no (PHS) 96-0017. Washington DC: Agency for Health Care Policy and Research.

Fingerhut LA, Cox CS (1998) Poisoning mortality, 1985–1995. Public Health Reports, Vol. 113, no. 3 May/June. Hyattsville, MD: National Center for Health Statistics, DHHS.

Fingerhut LA and Warner M (1997) Injury Chartbook. Health, United States, 1996–97. Hyattsville, MD: National Center for Health Statistics.

Fingerhut L, Cox C, Warner M et al. (1998) International comparative analysis of injury mortality: Findings from the ICE on Injury Statistics. In: Advance data from Vital and Health Statistics, no. 303. Hyattsville, MD: National Center for Health Statistics.

Hanzlick R (1997) Cause-of-death statements and certification of natural and unnatural deaths. Prepared by the Autopsy Committee and Forensic Pathology Committee of the College of American Pathologists in conjunction with the National Association of Medical Examiners.

Hanzlick R, Goodin J (1997) Mind your manners. Part III: Individual scenario results and discussion of the National Association of Medical Examiners Manner of Death Questionnaire, 1995. Am J Forensic Med Pathol 18:228–45.

Harel Y, Overpeck MD, Jones DH, Scheidt PC, Bijur PE, Trumble AC, Anderson J (1994) The effects of recall on estimating annual nonfatal injury rates for children and adolescents. Am J Public Health 84(4):599–605.

Injury Control and Emergency Health Services Section (ICEHS), American Public Health Association (1998) How States are collecting and using cause of injury data. A Report of the Data Committee of the ICEHS, APHA. http://www.tf.org/tf/injuries/apha4.html

Langley J, Smeijers J (1997) Injury mortality among children and teenagers in New Zealand compared with the United States of America. Injury Prev 3:195–9.

L'Hours ACP (1995) The ICD-10 Classification of Injuries and External Causes. In: Proceedings of the International Collaborative Effort on Injury Statistics, Vol. I. DHHS Pub no (PHS) 95-1252, pp. 22:1–16. Hyattsville, MD: National Center for Health Statistics.

Mackenzie SG, Pless IB (1999) CHIRPP: Canada's principal injury surveillance program. Injury Prev 5:208–13.

McLoughlin E, Annest, JL, Fingerhut LA, Rosenberg HM, Kochanek KD, Pickett D, Berenholz G (1997) Recommended framework for presenting injury mortality data. MMWR Recommendations and Reports 46 (no. RR-14):1–30.

Moyer LA, Boyle CA, Pollock DA (1989) Validity of death certificates for injury-related causes of death. Am J Epidemiol 130:1024–32.

Mulder S, Rogmans WHJ (1991) The Evaluation of the European Home and Leisure Accident Surveillance System. J Safety Res Vol. 22:201–10.

National Center for Health Statistics (1994) International Health Data Reference Guide, 1993. DHHS Pub no (PHS) 94-1007. Hyattsville, MD: National Center for Health Statistics.

National Center for Health Statistics (1998a) Division of Vital Statistics, Mortality Statistics-Instruction Manuals. http://www.cdc.gov/nchswww/about/major/dvs/im.htm

National Center for Health Statistics (1998b) Instruction manual, part 9-ICD-10 Cause-of-Death Lists for Tabulating Mortality Statistics, Effective 1999, and part 2A, Instructions for Classifying the Underlying Cause of Death.

National Center for Health Statistics (1998c) National Health Interview Survey. http://www.cdc.gov/nchswww/about/major/nhis/hisdesgn.htm

National Highway Traffic Safety Administration (1998) National Automotive Sampling System (NASS) General Estimates System (GES) Analytical User's Manual 1988–1997. Washington, DC: US Department of Transportation; National Center for Statistics and Analysis.

National Highway Traffic Safety Administration (1999) Fatality and Analysis Reporting System. http://www.nhtsa.dot.gov/people/ncsa/fars.html

NOMESCO (Nordic Medico-Statistical Committee) (1996) Classification of External Causes of Injury. Copenhagen: NOMESCO.

Parrish G (1995) Assessing and improving the quality of data from medical examiners and coroners. In: Proceedings of the International Collaborative Effort on Injury Statistics: Vol. I. Pub no (PHS) 95-1252, pp. 25:1–10. Hyattsville, MD: National Center for Health Statistics.

Rice DP et al. (1989) Cost of Injury in the United States: A Report to Congress. San Francisco, CA: Institute for Health and Aging, University of California and Injury Prevention Center, The Johns Hopkins University.

Robertson L (1998) Injury Epidemiology, 2nd edn. New York: Oxford University Press.

Rooney C (1996) Differences in the coding of injury deaths in England and Wales and the United States. In: Proceedings of the International Collaborative Effort on Injury Statistics, Vol. II. DHHS Pub no (PHS) 96-1252, pp. 15:1–23. Hyattsville, MD: National Center for Health Statistics.

Rosenberg H, Kochanek K (1995) The Death Certificate as a Source of Injury Data. In: Proceedings of the International Collaborative Effort on Injury Statistics, Vol. I. DHHS Pub no (PHS) 95-1252, pp. 8:1–17. Hyattsville, MD: National Center for Health Statistics.

Smith GS, Langlois JA, Buechner JS (1991) Methodological issues in using hospital discharge data to determine the incidence of hospitalized injuries. Am J Epidemiol 134:1146–58.

Smith GS, Langlois JA, Rockett IR (1995) International comparisons of injury mortality: hypothesis generation, ecological studies, and some data problems. In: Proceedings of the International Collaborative Effort on Injury Statistics, Vol. I. DHHS Pub no (PHS) 95-1252, pp. 13:1–15. Hyattsville, MD: National Center for Health Statistics.

Smith GS, Dannenberg AL, Amoroso PJ (2000) Hospitalization due to injuries in the military: evaluation of current data and recommendations on their use for injury prevention. Am J Prev Med 18-3S:41–53.

Toscano G, Windau J, Drudi D (1996) Using the Occupational Injury and Illness Classification System as a Safety and Health Management Tool. Compensation Working Conditions June:19–23.

Tursz A (1995) Injury mortality and morbidity reporting systems in France. In: Proceedings of the International Collaborative Effort on Injury Statistics. Vol. I. DHHS Pub no (PHS) 95-1252, pp. 15:1–16. Hyattsville, MD: National Center for Health Statistics.

World Health Organization (1977) Manual of the International Statistical Classification of Diseases, Injuries and Causes of Death, based on the recommendations of the Ninth Revision Conference, 1975. Geneva: World Health Organization.

World Health Organizaton (1992) International Statistical Classification of Diseases and Related Health Problems, 10th revision, Vol. 1. Geneva: World Health Organization.

World Health Organizaton (1993) International Statistical Classification of Diseases and Related Health Problems, 10th revision, Vol. 2. Geneva: World Health Organization.

World Health Organizaton Working Group on Injury Surveillance (1998) International Classification for External Causes of Injury (ICECI)-Draft.

Young TW, Pollock DA (1993) Misclassification of deaths caused by cocaine. An assessment by survey. Am J Forensic Med Pathol 14:43–7.

3

Measurement of Injury Severity and Co-morbidity

Grant O'Keefe and Gregory J. Jurkovich

Introduction

The purpose and need for injury severity scoring systems has changed with time, as has the needs of investigators and clinicians. The earliest effort at standardizing injury severity scoring is generally credited to the Abbreviated Injury Scale (AIS) Score, a scoring system initially developed to categorize injury type and severity following motor vehicle crashes; its primary purpose was to support multidisciplinary crash investigation (Committee on Medical Aspects of Automotive Safety, 1971). However, the evolution of trauma care and trauma systems has led to a need for more comprehensive injury recording, and thus, subsequent revision of the AIS. In contrast, the Glasgow Coma Scale (GCS) score was developed in the mid-1970s as a method to categorize the severity of traumatic brain injury (TBI) and has remained essentially unchanged (Teasdale and Jennett, 1974; Jennett and Teasdale, 1976). Over time this score has remained useful in predicting outcome following TBI, has been incorporated into other scores for predicting outcome, and is considered a critical component in the evaluation of trauma care systems (Boyd et al., 1987). These two scores provide examples of how changing needs over time have resulted in either a change in the actual scoring system or an application of the scoring system to a broader range of uses. The main purpose of scoring systems, however, largely remains the same: to grade injury severity to allow for comparisons between individual patients or groups of patients.

The objectives of this chapter are to describe existing measures of injury severity, to review the rationale for their development, and to discuss their use and important limitations. In addition, measures of co-morbidity, the term used to describe health status factors likely to influence the outcome after injury, will be reviewed.

Anatomic Scoring

Scoring systems based upon the anatomic injury are an important method of measuring injury severity and are critical to injury epidemiology, injury prevention, trauma system development and outcome analysis. A major potential advantage of anatomically based scoring systems is that they indicate the actual anatomic injury. In these systems, the score assigned to the anatomic injury is considered to be independent of any treatment, patient characteristics, or any post-injury variables.

32

Therefore, anatomic scoring systems have the advantage of being highly objective measures of injury severity and allow the comparison of individual patients or groups of patients with similar injuries.

Abbreviated Injury Severity Scale

The AIS scale was developed in 1971 as a joint venture of the Association for the Advancement of Automotive Medicine, the American Medical Association, and the Society of Automotive Engineers (Committee on Medical Aspects of Automotive Safety, 1971). The scale was designed to catalog anatomic injuries sustained in motor vehicle-related crashes and its primary role was to supplement crash investigations with detailed anatomical descriptions of occupant injury in order to correlate vehicular damage and crash mechanism with injury patterns. The AIS represents a numerical method for categorizing injuries both by anatomic location and severity. It provides a standard terminology, which was initially developed only for motor vehicle-related injuries, but has been used to describe injuries sustained by a variety of mechanisms and was most recently revised in 1990.

The AIS 90 incorporates a unique six-digit injury description code in addition to an AIS severity score (Association for the Advancement of Automotive Medicine, 1990). The severity component ranges from one to six and describes the relative severity of the injury. For each injury descriptor, the higher severity score indicates a progressively more severe injury than the preceding severity score (i.e., AIS 3 > AIS 2 > AIS 1). It is important to note that this description of relative injury severity only applies when comparing injuries within a single body region and that the individual severity scores are not necessarily related to any measure of outcome.

The AIS score has limitations. The AIS severity score assignment was based upon consensus expert opinion. Individual injuries were assigned scores from one to six, according to the relative degree of anatomic damage, but not in relation to their impact upon survival; although in many circumstances it would be logical to infer that more destructive injuries would have the most pronounced impact on mortality. The AIS severity score is not an interval scale, and each successive increase in score does not necessarily reflect a linear increase in injury severity. Moreover, AIS severity scores are not necessarily comparable across body regions, again, owing to the severity scores not being assigned in relation to outcome, such as mortality. For example, an AIS 4 severity score of the brain represents greater anatomic damage than an AIS 3 score of the brain. Likewise, an AIS 4 injury of a lower extremity is worse than an AIS 3 injury of the lower extremity. However, mortality risk or impact on long-term function is different (worse) for an AIS 3 head injury than an AIS 3 extremity injury. AIS injury scoring also does not address the effects of multiple injuries within one particular body region or the potentially adverse synergistic effects of injuries in multiple body regions.

While the AIS remains a useful tool in describing and numerically coding severity of individual anatomic injuries, the poor correlation between survival and severity scores has prompted the development of other scoring systems to assist in this area of injury research.

Injury Severity Score

The Injury Severity Score (ISS) attempts to address some of the limitations of AIS scoring by quantifying the effects of multiple injuries upon mortality (Baker et al., 1974; Baker 1997). Prior to its development, there was no method to relate multiple injuries to the likelihood of death. Although the AIS grade of the most severe injury was related to mortality, it was clear that the degree of injury in the next most severely injured body region also contributed to the risk of death. The ISS was an attempt to derive a summary score of injury severity that accounted for the variation in mortality associated with both the severity as well as the number of body regions injured. The authors who developed the ISS found that mortality did not increase linearly with an increasing AIS score for the most severe injury. They observed that the case fatality rate increased from 0.5% for injured victims with a maximum AIS of two to a 3.0% fatality rate for those with a maximum AIS of three. Further, the case fatality rate increased from 16% to 64% with an increase in the maximum AIS from four to five. It appeared that with increasing AIS scores, mortality increased to a greater degree for each AIS increase. The best estimate of mortality appeared to be represented by the sum of the squares of the AIS severity grades for the three most severely injured regions, thus forming the ISS (Baker et al., 1974). The ISS is the sum of the squares of the three highest body region AIS scores. No single region can be represented more than once, and a maximum of three AIS scores are used, regardless of the number of body regions injured. While the highest AIS severity score alone explains 25% of the variance in mortality, the ISS as described explains 49% of the variance in case fatality rate. By definition, the ISS ranges from one to 75, with one representing minor and 75 representing uniformly fatal injuries. Also by definition, any AIS body region score of six results in an ISS of 75, regardless of other body region injuries.

As the ISS is based upon the AIS severity assignments, it remains subject to the limitations of the AIS. Although not developed following rigorous statistical methods, the resultant ISS equation at least provided a better correlation with mortality than did more simple linear models. However, until recently, more complex models have not been evaluated for the ability to predict mortality in comparison with the ISS. Additional limitations of the ISS also exist. The ISS does not account for the effect of multiple injuries within a given body region, such as the combination of a liver and spleen injury, both of which are within the abdominal domain of AIS. Second, identical AIS severity scores for different body regions do not necessarily represent the same threat to survival. An injury to the brain with an AIS severity score of four is associated with a relatively greater mortality that an extremity injury with the same AIS score, and hence the ISS can also not account for this difference. Baker and colleagues have indicated that a revision of the ISS, which is based upon the AIS severity grades for the three most severe injuries, regardless of their body region, provides a better estimate of survival outcome than the original ISS (Baker, 1997). This score, termed the New ISS (NISS) retains the simplicity of

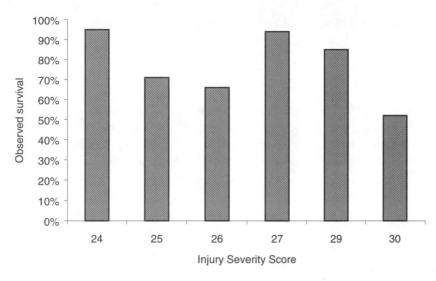

Figure 3.1 Mortality and Injury Severity Score in blunt trauma victims < 55 years of age. Data obtained from Harborview Medical Center Trauma Registry.

the ISS, but has not been widely applied. In two studies, the NISS performed only slightly better than the ISS in predicting mortality (Osler et al., 1997; Brenneman et al., 1998).

There is evidence of a non-linear relationship between the ISS and survival (Copes et al., 1988). Injured patients with a single AIS = 5 injury (ISS = 25) have a higher mortality than patients with three body region AIS = 3 injuries (ISS = 27) despite the later combination generating a higher ISS (see Figure 3.1). The implication of this observation is that while the impact of multiple injuries upon mortality is clear, a single severe injury (AIS = 5) carries a fivefold increase in mortality risk than multiple injuries of moderate severity (AIS = 3), despite being defined by a lower ISS. However, for the most part, increasing ISS correlates with increasing mortality.

Hospitals determine diagnoses at time of discharge based on the International Classification of Diseases, 9th Modification (ICD-9 CM) as a routine part of medical records coding and billing and these diagnosis codes can be converted to AIS codes, which allows calculation of an ISS. A conversion table, which relates ICD-9 CM diagnosis codes directly to AIS codes as recorded in the 1985 AIS modification has been developed, called the ICD-9 CM-MAP (MacKenzie et al., 1989). This has allowed investigators to evaluate large databases, and potentially avoid duplicate chart coding. However, ICD-Map scoring of AIS scores adds another level of variability, as ICD-9 CM diagnoses do not always correlate well with an AIS injury classification, and the subsequent ICD-9 CM-Map scores may not equal the AIS score assigned by a trained abstractor. Another important limitation of this technique applies to its use for large administrative databases such as statewide hospital discharge diagnosis coding. In many administrative databases the number of fields for diagnostic codes is limited, and injuries that would contribute to the calculation of the ISS may not be captured in the administrative database, underscoring injury severity.

Anatomic Profile

The anatomic profile (AP) was developed in an attempt to overcome limitations of the ISS and to increase precision in quantifying multiple injuries. The AP uses the AIS severity code as its building blocks but differs from the ISS by including multiple injuries from individual body regions in its calculation (Champion et al., 1990a). The score provides four components in its description of injury indicated by A, B, C, and D. All serious injuries (AIS $\geq$ 3) are summarized by the first three components of the anatomic profile. The developers of the AP scoring system suggest that it does provide better precision in predicting mortality than the ISS, but it has not been widely adopted. This is likely due to its complexity and lack of a single summary score.

Physiologic Scoring

ISS systems based upon physiologic data have a number of potential advantages in many areas of injury research. In addition to the information captured by scales of anatomic injury severity, measures of the physiologic response to injury such as heart rate (HR), systolic blood pressure (SBP), respiratory rate (RR), and level of consciousness are also important indicators of the severity of an injury.

However, physiologic measurements change over time, in response to the evolution of an injury such as an increase in size of intracranial mass lesion and also in response to treatment such as fluid resuscitation and endotracheal intubation. While representing an advantage when monitoring individual trauma patients, this inherent variability is a limitation of scoring systems based upon physiologic measurements.

Glasgow Coma Scale Score

The GCS score was first reported in the early 1970s as an objective method to describe the level consciousness in patients with acute traumatic, vascular or infective brain injury. The GCS score is an objective estimate of central nervous system function based upon observation of the following functions: motor response, verbal response, and eye-opening. The total GCS score ranging from a minimum of three to a maximum of 15. The scale for each of the three components is based on an assumed hierarchical relationship between each response and the level of central nervous system function. Advantages of the GCS include its relative simplicity and reproducibility and early in its development interobserver variability was considered to be quite low (Teasdale and Jennett, 1974). The authors who originally described the GCS were the first to relate the sum score to outcome following TBI and their findings are indicated in Figure 3.2 (Jennett and Teasdale 1976; Jennet et al., 1979).

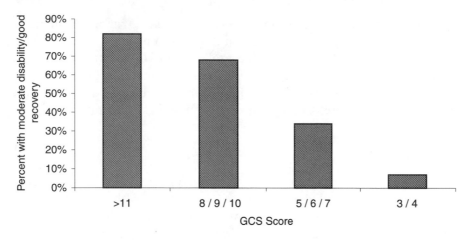

Figure 3.2 Outcome and GCS Score in Severe Traumatic Brain Injury. Data obtained from Jennett (1979, p. 283).

Recent studies have confirmed a strong relationship between the GCS score and survival following TBI (Pal et al., 1989). However, the GCS has a number of limitations. Only patients who were comatose for at least 6 hours after injury were included in the study describing the GCS as a prognostic index following severe head injury, and therefore, the prognostic information is derived from patients with moderate to severe TBI. Subsequent studies have utilized the GCS in a wider range of TBI severity and have not been as explicit as the original investigators in defining the time point following injury or treatment at which the GCS was measured (e.g., Foulkes et al., 1991). The verbal response component of the GCS is often unavailable, most often due to endotracheal intubation, and in these circumstances, the GCS score cannot be used in outcome prediction or for severity adjustment. The Major Trauma Outcome Study (MTOS) reported that 11% of the patients could not be included in the final analysis because of missing physiologic variables, primarily the GCS score (Champion et al., 1990b). Up to 25% of trauma patients in the emergency department may be endotracheally intubated, and therefore unavailable for GCS scoring (Offner et al., 1992). Options for overcoming this limitation of the GCS score have been evaluated, and include statistical modeling using the eye opening and best motor response to estimate the often missing verbal component (Rutledge et al., 1996). Based upon 2521 GCS scores from 665 nonintubated patients the authors suggest that the verbal component can be estimated by a second-order regression equation using the available eye and motor component scores. Unfortunately, this proposed approach has a number of limitations. The authors excluded 13% of the GCS measurements as "outliers" and therefore have not completely overcome the problem of excluding subjects. Moreover, the use of multiple GCS measurements over time from individual subjects, as done in this study will artificially increase the statistical strength of the relationship, as the GCS scores taken from the same individual are not independent.

Despite these important limitations, the GCS provides the best estimate of outcome following TBI and has been shown to perform better in correctly categorizing survival or mortality than other general measures of outcome, such as the simplified acute physiology score (Rocca et al., 1998). Others have found the GCS to be a better predictor of outcome following TBI than anatomic measures such as the head AIS severity score (Coplin, personal communication).

Revised Trauma Score

The Revised Trauma Score (RTS) is the most commonly used physiologic severity scoring system and is not limited to the evaluation of patients with TBI as is the GCS score. The initial Trauma Score was a physiologic injury severity score that numerically summarized circulatory, respiratory, and central nervous system function following trauma (Champion et al., 1981). This score had been used for a number of years as a field triage tool and also in outcome evaluations. The RTS is restricted to the three least subjective components of the original Trauma Score and was shown to provide the equivalent outcome predictions with less intraobserver variability (Champion et al., 1989). The RTS is based upon the GCS score, systolic blood pressure (SBP), and respiratory rate (RR). When used for outcome evaluation, the RTS is based upon a weighted sum of the interval-coded values for the GCS score, SBP and RR. The associated weights were determined by logistic regression with survival as the outcome variable and are based upon data from the MTOS (Champion et al., 1989). The RTS shares limitations with the GCS as a physiologic measure. All three components are time and treatment dependent and the RTS is also subject to limitations associated with missing values for the GCS verbal component and the RR that are often unavailable.

Combined Scoring Systems Estimating Survival Outcome after Trauma

By combining measures of the severity of anatomic injury with those of acute physiologic derangement and age (as an estimate of physiologic reserve), it has been possible to provide statistically strong estimates of survival probability following trauma. Multiple factors contribute to death following injury, and combining the advantages of physiologic and anatomic classification systems has provided better estimates of outcome. These combined scoring systems presently are the standard measures of adjustment for case-mix and injury severity. However, the advantage of improved prediction with these composite scoring systems is accompanied by the limitations of each of the scores upon which they are based.

Trauma and Injury Severity Score (TRISS)

TRISS is a method for assigning an individual patient a probability of survival $P_{(s)}$ based upon the presenting RTS, mechanism of injury (blunt vs. penetrating), age, and ISS. The TRISS method was initially developed and validated on the MTOS study database (Boyd et al., 1987). Logistic regression coefficients were estimated and two models estimating expected mortality were developed, one for blunt trauma and one for penetrating trauma patients. The logistic model and the coefficient weights based upon the MTOS study sample are shown in Figure 3.3. The TRISS method is presently the most widely use scoring system in injury control research and trauma system evaluation, and continues to use the coefficient weights from the MTOS patients who were injured between 1982 and 1988. Other investigators have developed and attempted to validate newer coefficients based upon more contemporary data sets and this approach leads to less misclassification (Hannan et al., 1995). Some have developed new coefficients for TRISS analysis and found them to differ from those derived from the MTOS (Lane et al., 1996). These authors reported that the new coefficients better predicted survival outcome than those derived from the MTOS, which may, in part, reflect the bias of applying a predictive model to the same cohort upon which it was developed.

While the TRISS method incorporates advantages of anatomic and physiologic scoring systems and does provide more accurate estimates of expected survival, it also is subject to the limitations of the ISS and RTS from which it is derived. Overall the misclassification rates of TRISS have been reported to be less than 5% in non-MTOS patient samples, and predicted versus actual survival rates are not markedly different (Offner et al., 1992; Lane et al., 1996). However, in more severely traumatized patients the misclassification range has been reported to be greater than 30% (Demetriades et al., 1998). TRISS has a high misclassification rate in patients with abdominal gunshot wounds (Cornwell et al., 1998). In this study, 39 of 108 patients with fatal abdominal gunshot wounds had TRISS $P_{(s)}$ estimates of greater than 50%. Peer review of these 39 deaths suggested that only one was potentially preventable. This suggests that the components of TRISS do not adequately capture overall injury severity in patients with penetrating abdominal injuries. The high frequency of multiple organ injuries within a single body region in gunshot wound victims suggests that misclassification is due to the limitations of the ISS in these patients. In addition, the limitations of physiologic measures apply to TRISS and a number of methods have been proposed to address such limitations, specifically regarding their impact upon TRISS scoring. A method for estimating probability of survival similar to TRISS has been developed, which overcomes the problem of endotracheal intubation by including the GCS motor response, SBP, ISS, and age; excluding the often missing GCS verbal component and RR (Offner et al., 1992). These authors developed new coefficients for estimating $P_{(s)}$ using logistic regression, including only the predictor variables indicated above. However, this solution did not completely solve the problem of missing data, as 19% of eligible subjects were excluded. However, they were able to include the 23% of patients who had been intubated and would not be available for standard TRISS analysis. One additional option is to provide a range of scores by including the highest and lowest possible values for the missing variable (Harviel et al., 1989).

Interobserver variability has been demonstrated in the assignment of individual TRISS survival probabilities and represents another limitation of this and other scoring systems (Brennan and Silman, 1992). The extent of the variability in TRISS scoring has been shown to lead potentially to a high frequency of misclassification. Patients receiving TRISS survival probability scores in the 0.05–0.95 range demonstrated significant interobserver variability, potentially limiting the validity of the TRISS method as a research and evaluation tool (Zoltie and deDombal, 1993). Aside from a few studies, the importance of variation in the assignment of various scoring systems has not been evaluated.

Age is an indirect measure of injury co-morbidity and also reflects an overall decrease in physiologic reserve. TRISS controls for the effects of age by assigning a indicator of one where age is ≥ 55 years and an indicator of zero where age is ≤ 54 years. Therefore, all ages 55 years and above are considered to have the same impact upon survival, which is likely not the case. This feature suggests that TRISS may not provide accurate estimates in the most elderly injury victims.

A Severity Characterization of Trauma

In an attempt to address the limitations of the TRISS method, a scoring system termed A Severity Characterization of Trauma (ASCOT) has been developed (Champion et al., 1990a). The ASCOT replaces the ISS with the anatomic profile and breaks down age into 10-year periods. The ASCOT, like TRISS uses anatomic and physiologic measures of injury severity, age, and the mechanism of injury to generate an expected probability of survival. Where the TRISS method has three predictor variables, ASCOT includes seven. The ASCOT separates the RTS into its component GCS, SBP, and RR, places age into one of five categories and includes the A, B, and C components of the anatomic profile. The ASCOT has not achieved wide use. This may be due to its relative complexity and absence of a single summary severity statistic.

The ICISS System for ISS

A series of studies by one group of investigators has evaluated an ICD-9 CM based injury severity score (ICISS) and compared its ability to predict mortality with the ISS and TRISS. They initially incorporated information based upon mortality for each of the 2034 individual injury ICD-9 CM codes (800.00–959.9) and actual patient survival (at hospital discharge) from a statewide trauma registry (Rutledge et al., 1993). It is based on the calculation of the mortality risk initially termed the mortality risk ratio (MRR) for each individual ICD-9 CM injury code. The results of the initial work suggested that injury ICD-9 CM codes are better predictors of mortality than the ISS. The score has evolved through a number of iterations, which have included the addition of the RTS, cause of injury, ICD-9 CM procedure codes and age. The ICISS approach has been applied to a number of large databases and appears to predict survival as accurately as ISS or TRISS (Rutledge et al., 1997). The present iteration of this method, like TRISS, incorporates the patient's age and RTS, but replaces the ISS with the product of the MRRs for each of the patients ICD-9 CM diagnosis and procedure codes (Rutledge and Osler, 1998). As was done with TRISS, a logistic model was developed and an estimated $P_{(s)}$ determined for each patient. The addition of the RTS and age to the ICISS resulted in the best statistical fit based upon the Hosmer–Lemeshow Goodness-of-Fit statistic in comparison with TRISS, ISS, and ICISS alone, but the limitations of physiologic scores again emerge.

Harborview Assessment for Risk of Mortality Score (HARM)

Investigators at Harborview Injury Prevention and Research Center have recently developed another method of predicting in-hospital mortality following injury. Like the ICISS score, the HARM score was developed to better estimate the probability of mortality following injury, based on information available from hospital discharge codes without relying on physiologic data. The unique feature of this scoring system is the inclusion of two-way interaction terms for several combinations of injuries demonstrated to impact survival synergistically. The resultant regression model takes into account ICD-9 CM codes for anatomic injury, mechanism, intent, pre-existing medical conditions, and age, data available on over 98% of hospital discharge coding charts. Compared with TRISS and ICISS predictions of survival, the HARM scores provides improved sensitivity, specificity, and increased area under the receiver operator characteristic (ROC) curve (HARM = 0.9592; TRISS $P_{(s)}$ = 0.9473; ICISS = 0.9402). Physiologic data were unavailable on 38% of the charts in which a HARM score could be calculated (West TA, personal communication). The HARM score requires validation on other databases, but represents a promising example of a combined scoring system, which avoids the limitations imposed by using physiologic data.

Measurement of Co-morbidity

The severity of anatomic injury and degree of acute physiologic derangement are important, but not exclusive determinants of outcome after trauma. The patient's physiologic reserve is an important contributor and must be considered when conducting injury outcome research and evaluating trauma systems and trauma care effectiveness. The obvious impact of age upon the relationship between injury severity and survival prompted the inclusion of age in the TRISS scoring system and has also stimulated investigation to determine other estimates of pre-existing health status that contribute to mortality and alter the relationship between injury severity and survival. Enumerating the existence and number of pre-existing medical conditions has been used as a method to evaluate and control for baseline health status when evaluating survival outcome following injury. However, more rigorous methods defining the existence and severity of underlying medical conditions and physiologic reserve have been developed and can be applied to the evaluation of survival and other outcomes following injury.

Pre-existing Medical Conditions

Pre-existing medical conditions affect survival after injury. Ischemic heart disease, cirrhosis, coagulopathy, chronic obstructive pulmonary disease, and diabetes significantly increase the risk of mortality during hospital admission for an injury (Morris et al., 1990). These conclusions have been supported by results of other investigations in which in-hospital mortality after trauma is related to the presence of one or more of these pre-existing conditions (Milzman et al., 1992). Although important in determining individual patient mortality, pre-existing conditions are reported to be uncommon in trauma patients and have been considered to have little overall impact upon outcomes of large groups of patients (Sacco et al., 1993). The frequency of one or more pre-existing conditions has been identified in between 4.6% and 16% of trauma patients. This 16% estimate, from a single regional trauma center indicates that important medical conditions may be seen more commonly at some institutions, but, alternatively, it may represent differences in chart recording and coding practices (Milzman et al., 1992).

Of the three major studies examining pre-existing conditions and trauma outcome, two were retrospective cohort studies and one a retrospective case–control study. All have been based upon data from existing databases, two were specific for trauma patients and the third was based upon computerized hospital discharge abstract data. There has been no prospective study in trauma patients of a sufficient size to address potentially more complex relationship between pre-existing conditions and survival following trauma.

Charlson Co-Morbidity Index

The Charlson Co-Morbidity Index is a weighed sum of co-morbid conditions and age, the weights for individual co-morbid diseases were derived from the adjusted relative risk (hazards ratio) for 1-year mortality (Charlson et al., 1987; Pompei et al., 1988, p. 275). Conditions assigned a weight of one include diabetes without end-organ damage, previous myocardial infarction, peripheral vascular disease, and other conditions. Moderate to severe liver disease is assigned a weight of three and metastatic cancer or acquired immune deficiency syndrome are assigned a weight of six. The effect of age upon survival was examined in a 10-year follow-up of patients with breast cancer. Each decade in age above 40 is assigned a sequentially higher co-morbidity ranking. For instance, a 50-year old patient with a co-morbidity index of two would have a total or combined age-co-morbidity score of three. This index has also been used in adjusting for the effects of co-morbid illness when using administrative data sets and appears to function well (D'Hoore et al., 1996). Unfortunately, the Charlson Co-Morbidity Index does not appear to be useful in predicting short-term mortality (Pompei et al., 1991; Cleves et al., 1997).

The Charlson Co-Morbidity Index has been used to control for the effects of co-morbid conditions in a follow-up study of elderly injury victims (Gubler et al., 1997, p. 1010). The impact of the Charlson index rating upon long-term survival was similar to other reports in the literature.

Other Methods to Measure Co-morbidity

Other scales have been developed which may be less complicated than the Charlson Co-Morbidity Index and have been derived specifically for use with administrative data sets. The scale developed by Von Korff et al. (1992) includes age, gender, co-morbid conditions such as diabetes and heart disease and a history of hospitalization and physician visits (Coleman et al., 1998, p. 419). The more complex methods for estimating intermediate and long-term survival have not been used in injury victims but may provide well validated methods for controlling the effects of co-morbidity upon mortality and possibly other outcomes following injury, and warrant study in trauma victims.

Future Needs in the Development and Use of Injury Scoring Systems

As injury control investigations span a wide range of activities and objectives, a comprehensive scoring system suited for all applications may never be realized. However, the development of a system which functions well, with minimal modifications, based upon a limited number of easily obtainable data points is an important goal for injury control research. The AIS, ISS, GCS, and TRISS are presently the most widely used measures. The AIS combines specific information about individual injuries with an arbitrary scale of severity, and severity scores for individual injuries correlate poorly with mortality. Whether future AIS modification would benefit from assigning severity scores consistently across body regions, using a method similar to that used to develop the ICISS, remains to be proven. Future modification of the AIS may also decrease some of the limitations associated with the ISS and TRISS methods of assigning survival probabilities.

The deficiencies of the ISS have been described in relation to the inability of this summary score to incorporate the effects of multiple injuries to a given body region, to its nonlinear relationship with survival, and to interobserver variability in AIS severity scoring and ISS calculation. The NISS, which considers the most severe injuries regardless of body region, has not provided better estimates and has not solved the problem of capturing the cumulative effects of multiple injuries. The approach used in developing the HARM score is appealing in that interactions between individual injuries are directly examined for their impact upon mortality.

Physiologic scoring systems remain important in many aspects of the initial care of injury victims and therefore in research evaluating trauma care. Trauma care research, trauma system development, and outcome evaluation requires valid severity measures that reflect the physiologic response to individual injuries or a combination of injuries. Physiologic variables have been shown to explain significant variability in mortality outcomes and have played an important part in injury control research. However, their inherent variability coupled with the high frequency of these measures not being recorded, may limit their use in future scoring systems.

The development of scoring systems has primarily addressed hospital mortality as the primary outcome measure. However, other measures of outcome after injury are of considerable importance in evaluating the effectiveness of trauma care. Functional outcome is a critical measure of the impact of injuries and of their treatment, and represents an important area of future research. It will be important to adjust for injury severity and pre-existing conditions when evaluating which components of trauma care and trauma systems affect functional outcomes. Moreover, resource utilization has become an important consideration in the field of injury control. Measures of injury severity and co-morbidity will need to be validated in reference to these measures of outcome that now represent a considerable component of injury control research and practice.

References

Association for the Advancement of Automotive Medicine (1990) The Abbreviated Injury Scale. Des Plaines, IL: AAAM.
Baker SP (1997) Advances and adventures in injury prevention. J Trauma: Injury Infect Crit Care 42:369–73.
Baker SP, O'Neill B, Haddon W, Long WB (1974) The Injury Severity Score: a method for describing patients with multiple injuries and evaluating emergency care. J Trauma 14:187–96.
Boyd CR, Tolson MA, Copes WS (1987) Evaluating trauma care: The TRISS method. J Trauma 27:370–8.
Brennan P, Silman (1992) A Statistical methods for assessing observer variability in clinical measures. Br Med J 304:1491–4.
Brenneman FD, Boulanger BR, McLellan BA, Redelmeier DA (1998) Measuring injury severity: time for a change? J Trauma: Injury Infect Crit Care 44:580–2.
Champion HR, Sacco WJ, Carnazzo AJ, Copes W, Fouty WJ (1981) Trauma score. Crit Care Med 9:672–6.
Champion HR, Sacco WJ, Copes WS (1989) A revision of the trauma score. J Trauma 29:623–9.
    (1990a) A new characterization of injury severity. J Trauma 30:539–46.
    (1990b) The Major Trauma Outcome Study: establishing national norms for trauma care. J Trauma 30:1356–65.
Charlson ME, Pompei P, Ales KL, MacKenzie CR (1987) A new method of classifying prognostic comorbidity in longitudinal studies: development and validation. J Chronic Dis 40:373–83.
Cleves MA, Sanchez N, Draheim M (1997) Evaluation of two competing methods for calculating Charlson's comorbidity index when analyzing short-term mortality using administrative data. J Clin Epidemiol 50:903–8.
Coleman EA, Wagner EH, Grothaus LC, Hecht J, Savarino J, Buchner DM (1998) Predicting hospitalization and functional decline in older health plan enrollees: Are administrative data as accurate as self-report? Geriatric Soc 46:419–25.
Committee on Medical Aspects of Automotive Safety (1971) Rating the severity of tissue damage; I. The Abbreviated Scale. J Am Med Assoc 2152:277–80.
Copes WS, Champion HR, Sacco WJ (1988) The Injury Severity Score revisited. J Trauma 28:69–77.

Cornwell EE, III, Velmahos GC, Berne TV, Tatevossian R, Belzberg H, Ecksstein M, Murray JA, Asensio JA, Demetriades D (1998) Lethal abdominal gunshot wounds at a level I trauma center: analysis of TRISS (Revised Trauma Score and Injury Severity Score) fallouts. J Am Coll Surg 187:123–9.

Demetriades D, Chan LS, Velmahos G, Berne TV, Cornwell EE III, Belxzberg H, Asensio JA, Murray J, Berne J, Shoemaker W (1998) TRISS methodology in trauma: the need for alternatives. Br J Surg 85:379–84.

D'Hoore W, Bouckaert A, Tilquin C (1996) Practical considerations on the use of the Charlson comorbidity index with administrative data bases. J Clin Epidemiol 49:1429–33.

Foulkes MA, Eisenberg HM, Jane JA, Marmarou A, Marshall LF, The Traumatic Coma Data Bank Research Group (1991) The Traumatic Coma Data Bank: design, methods, and baseline characteristics. J Neurosurg 75:S8–13.

Gubler KD, Davis R, Koepsell T, Soderberg R, Maier RV, Rivara FP (1997) Long-term survival of elderly trauma patients. Arch Surg 132:1010–14.

Hannan EL, Mendeloff J, Farrell LS, Cayten CG, Murphy JG (1995) Validation of TRISS and ASCOT using a non-MTOS trauma registry. J Trauma 381:83–8.

Harviel JD, Landsman I, Greenberg A, Copes WS, Flannagan MF, Champion HR (1989) The effect of autopsy on injury severity and survival probability calculations. J Trauma 296:766–73.

Jennett B, Teasdale G (1976) Predicting outcome in individual patients after severe head injury. Lancet 5:1031–4.

Jennett B, Teasdale G, Braakman A, Minderhoud J, Jeiden J, Kurz T (1979) Prognosis of patients with severe head injury. Neurosurgery 4:283–9.

Lane PL, Doig G, Mikrogianakis A, Charyk ST, Stefanits T (1996) An evaluation of Ontario trauma outcomes and the development of regional norms for trauma and Injury Severity Score (TRISS) analysis. J Trauma Injury Infect Crit Care 41:731–4.

MacKenzie EJ, Steinwachs DM, Shankar B (1989) Classifying trauma severity based on hospital discharge diagnosis. Validation of an ICD-9 CM to AIS-85 conversion table. Med Care 27:412–22.

Milzman DP, Boulanger BR, Rodriguez A, Soderstrom CA, Mitchell KA, Magnant CM (1992) Pre-existing disease in trauma patients: a predictor of fate independent of age and injury severity score. J Trauma 32:236–44.

Morris JA, MacKenzie EJ, Edelstein SL (1990) The effect of preexisting conditions on mortality in trauma patients. J Am Med Assoc 263:1942–6.

Offner PJ, Jurkovich GJ, Gurney J, Rivara FP (1992) Revision of TRISS for intubated patients. J Trauma 32:32–5.

Osler T, Baker SP, Long W (1997) A modification of the injury severity score that both improves accuracy and simplifies scoring. J Trauma Injury Infect Crit Care 43:922–5.

Pal J, Brown R, Fleiszer D (1989) The Value of the Glasgow Coma Scale and Injury Severity Score: predicting outcome in multiple trauma patients with head injury. J Trauma 29:746–8.

Pompei P, Charlson ME, Ales K, MacKenzie CR, Norton M (1991) Relating patient characteristics at the time of admission to outcomes of hospitalization. J Clin Epidemiol 44:1063–9.

Pompei P, Charlson ME, Douglas RG Jr (1988) Clinical assessments as predictors of one year survival after hospitalization: implications for prognostic stratification. J Clin Epidemiol 41:275–84.

Rocca B, Martin C, Viviand X, Bidet P-F, Saint-Gilles HL, Chevalier A (1998) Comparison of four severity scores in patients with head trauma. J Trauma Injury Infect Crit Care 29:299–305.

Rutledge R, Osler T (1998) The ICD-9-based illness severity score: a new model that outperforms both DRG and APR-DRG as predictors of survival and resource utilization. J Trauma Injury Infect Crit Care 45:791–9.

Rutledge R, Fakhry S, Baker C, Oiler D (1993) Injury severity grading in trauma patients: a simplified technique based upon ICD-9 coding. J Trauma 35:497–506.

Rutledge R, Lentz CW, Fakhry S, Hunt J (1996) Appropriate use of the Glasgow Coma Scale in intubated patients: a linear regression prediction of the Glasgow Verbal Score from the Glasgow Eye and Motor Scores. J Trauma Injury Infect Crit Care 41:514–22.

Rutledge R, Hoyt DB, Eastman AB, Sise MJ, Velky T, Canty T, Wachtel TM, Osler TM (1997) Comparison of the Injury Severity Score and ICD-9 diagnosis codes as predictors of outcome in injury: analysis of 44,032 patients. J Trauma Injury Infect Crit Care 42:477–89.

Rutledge R, Osler T, Emery S, Kromhout-Schiro S (1998) The end of the Injury Severity Score (ISS) and the Trauma and Injury Severity Score (TRISS, ICISS, and International Classification of Diseases, Ninth revision-based prediction tool, outperforms both ISS and TRISS as predictors of trauma patient survival, hospital charges, and hospital length of stay. J Trauma Injury Infect Crit Care 44:41–8.

Sacco WJ, Copes WS, Bain LW, MaKenzie EJ, Frey CF, Hoyt DB, Weigelt JA, Champion HR (1993) Effect of preinjury illness trauma patient survival outcome. J Trauma 35:538–43.

Teasdale G, Jennett B (1974) Assessment of coma and impaired consciousness – a practical scale. Lancet 7:81–3.

Von Korff M, Wagner EH, Saunders K (1992) A chronic disease score from automated pharmacy data. J Clin Epidemiol 45:197–203.

Zoltie N, deDombal FT (1993) The hit and miss of ISS and TRISS. Br Med J 307:906–9.

4

Data Linkages and Using Administrative and Secondary Databases

Beth A. Mueller

Introduction

Administrative and other databases originally created for purposes other than research are increasingly being considered for use in injury research. This is not surprising – those conducting health research or surveillance have always considered the potential uses and benefits of secondary data. This chapter attempts to provide an overview of the benefits and limitations of use of these electronic databases, categories of uses, types of databases that have been employed in injury research, and some of the methods used. It is by no means an exhaustive description of all such uses, nor is it intended as a text for conducting data linkages. Based on our experience, we have attempted to provide a framework for considering use of these databases or conducting linkages, and to raise awareness of some of the important issues that need to be considered.

For some research projects, there are several benefits associated with using administrative or secondary data. For purposes of this chapter, administrative data include data (not necessarily related to health status) routinely collected as part of the administrative operations of some organization. Examples of administrative data are drivers' license records, employment rosters, vital records such as birth or death certificates, and insurance claims. "Secondary" databases typically encompass the administrative databases mentioned above as well as research or surveillance data that have been collected for purposes other than your own project. Issues to be discussed here that are related to data access, linkage, and use apply to both administrative and non-administrative, secondary databases and thus, the latter, more general term will be used to refer to both.

In general, collection of primary data for research is relatively more costly and time consuming than accessing existing data. Administration of research questionnaires or surveys, review of medical records, standardized observation of behavior, and obtaining and processing laboratory specimens do not need to be attempted within the context of a research study if reliable related or surrogate information, available for the population and time period of interest, already exists in another form. Advantages of using some existing databases include access to information for a larger number of people than would be possible to otherwise identify, or the ability to learn information about or to calculate rates of events for an underlying population, if the data are population-based (as with death certificates, and some hospital discharge or trauma registry databases). Even research studies that do require primary data collection frequently benefit from linkages to data available through another source. Existing databases may provide information about potential confounders (such as the presence of co-morbid conditions), or provide a means of validating some aspect of the research data. For example, self-reported information on alcohol use among people with injuries treated in an emergency department might be compared with trauma registry data from a facility where blood alcohol measurements are routinely made for all injured patients. Many rich databases exist, and there is a growing realization that secondary data may provide valuable information either alone, or in combination with other sources (Copes et al., 1996; Huff et al., 1996; Lillard and Farmer, 1997; Nasca, 1997; Sorock et al., 1997). Sometimes the fact that the data contained in a secondary database were not collected for research purposes is a strength, because they lack biases that might exist in data (especially self-reported data) collected for a specific research purpose. For example, one could validate self-reported motor-vehicle collision history of study subjects by linkage with a drivers' license database. Secondary data may also comprise an independent measure of exposures or incidents occurring prior to the outcomes of interest. An example of this is the use of drivers' license records to control for prior driving record in an assessment of the extent to which a brain injury or stroke may adversely affect an individual's ability to drive (Haselkorn et al., 1998).

Recent improvements in information technology have made access to and use of secondary databases even more feasible. Transferring electronic information between machines, or from one data format to another, is no longer the onerous task it once was, particularly in view of the increased use of electronic records. As standard formats for police, medical, or other records (most notably the adoption of standard medical record formats) also increase in use, this ability will be enhanced even further. The abilities to conduct data linkages, and to screen large volumes of data or text for "keywords" that might identify target populations, are constantly being refined to the extent that software packages currently exist to conduct at least some of the complex programming activities necessary to create or augment a research database from other data sources (Newman and Brown, 1997).

Categories of Secondary Data Use

One might classify the ways secondary databases are used for injury (and other) research purposes in three general ways. First, there is the use of an existing database to identify events. For databases in which each event represents a unique individual (such as a death certificate file) identification of an event is equivalent to identifying a person, and case-finding for research in this manner probably represents the most common use of secondary databases. Although injury-related databases such as the National Electronic Injury Surveillance System (NEISS) in the United States, the Canadian Hospital Injury Reporting and Prevention Program in Canada, and the European Home and Leisure Accident Surveillance System (EHLASS) in Europe have been used for this purpose for many years, the use of other secondary databases to provide injury surveillance information, or as a starting point for further research is being increasingly explored. One example of this is the use of a hospital discharge database to measure the number of hospitalizations occurring within a year that are related to hip fracture, and to describe the associated characteristics such as frequency of different procedures performed, mean number of days hospitalized, or the mean hospital charges billed (Alexander et al., 1992). If the database contains E-codes (external causes), then the evaluation may be refined to include only those hip fractures due to falls. The counting of events in this manner typically does not require the use of patient identifying information such as name, social security number, or other personal identifier. Use of these data however, to identify subjects so that they might be invited to participate in a research study, or for a review of medical records, would obviously require some means of identifying individuals (and thus, would necessitate a more rigorous level of review by a human subjects protection review board).

If a secondary database consists of event or episode records in which individuals may be represented more than once (for example, an outpatient clinic visit register, hospital discharge database, or work injury claims file), one has the potential to examine the data longitudinally. This may be considered a second category of usage, in which linkages within the same database are conducted in order to identify individuals with specific conditions at their initial appearance in the data (e.g., at their initial clinic visit for an injury), or to create a chain of events occurring to the same individual. This type of use typically involves a data linkage procedure often referred to as unduplication or internal linkage, similar to the matching of two similarly formatted files (Alsop and Langley, 1998). Again, using a hospital discharge database as an example, linkage of records could be conducted to identify all hospitalizations occurring to the same person. Note that distinguishing individuals (as opposed to hospitalizations) within the database requires this type of linkage. This difference (between events and individuals), and the steps necessary to unduplicate a file, are frequently overlooked in planning use of a secondary database. Such an oversight results in an overestimate of the number of individuals with a specific condition (which may result in erroneous assumptions about the number of cases potentially available for a research project), and an underestimate of the programming resources necessary to conduct a research project.

The results of unduplication may include identification of an individual's first hospitalization (or for some, their only hospitalization) for a specific condition (e.g., in order to identify potential subjects for a case-control study) or identification of multiple hospitalizations experienced by an individual as a result of a single injury event (e.g., so that related morbidity and costs of case may be measured). Thus, one could describe patterns of hospitalization and re-hospitalization of individuals (Samsa et al., 1996; Gubler et al., 1996). One might describe, for example, the number of individuals hospitalized for a hip fracture repair who require re-hospitalization within a specified period of time (Hudson et al., 1998). Unduplication may identify multiple hospitalizations experienced by an individual for any reason (i.e., for different injury events or for injury and non-injury related reasons); or, in some instances identification of all hospitalizations related to a multiperson injury event. An example of the latter would be linkage of records to identify all those hospitalized due to a multivehicle collision.

Although the use of some unique identifier or personal information within an events database is required to conduct unduplication, frequently the researchers themselves may not require any personal or unique identifying information if the linkage is performed by the entity "owning" the data. (For example, the data manager within a health agency or organization that creates and manages a hospital discharge database may be able to perform the linkage prior to releasing to a non-affiliated investigator a research data file that is stripped of all identifying information.) If the owner of the data is unable to perform such a linkage for research purposes (as may be the case in a busy health agency with limited resources), it may be possible to create a unique identifier for each individual that does not contain identifying information, or which is encrypted in some fashion, so the data file released can subsequently be linked by the investigators themselves without accessing personal identifying information. For example, substitution of a medical records number with a sequential unique identification number within the database, conducted prior to release of a public use file that is stripped of identifiers, will allow researchers to unduplicate data as necessary for specific projects.

A third use of secondary data is the linkage of two or more different databases resulting in a new, enriched, database. This may consist of linkages of one or more administrative databases with a separate data file collected for research purpose; linkage of an administrative file to a trauma or other registry (Mueller et al., 1998); or linkages of several secondary or large survey data files created for entirely different purposes (Patterson et al., 1996; Herrchen et al., 1997; Lillard and Farmer, 1997). Examples include a linkage of trauma registry data to drivers' license data to compare police assessment of alcohol use with blood alcohol measurements (Grossman et al., 1996) and linkage of drivers' license data to hospital discharge data to examine the possible decreased ability to drive following traumatic brain injury (Haselkorn et al., 1998). The methodological and logistical challenges of this type of linkage generally exceed those of the other two types of database use mentioned earlier, particularly when attempting linkages of data sources held by different agencies. Issues that must be dealt with, in addition to those of privacy/confidentiality of information, may include the lack of a unique (or in some instances, any) identifier across all databases, handling of diverse file formats, and the final ownership of the linked product.

Information from Secondary Databases of Potential Use for Injury Research

Many types of databases have been used or considered for use in health research, including police and traffic safety reports (Rosman, 1996), insurance databases and automated records from health-care organizations (Gilmore et al., 1996; Lipowski and Bigelow, 1996; Cummings et al., 1997b; Selby, 1997; Lillard and Farmer, 1997), vital statistics (Wolf et al., 1993; Herman et al., 1997) hospital discharge records (Alsop and Langley, 1998; Mullins et al., 1998), hospital billing records (Weiss et al., 1997), pharmacy records (Gilmore et al., 1996; Garcia Rodriguez and Perez

Gutthann, 1998; Thapa et al., 1998), criminal justice records (Rivara et al., 1995; Conseur et al., 1997a); emergency medical service (Walen, 1997) and emergency department records (Williams et al., 1996), and employment or other rosters identifying individuals (Sugarman and Grossman, 1996; Hertzman et al., 1997). Use of these data in health research, which is typically not the original purpose for which they were collected, is never undertaken lightly. In our experience, such use is generally contingent upon the approval of both the gate keeper or administrator of the database, and of the institutional review boards charged with reviewing human subjects research protocols within all institutions involved. Both entities require that there be sufficient merit in the research use of the database, and that the data handling procedures be conducted with strict regard to patient or subject confidentiality.

Some general types of secondary databases for injury research are shown in Table 4.1, along with descriptions of how the information was used, and references to relevant examples in the literature.

Considerations for Use of Secondary Data and Database Linkages

A framework for considering use of secondary databases for research has been proposed by Sorenson et al. (1996). A brief presentation of the issues they raised follows (Table 4.2) with a view to some of the logistic and scientific considerations that should be considered in planning. These are further expanded to include logistic and scientific issues related to record linkage studies in which not only should these same items be considered for each parent database, but the relative relationships of these characteristics across the two (or more) databases be considered.

Data Linkage Strategies

The level of time and effort required to conduct data linkages depends on the amount and type of information available to conduct a linkage, but always seems to be underestimated in the planning stages of a project. Linkage strategies are generally classified as deterministic or probabilistic. Deterministic linkage is a matching process which may consist of a fairly straightforward matching of a single identifier (as is possible if each record contains a unique subject identification number) or a complex series of steps in which several variables in both databases are matched hierarchically. In the absence of custom software or use of commercial data linkage software, deterministic linkage is most often used by researchers, as it can be conducted with standard statistical software packages. Probabilistic linkage is a multistage process in which evaluation of linkages is based on probability theory, with calculation of a weighted score for every possible pair of records that reflects the likelihood that they belong to the same person (Jaro, 1995). A limited number of commercial software products specifically designed to conduct data probabilistic linkages are available. Occasionally, linkages may utilize a combination of both procedures (Kendrick et al., 1998). A few comparisons of linkage

Table 4.1 Summary of secondary databases that have been used for injury research

Database source	Information contained of relevance to injury research	Examples of use for injury research
Vital records (birth, death, fetal death)	Survival status, death after injury occurrence, occurrence of injury-related deaths; identification of parental and birth characteristics (from linked birth–death records)	Linked death and fetal death certificates to police crash reports to evaluate adverse pregnancy outcomes to pregnant women involved in auto crashes (Wolf et al., 1993); linked death certificates – hospital discharge records to evaluate trends in firearm injuries (Cummings et al., 1998); linked birth–death certificates to examine risk factors for infant injury death (Cummings et al., 1994) or childhood mortality from fires (Scholer et al., 1998); evaluated pre- and postlegislation mortality due to firearms (Cummings et al., 1997a)
Hospital discharge or billing data	Comorbidity status (from diagnosis or procedure codes); injury severity, type, and mechanism; occurrence of hospitalization or re-hospitalization; use of resources, patterns of care, injury outcomes (length of stay, need for surgical intervention from procedure codes) or hospital charges billed; insurance coverage status	Linked hospitalization–justice reports to evaluate trauma hospitalizations to juvenile offenders (Conseur et al., 1997a); linked police crash reports–hospital discharge records to evaluate costs/outcomes from motorcycle crashes (Rowland et al., 1996); follow-up of children with head trauma to determine rehospitalization (Davis et al., 1995); cost, frequency of falls in elderly (Alexander et al., 1992); prior injury as risk for assaultive injury (Dowd et al., 1996); hospital charges for injury (Unwin and Codde, 1998)
Police reports (crash reports, justice system reports)	Crash reports: Identification of motor vehicle crashes, pedestrian–vehicle collisions; alcohol use status of drivers; crash or driver characteristics. Justice reports: contacts with justice system	Linked police crash reports–EMS–hospital discharge records to evaluation crash outcomes (Johnson and Walker, 1996); linked police crash reports–hospital discharge records to estimate hospital charges to drinking drivers (Mueller et al., 1998); linked birth records–justice reports to evaluate maternal/perinatal risk factors for juvenile delinquency (Conseur et al., 1997b); identified motorcycle crashes to evaluate pre- and posthelmet use legislation injury severity (Peek-Asa and Kraus, 1997)
Government regulatory agency records	Civil aviation incident reports, consumer protection agency reports, labor bureau records	Pilot and plane factors in civil aviation reports (Rostykus et al., 1998); farm injuries identified in product safety database (Rivara, 1997); work injury and illness identified by labor bureau (Murphy et al., 1996)

Source	Data Contents	Uses
EMS Reports	Ambulance reports: reason for response, medical care given, patient characteristics	Linked EMS–hospital discharge–police crash reports–coroner reports to evaluate patterns of emergency care (Grossman et al., 1995); Identified children intubated in prehospital setting (Brownstein et al., 1996)
Coroner's Reports	Identification of fatalities, patient and event characteristics	Identified homicide/suicide cases (Kellermann et al., 1998)
Departments of Licensing (drivers or other licensing bureaus)	(Drivers' licenses): Driver characteristics, licensing actions. (Gun registration): Characteristics of purchasers, dates of purchase, numbers and types purchased	Linked drivers' license–hospital discharge data to evaluate driving record after head injury (Haselkorn et al., 1998); linked death certificates–drivers' licenses–hospital discharge to evaluate prior injury as risk for youth suicide (Grossman, et al., 1993); evaluated trends in handgun purchases (Dowd et al., 1998)
Employment records	Job status, occupation, identification of work-related injuries	
Pharmacy records	Prescriptions dispensed (prior to or after injury)	Linked to injury data to evaluate risk of falls in elderly associated with antidepressants (Thapa et al., 1998).
HMO records	Identification of individuals with specific conditions (hospitalized or treated at outpatient visit) or who require certain treatments or medications.	Linked work injury reports from HMO–pharmacy records to evaluate potential association of occupational injuries with medication use (Gilmore et al., 1996)
Trauma Registries	Identification of injury events or cases, type of injuries, injury severity, medical care required	
Insurance, Workers' Compensation reports	Identification of injuries, extent of care required, costs of care required	Evaluation of farm work injuries to children (Heyer et al., 1992); trauma recidivism and long-term survival following trauma in the elderly (Gubler et al., 1996, 1997); see also Pharmacy records above.

EMS, Emergency Medical Services; HMO, Health Maintenance Organization.

Table 4.2 Considerations for use of secondary data and conducting record linkages

Planning considerations for: *Use of secondary or administrative data*	*Conducting data linkages*
1 Completeness of population coverage. What are possible reasons for underregistration or coverage and how would this impact results? Is it possible that there are duplicate records for the same individual? Is unduplication (internal linkage) necessary to achieve a count of individuals, rather than events?	Membership of individuals in the databases to be used. Are all the same individuals in both databases? Is complete overlap expected in membership of both databases to be linked? If not, what % of subjects are expected to be present in both?
2 Accuracy of information. How were the data originally collected? Are the data reliable enough for research purpose? Has anyone previously examined these data for accuracy?	(a) The quality of the data items used in linkage (name changes occur, as do key entry errors and misspellings) (b) The relative quality of other relevant data items in the various files. (Can one file be used as the "gold standard"?)
3 Completeness of information. What if a key data item is available for only 20% of subjects? It is a mistake to assume that if a variable is listed in a data layout, it is either accurate or complete enough for the research purpose.	What to do if information used in linkage is missing for some individuals? Are there other data items that might be used?
4 Time period covered. Is it relevant to the research question? Is the level of reporting consistent throughout the entire time period, or are there reporting or coding changes to be considered?	The relative periods of coverage of the files, i.e., Are you augmenting data that reflects a characteristic that is not time-related, or trying to obtain follow-up information (e.g., survival) for a period of time following an event?

5 Accessibility. Some secondary databases are marketed or routinely made available for *bona fide* research. Usually, it is necessary to identify two contacts within the organization holding the data: the person with administrative oversight, and the programmer or data manager.

Databases that are available for research use without linkage may not be available if a linkage is proposed. All agencies involved must fully understand and support the research purpose for the linkage. Who conducts the linkage? Who will have access to the final product?

6 Cost. May include purchase of the database and/or programmer time necessary to format and release database or subfile to researcher.

The cost of the linkage process is not trivial and is always underestimated in the planning process. This includes data handling to format databases, computer programming for linkages, evaluating linkage yield (which typically involves some manual review and checking), and creation of the statistical research file.

7 Data format. Database may require translation into a format that can be accessed by the statistical software package of choice. This may be an extra cost to the project.

Databases may need to be translated into common format that can be used by linkage programs. (Often, further translation necessary to turn final file into statistical format.)

8 Database size. Secondary databases are often quite large. Will a subset of records suffice?

Linkage of several large databases may require special handling.

yields or accuracy using different strategies have been conducted with varying results (Clark and Hahn, 1995; Adams et al., 1997; Alsop and Langley, 1998). It is likely that different methods suit different circumstances. At present, most researchers embarking on a record linkage study probably use whatever method is most readily available to them, and in fact may not even have a choice in some circumstances when the programming is performed by the agency with oversight of the relevant database. In the simplest case, as when linking two files containing a common type of unique identifier (which may also occur when unduplicating records or conducting internal linkage within a single file), a deterministic method may be used consisting of matching up records with the same identifier. In our experience (which is perhaps representative of conducting data linkages in the United States), it is rare to have the same unique identifier common to both databases. In other countries (e.g., in Scandinavian countries), linkages of secondary and health surveillance databases often utilize a national identification number that references all medical contacts within a national system of health care (Gissler et al., 1998).

If several data items are required to conduct the linkage (e.g., if the linkage will be based on the last name, first initial of the first name, gender, and date of birth of individuals within a database), a more complex method is needed. Such linkages might still be conducted using a deterministic procedure; however, they may involve a series of steps undertaken in some hierarchical fashion. For example, if this set of data items is available in both databases, and will be used in conducting a linkage, then as a first pass through the data, the records of individuals with equivalent information contained in all fields (in other words, the exact matches) might be identified. A second pass through the remaining records might identify those with exact matching of the name variables and all other variables but one. Subsequent passes through the remaining unmatched records with successively relaxed matching criteria could follow. This approach has been described as a sequential deterministic method (Herman et al., 1997).

Another approach to dealing with the lack of a common unique identifier across databases would be to try to create a virtual identifier based on some combination of information available within both files. This might be a construct of year of birth, gender, and the first three letters of the last name. Such a method might be used if one file contains such a personal identifier code and the other contains a full name, age (rather than date of birth), and gender, with the year of birth calculated based on subject's age and reference year of the database. If a sequential deterministic approach were used, decisions about which elements of the virtual identifier might be relaxed sequentially would need to be made. For example, a "match" might be considered to have occurred if the birth years in the two files were within 1 year of each other. Obviously, the greater the extent of information available with which to perform linkages, the more accurate the results; however sufficient yields for many research projects are possible with less than complete information. The extent to which various data elements contribute to the success of a linkage is just beginning to be evaluated (Roos et al., 1996). One evaluation found that, compared with a gold standard linkage performed between police road crash reports and hospital records using full name, date of birth, gender, and other variables, 90% of linkages were successfully identified based on partial information (phonetic code of family name, age, gender, crash date, and road user type). When the linkage was attempted without the name or partial name code, 50% of linkages were successfully identified (Rosman, 1996).

If no identifying information is available in one or both of the files to be linked, the virtual identifier could be created based on other available information. For example, if one were attempting to link a non-identified police file of crash reports with an emergency medical services or hospital discharge database (which may also be non-identified), the date and time the incident occurred, and subject's gender, could be used as a proxy identifier for records linkage. Use of such a virtual identifier alone to link birth and hospital discharge records in California resulted in linkage of 91% of eligible births. Addition of secondary health information available (low birth weight status on the birth certificate and similar status in the hospital discharge data) increased this yield to 98% (Herrchen et al., 1997).

The results of the linkage procedure typically generates a crosswalk file, which contains record identifiers from each database for linked individuals. Once the linkage is complete, this file may be used to abstract the relevant information from the database(s) in order to create the final research database. In many instances, this file will contain personal identifying information which is not necessary for the conduct of the research. For example, a linkage of police reports and hospital discharge records may be based on a subset of variables including a partial name code, age, gender, and date of crash/hospitalization. These items are drawn from each database into two separate subfiles, one for each database, as well as the unique report number from the police report, and the unique record number from the hospital discharge database. Although the latter two items are not necessary for the linkage, they are necessary to retrieve the required data from the databases once the linkage is performed to satisfaction. This crosswalk file represents the sole link between the entire contents of each database, and can be destroyed after the linkage is performed and the research data file has been created containing only the information necessary for the project. In our experience, destruction of the cross-walk file at the close of the project is required by the human subjects protection committees overseeing the research protocol.

Other Issues in Data Linkage

In instances where both files contain a full identifier or name, exact matching may still not result in the identification of all linkages. Some of the reasons for this include the possibility of key entry errors (e.g., changing one digit of a unique identifier, or altering the spelling of a name), the occasional use of aliases or nicknames, and the fact that name changes may have occurred in the elapsed time between the creation of the two databases. Depending on the resources available for a record linkage, the yield after the initial pass through the data, and the characteristics of the databases, further evaluation of the remaining, unmatched records is usually attempted. With any linkage strategy however, it is important to create a variable indicating the confidence of the match. Probabilistic matches using a weighting scheme typically generate such a variable, based on a weighting score to indicate the certainty of the match. However, even with a simple deterministic linkage one should be able to generate a variable to indicate if the match is exact (in all fields); close (matched in all fields except one); definitely not matched (no fields match), etc. Regardless of the linkage strategy used, information about the matching process should be routinely reported as part of the study results (Brenner and Schmidtmann, 1996). This may include the number of records within each database submitted to the linkage procedure, a description of either the certainty or closeness of the match that was deemed good enough for inclusion in the analysis (e.g., were exact matches only included, or were close matches also included), and the final yield (number of subjects included in the analysis as a result of the linkage). This information may be used to assess the possible effect of potential bias due to the non-inclusion of subjects in the analysis because they were not identified in the linkage. By comparing results before and after restricting the population to those with the greatest degree of certainty concerning the linkage (or the exact matches only), one can also assess to some extent, bias that may be present.

Of relevance to registry databases, but also of relevance to the reporting of rates based on certain secondary databases (e.g., hospital discharge databases) in which internal linkage may be performed to unduplicate records, two measures of potential linkage errors have been proposed (Brenner and Schmidtmann, 1996, 1998). The homonym rate is the proportion of subjects not counted due to erroneous linkage with other subjects. This would have the effect of underestimating an incidence rate. The synonym rate is the proportion of subjects overcounted due to a failure to link records on the same individual. This would lead to overestimation of an incidence rate. The effects of these errors on registry based follow-up studies is also beginning to be examined (Brenner et al., 1997).

Depending on the databases being used, and the purpose of the research, it is important to recognize that failure of a subject to link between two data files may be due to several reasons. For example, linkage of 1 year of birth certificates to the same year and 5 subsequent years of hospital discharge records for the same state might be performed to identify children who were hospitalized with injuries during their early childhood. Hopefully, the major reason for nonlinkage of a birth certificate with subsequent years of hospital records is because the child was not hospitalized; in fact, the investigator would likely assume so. However, most investigators would agree that some portion of records that should have matched, will not, possibly due to miscoding or spelling errors in one database, and resulting in an underestimate of the number of children hospitalized with injuries. Depending on the nature of the databases, some sense of the extent of linkage error occurring might be gained. Sometimes it may be possible to use an external benchmark (e.g., a rate calculated from a different data source). In this example, if the rate of injury hospitalization among children based on the linkage was similar to injury hospitalization rates reported in other populations, or based on follow-up studies, then one would have greater confidence that the linkage yield was appropriate. In some instances, information from other external databases may be available for comparison (Shevchenko et al., 1995; Roos et al., 1996; Ellekjaer et al., 1999), or it may be possible to compare data from a secondary database with self-reported data collected from a portion of the same subjects (Robinson et al., 1997). However, many investigators may also fail to consider that children are one of the most mobile population groups and that a child who has moved to another state might have hospitalizations that occurred elsewhere. This would also result in an underestimate of the true occurrence of injury hospitalizations. If children who are at greatest risk of hospitalization are also the most mobile (as might be the situation for low-income families who relocate frequently in search of jobs), then the results may be further biased. It may be possible to obtain migration information from regional census data for the age group of interest to help assess the possible effect of migration on the results of a data linkage. Another commonly overlooked reason for nonlinkage (although this has greater relevance for older populations) is that the child is deceased. If one were concerned enough about this possibility, or wanted to also identify injuries resulting in deaths without hospitalization, then linkage to death certificates for the same 6-year period covered by the hospital discharge records would be in order. At a minimum, one should consider the potential biases caused by these factors, and their possible effects on any results.

Finally, it should be remembered that the accuracy of the research database resulting from a record linkage is dependent upon the accuracy of the parent databases. In record linkages, the effects of inaccuracies in the original data are compounded, as missing or inaccurate data will affect the quality of the record linkage as well as decrease reliability of the other data items. Knowing the limitations of the underlying databases is important, for example, the biases that may be due to referral patterns for trauma registries (Layde et al., 1996; Waller et al., 1995); underassessment or inaccuracies in injury identification based on hospital discharge data (MacIntyre et al., 1997; Mullins et al., 1998); or underestimation of injury severity or levels of hospitalized injuries based on police reports (Cercarelli et al., 1996; Steinwachs et al., 1998).

Confidentiality and Privacy Concerns

Many research studies are possible without any knowledge of personally identifying information and, in fact, many of the administrative databases used in surveillance or other programs do not contain identifying information, yet they provide a means of measuring injury occurrence, associated costs, temporal trends, etc. Agencies controlling administrative databases that do contain personally identifying information may be restricted to only releasing unidentified, or "stripped" subfiles. If a research project requires a records linkage using identifiers, however, occasionally the agency may be able to perform the linkage procedure (so that no identifiers are released to the investigator) in order to create an appropriate research data file. In some instances, files containing identifiers may be released by the agency so that record linkage can be conducted by the investigator. The latter situation generally affords researchers the greatest level of control over the linkage strategy and the best sense of how accurately the linkage is performed. It also, however, carries with it the greatest responsibility. Currently, there is national recognition that health information is increasingly being stored electronically, and a re-evaluation of legislation with respect to protection of privacy is underway (Gostin, 1997). In balancing issues of personal privacy versus the public health benefits to society that may be realized from appropriate use of health care data, many difficult issues need to be addressed as new policy is being developed.

Presently, use of health care data for research is addressed locally by the human subjects protection committees (Institutional Review Boards) of the investigator's institution, and those of the agency overseeing the database (see chapter by McGough and Wolf, this volume). In addition to ensuring that no results are released in any fashion that might allow identification of individuals, data handling must be conducted with a high level of security, which may include creation of password protected files; firewalls, and other strategies to protect the electronic information; keeping of all paper records in locked files; destruction of crosswalk files in record linkage projects, and prohibition of data redistribution, or of use of the data for other than the research purpose for which it was accessed.

In summary, many rich administrative and secondary databases exist that could potentially supplement or form the basis of injury research projects. With the rapid developments in information technology that are currently underway, and a move towards standardization of medical record and other data formats, the ability to access databases that perform linkages for research will continue to improve. Use of these data should not occur, however, without a full understanding of the responsibilities related to handling of confidential information, and of the limitations of both the parent and resultant linked databases.

References

Adams MM, Wilson HG, Casto DL, Berg CJ, McDermott JM, Gaudino JA, McCarthy BJ (1997) Constructing reproductive histories by linking vital records. Am J Epidemiol 145:339–48.

Alexander BH, Rivara FP, Wolf ME (1992) The cost and frequency of hospitalization for fall-related injuries in older adults. Am J Public Health 82:1020–3.

Alsop JC, Langley JD (1998) Determining first admissions in a hospital discharge file via record linkage. Methods Info Med 37:32–7.

Brenner H, Schmidtmann I (1998) Effects of record linkage errors on disease registration. Methods Info Med 37:69–74.

Brenner H, Schmidtmann I, Stegmaier C (1997) Effects of record linkage errors on registry-based follow-up studies. Stat Med 16(23):2633–43.

Brenner H, Schmidtmann I (1996) Determinants of homonym and synonym rates of record linkage in disease registration. Methods Info Med 35:19–24.

Brownstein D, Shugerman R, Cummings P, Rivara FP, Copass M (1996) Prehospital endotracheal intubation of children by paramedics. Ann Emerg Med 28:34–9.

Cercarelli LR, Rosman DL, Ryan GA (1996) Comparison of accident and emergency with police road injury data. J Trauma 40(5):805–9.

Clark DE, Hahn DR (1995) Comparison of probabilistic and deterministic record linkage in the development of a statewide trauma registry. Proc Annu Symp Comput Appl Med Care 397–401.

Copes WS, Stark MM, Lawnick MM, Tepper S, Wilkerson D, DeJong G, Brannon R, Hamilton BB (1996) Linking data from national trauma and rehabilitation registries. J Trauma 40(3):428–36.

Conseur A, Rivara FP, Emanuel I (1997a) Juvenile delinquency and adolescent trauma: how strong is the connection? Pediatrics 99:E5.

Conseur A, Rivara FP, Barnoski R, Emanuel I (1997b) Maternal and perinatal risk factors for later delinquency. Pediatrics 99:785–90.

Cummings P, Theis MK, Mueller BA, Rivara FP (1994) Infant injury death in Washington State, 1981 through 1990. Arch Pediatr Adolesc Med 148:1021–6.

Cummings P, LeMier M, Keck DB (1998) Trends in firearm-related injuries in Washington State, 1989–1995. Ann Emerg Med 32:37–43.

Cummings P, Grossman DC, Rivara FP, Koepsell TD (1997a) State gun safe storage laws and child mortality due to firearms. JAMA 278:1084–6.

Cummings P, Koepsell TD, Grossman DC, Savarino J, Thompson RS (1997b) The association between the purchase of a handgun and homicide or suicide. Am J Public Health 87:974–8.

Cummings P, LeMier M, Keck DB (1998) Trends in firearm-related injuries in Washington State, 1989–1995. Ann Emerg Med 32:37–43.

Davis RL, Hughes M, Gubler KD, Waller PL, Rivara FP (1995) The use of cranial CT scans in the triage of pediatric patients with mild head injury. Pediatrics 95:345–9.

Dowd MD, Langley J, Koepsell T, Soderberg R, Rivara FP (1998) Hospitalizations for injury in New Zealand: prior injury as a risk factor for assaultive injury. Am J Public Health. 86:929–34.

Ellekjaer H, Holmen J, Kruger O, Terent A (1999) Identification of incident stroke in Norway: hospital discharge data compared with a population-based stroke register. Stroke 30:56–60.

Garcia Rodriguez LA, Perez Gutthann S (1998) Use of the UK General Practice Research Database for pharmacoepidemiology. Br J Clin Pharmacol 45:419–25.

Gilmore TM, Alexander BH, Mueller BA, Rivara FP (1996) Occupational injuries and medication use. Am J Ind Med 30:234–9.

Gissler M. Hemminki E. Louhiala P. Jarvelin MR (1998) Health registers as a feasible means of measuring health status in childhood – a 7-year follow-up of the 1987 Finnish birth cohort. Paediatric Perinat Epidemiol 12(4):437–55.

Gostin L (1997) Health care information and the protection of personal privacy: ethical and legal considerations. Ann Intern Med 127:683–690.

Grossman DC, Hart LG, Rivara FP, Maier RV, Rosenblatt R (1995) From roadside to bedside: the regionalization of trauma care in a remote rural county. J Trauma 38:14–21.

Grossman D, Mueller BA, Kenaston T, Salzberg P, Cooper W, Jurkovich GJ (1996) The Validity of police assessment of driver sobriety. Accid Anal Prev 28:435–442.

Grossman DC, Soderberg R, Rivara FP (1993) Prior injury and motor vehicle crash as risk factors for youth suicide. Epidemiology 4:115–19.

Gubler KD, Maier RV, Davis R, Koepsell T, Soderberg R, Rivara FP (1996) Trauma recidivism in the elderly. J Trauma 41:952–6.

Gubler KD, Davis R, Koepsell T, Soderberg R, Maier RV, Rivara FP (1997) Long-term survival of elderly trauma patients. Arch Surg 132:1010–14.

Haselkorn J, Mueller BA, Rivara FP (1998) Characteristics of drivers and driving record after traumatic and nontraumatic brain injury. Arch Phys Med Rehab 79:738–42.

Herman AA, McCarthy BJ, Bakewell JM, Ward RH, Mueller BA, Maconochie NE, Read AW, Zadka P, Skjaerven R (1997) Data linkage methods used in maternally-linked birth and infant death surveillance data sets from the United States (Georgia, Missouri, Utah and Washington State), Israel, Norway, Scotland and Western Australia. Paediatric Perinat Epidemiol 11 (Suppl 1):5–22.

Herrchen B, Gould JB, Nesbitt TS (1997) Vital statistics linked birth/infant death and hospital discharge record linkage for epidemiological studies. Comput Biomed Res 30(4):290–305.

Hertzman C, Teschke K, Ostry A, Hershler R, Dimich-Ward H, Kelly S, Spinelli JJ, Gallagher RP, McBride M, Marion SA (1997) Mortality and cancer incidence among sawmill workers exposed to chlorophenate wood preservatives. Am J Public Health 87:71–9.

Heyer NJ, Franklin G, Rivara FP, Parker P, Haug JA (1992) Occupational injuries among minors doing farm work in Washington State: 1986–1989. Am J Public Health 82:557–60.

Hudson JI, Kenzora JE, Hebel JR, Gardner JF, Scherlis L, Epstein RS, Magaziner JS (1998) Eight-year outcome associated with clinical options in the management of femoral neck fractures. Clinical Orthopaed Rel Res 348:59–66.

Huff L, Bogdan G, Burke K, Hayes E, Perry W, Graham L, Lentzner H (1996) Using hospital discharge data for disease surveillance. Public Health Rep 111:78–81.

Jaro MA (1995) Probabilistic linkage of large public health data files. Stat Med 14:491–8.

Johnson SW, Walker J (1996) NHTSA Technical Report: The Crash Outcome Evaluation System (CODES). DOT HS 808 338. Washington, DC: Department of Transportation, National Highway Traffic Safety Administration.

Kendrick SW, Douglas MM, Gardner D, Hucker D (1998) Best-link matching of Scottish health data sets. Methods Info Med 37:64–8.

Kellermann AL, Somes G, Rivara FP, Lee RK, Banton JG (1998) Injuries and deaths due to firearms in the home. J Trauma 45:263–7.

Layde PM, Stueland DT, Nordstrom DL (1996) Representativeness of trauma center registries for farm injury surveillance. Accid Anal Prev 28:581–6.

Lillard LA, Farmer MM (1997) Linking Medicare and national survey data. Ann Intern Med 127(8 Pt 2):691–5.

Lipowski EE, Bigelow WE (1996) Data linkages for research on outcomes of long-term care. Gerontologist 36(4):441–7.

MacIntyre CR, Ackland MJ, Chandraraj EJ (1997) Accuracy of injury coding in Victorian hospital morbidity data. Aust NZ J Public Health 21:779–83.

Mueller BA, Kenaston T, Grossman, D, Salzberg, P (1998) Hospital charges for injured drinking drivers in Washington State: 1987–1993. Accid Anal Prev 30:597–605.

Mullins RJ, Mann NC, Hedges JR, Worrall W, Helfand M, Zechnich AD, Jurkovich GJ (1998) Adequacy of hospital discharge status as a measure of outcome among injured patients. JAMA 179:1727–31.

Murphy PL, Sorock GB, Courtney TK, Webster BS, Leamon TB (1996) Injury and illness in the American workplace: a comparison of data sources. Am J Indust Med 30:130–41.

Nasca PC (1997) Current problems that are likely to affect the future of epidemiology. Am J Epidemiol 146:907–11.

Newman TB, Brown AN (1997) Use of commercial record linkage software and vital statistics to identify patient deaths. J Am Medical Informatics Assoc 4(3):233–7.

Patterson L, Weiss H, Schano P (1996) Combining multiple data bases for outcomes assessment. Am J Med Qual 11(1):s73–7.

Peek-Asa C, Kraus JF (1997) Estimates of injury impairment after acute traumatic injury in motorcycle crashes before and after passage of a mandatory helmet use law. Ann Emerg Med 29(5):630–6.

Rivara FP, Shepherd JP, Farrington DP, Richmond PW, Cannon P (1995) Victim as offender in youth violence. Ann Emerg Med 24:609–14.

Rivara FP (1997) Fatal and non-fatal farm injuries to children and adolescents in the United States, 1990–3. Injury Prev 3:190–4.

Robinson JR, Young TK, Roos LL, Gelskey DE (1997) Estimating the burden of disease. Comparing administrative data and self-reports. Med Care 35(9):932–47.

Roos LL, Walld R, Wajda A, Bond R, Hartford K (1996) Record linkage strategies, out-patient procedures, and administrative data. Med Care 35(6):570–82.

Rosman DL (1996) The feasibility of linking hospital and police road crash casualty records without names. Accid Anal Prev 28(2):271–4.

Rostykus PS, Cummings P, Mueller BA (1998) Risk factors for pilot fatalities in general aviation airplane crash landings. JAMA 280:997–9.

Rowland J, Rivara FP, Salzberg P, Soderberg R, Maier R, Koepsell T (1996) Motorcycle helmet use and injury outcome and hospitalization costs from crashes in Washington State. Am J Public Health 86:41–5.

Samsa GP, Landsman PB, Hamilton B (1996) Inpatient hospital utilization among veterans with traumatic spinal cord injury. Arch Phys Med Rehab 77(10):1037–43.

Scholer SJ, Hickson GB, Mitchel EF Jr, Ray WA (1998) Predictors of mortality from fires in young children. Pediatrics 101(5):E12.

Selby JV (1997) Linking automated databases for research in managed care settings. Ann Intern Med 127(8 Pt 2):719–24.

Shevchenko IP, Lynch JT, Mattie AS, Reed-Fourquet LL (1995) Verification of information in a large medical database using linkages with external databases. Stat Med 14:511–30.

Sorenson MT, Sabroe S, Olsen J (1996) A framework for evaluation of secondary data sources for epidemiological research. Int J Epidemiol 25(2):435–42.

Sorock GS, Smith GS, Reeve GR, Dement J, Stout M, Layne L, Pastula ST (1997) Three perspectives on work-related injury surveillance systems. Am J Indust Med 32:114–28.

Steinwachs DM, Stuart ME, Scholle S, Starfield B, Fox MH, Weiner JP (1998) A comparison of ambulatory Medicaid claims to medical records: a reliability assessment. Am J Med Quality 13:63–9.

Sugarman JR, Grossman DC (1996) Trauma among American Indians in an urban county. Public Health Rep 111:320.

Thapa PB, Gideon P, Cost TW, Milam AB, Ray WA (1998) Antidepressants and the risk of falls among nursing home residents. N Engl J Med 339(13):875–82.

Unwin E, Codde J (1998) Estimating the cost of hospital treatment for injuries using linked morbidity data. Aust NZ J Public Health 22(5):624–6.

Walen SA (1997) Linking large administrative databases: a method for conducting emergency medical services cohort studies using existing data. Acad Emerg Med 4(11):1087–96.

Waller JA, Skelly JM, Davis JH (1995) Trauma center-related biases in injury research. J Trauma 38:325–9.

Weiss HB, Dill SM, Garrison HG, Coben JH (1997) The potential of using billing data for emergency department injury surveillance. Acad Emerg Med 4(4):282–7.

Williams JM, Furbee PM, Prescott JE (1996) Development of an emergency department-based injury surveillance system. Ann Emerg Med 27:59–65.

Wolf ME, Alexander BH, Rivara FP, Hickok DE, Maier RV, Starzyk PM (1993) A retrospective cohort study of seatbelt use and pregnancy outcome after a motor vehicle crash. J Trauma 34:116–19.

5

Rates, Rate Denominators, and Rate Comparisons

Peter Cummings, Robyn Norton, and
Thomas D. Koepsell

Introduction

In the conduct of injury research, we often wish to measure the frequency of injury occurrence, of events that might produce injuries, or of injured persons. Counts alone are inadequate for many purposes, as they include no information about the size of the population or period of time from which the counts arose. Rates, which can account for population size and time intervals, are the topic of this chapter.

Basic Concepts
Counts

Two types of counts may be defined. Incident cases are newly injured persons counted over a period of time. Prevalent cases are persons with an injury-induced condition counted at a single point in time. In injury research, incident events are sometimes counted, rather than persons; for example, traffic crashes in a year, or falls in a nursing home in one month. Note that a crash event may include several people, and a single person might fall several times.

Counts, without a denominator, are often inadequate for research purposes. Imagine we are told that there were 100 deaths due to fires in community A and 1000 deaths due to fires in community B. Without information about the size of the populations in A and B, and the time periods over which the deaths were counted in each region, we are unable to compare the hazards for death by fire in the two areas. A denominator can provide the needed information.

What is a Rate?

A rate is a count divided by a denominator. Some have expressed the view that the term rate should be reserved for incidence rates, which have incident counts in the numerator and person-time in the denominator (Rothman, 1986, pp. 23–34). We sympathize with this view, as this practice would prevent the confusion that often arises between incidence rates and other rates which are actually proportions. However, we shall discuss other common uses of the term rate in this chapter.

The key concept here is that there are two common uses of the word rate which are sometimes confused. The two can be kept distinct by paying careful attention to the correct units for both numerator and denominator. When a count is divided by another count of the same units, this is a proportion, a unitless measure which ranges from zero to one. Thus if 40 persons in a region died in traffic crashes, and the total number, or count, of persons who were in those crashes was 10,000, we can compute that the proportion who died was 40 persons ÷ 10,000 persons = 0.004 (which is commonly called a case-fatality rate). When a count is divided by some denominator other than a count of the same units, such as dividing total incident cases by person-time, the resulting ratio, which still has units, is not a proportion. Thus if a nursing home accumulated 10,000 person-years of patient residence (which could come from 10,000 patients who were residents for one year, or 1000 who lived there for 10 years), and if 40 patients died of falls during that person-time, the incidence rate would be calculated as 40 deaths ÷ 10,000 person-years = 0.004/ year, which is commonly expressed as a mortality of 400 per 100,000 person-years.

Defining Populations

To generate a rate, the population from which the counts arose must be defined. This could be the residents of New Zealand, the members of the Kaiser Permanente health maintenance organization, all Toyota factory workers, the licensed drivers of France, or the patients admitted to the Mayo Clinic. We need not know the name of each individual, but we must be able to define who belongs to the group we are studying.

Subpopulations (Categories)

Within a given population or study base that we have defined, we may wish to identify subpopulations for which we will generate rates. Common classification schemes are based on age or sex, but the number of possible subgroups is limited only by our imagination and the information that we have available to define categories.

Denominators

Population size is a common choice for a denominator. Many geopolitical regions, such as cities or countries, create estimates of the population during a given year. These are counts, derived in part from a periodic census, that approximate the number of area residents who would have been enumerated had an actual count been done on one day in the middle of the year. As we shall see, population size is precisely the denominator we want for some rates.

Person-time is the other common denominator, and is the one that is usually needed for incidence rates. When estimating a mortality incidence rate, the investigator often divides the count of the dead in one year by the estimated size of the population in that year; superficially, it appears that one count is being divided by another, to create a proportion. However, most populations are dynamic, with people moving in and out of the population. In 1994, the estimated count of the

Swedish population was 8,745,109. However, during January 1, 1994 through December 31, 1994, there were more than that number of people who were residents of Sweden for at least part of 1994. Some people were born into the Swedish population during that year and others moved to Sweden. Some Swedish residents died part way through 1994, and others left the country. When the observation period is one-year, the estimated population count is used as a good estimate of the person-years of time lived by Swedish citizens in that year.

The difference between person-years and population counts will be seen easily if we use 2 years of data. Sweden's population was about 8,816,381 in 1995. The average size of the Swedish population in 1994–95 is calculated by adding the two annual population counts and dividing by two, or about 8.8 million persons. However, the estimated person-years for 1994–95 is calculated by adding the two population counts, or about 17.6 million person-years. Sweden did not have 17.6 persons in 1994–95, but about 17.6 million person-years were lived by people in Sweden during that period.

Failure to distinguish between persons and person-time can result in incorrectly calculated rates. In a study of fractures arising from a population of 20 million people, investigators counted all the fractures among hospitalized patients during a 4-year period. To estimate the fracture rate, they mistakenly averaged the population over the 4 years, and therefore used a denominator of about 20 million persons. Fortunately, a reviewer pointed out that the correct denominator was about 80 million person-years and the rates were properly recalculated.

Special Denominator Choices

In injury research, we sometimes use measures other than the total amount of time that was lived by each person during some period. These measures of the at-risk time may include time lived as a licensed driver or time spent at a job. Furthermore, the injury field uses denominators other than person-time, such as passenger-miles of car or airline travel.

To assess the role of age in traffic crashes, for example, we can choose among several numerators and denominators. Let us select, as the numerator, the count of U.S. crash events in 1990 in which one or more persons died. We will categorize these fatal crashes according to the age of the involved driver(s) and give estimates here for middle-age persons age 45–49 years, and the elderly, persons age 75 years or older (Insurance Institute for Highway Safety, 1992). Our first denominator is estimated person-years, by age group, that U.S. residents lived in 1990. The incidence of crash events per 10,000 person-years was 2.0 for middle-age persons and 2.2 for the elderly. But many elderly persons do not drive, either because they never learned, or because they stopped due to failing health. Using licensed drivers as the denominator, the respective rates were 2.0 and 3.5 per 10,000 licensed driver-years. When the elderly do drive, they drive fewer miles compared with others. Per 100 million driver-miles, the middle-age group was involved in fatal crashes as drivers at a rate of 2.0, compared with 11.5 for the elderly. Examining these rates suggests that older drivers help to reduce their risk for a serious crash by reducing their driving.

However, if you are planning a trip and can choose your driver from among persons age 40 or 80 years, you should probably select a 40-year-old, all else being equal.

Types of Rates
Prevalence Rates or Proportions

The prevalence of an injury-induced condition is estimated by counting living cases at one point in time and dividing by the population count at that same time. Prevalence is a proportion that has no units.

Prevalence is typically used to estimate the health-care needs of a population for chronic conditions. Murray and Lopez (1996) estimated that in 1990 there were 1,314,000 persons living with spinal cord injury due to traffic crashes in the established market economies, the countries of western Europe, the United States, Canada, Australia, New Zealand, and Japan. The combined populations of these nations were 798 million and the estimated prevalence was therefore 165 per 100,000. In contrast, the prevalence of this condition was 79 per 100,000 in India.

Prevalence is rarely of interest in studies of injury etiology, because it is affected not only by incidence, but also by the length of time that persons have the condition. If incidence remained unchanged, the prevalence of spinal cord injury would increase if people with these injuries lived longer due to better medical care. Furthermore, prevalence would decrease if the proportion of cases that recovered completely were to increase, or the time to recovery decreased, or more of these people died quickly from their condition. Rather than tease out these factors, investigators studying injury etiology and prevention usually want estimates of incidence.

As prevalence is a proportion, estimates of precision use binomial methods (Fisher and van Belle, 1993, p. 183–5; Armitage and Berry, 1994, pp. 118–125; Rosner, 1995, pp. 174–8). If C is the count of cases and N is the total population, the 95% confidence limits for the proportion, C/N, are approximated by $(C/N) \pm 1.96 \times \sqrt{(C/N) \times (1 - (C/N))/N}$. This is a large-sample method which works well if the counts of both cases and non-cases are at least 10. When this condition is not met, exact methods are described in the textbooks just cited and are available in many software packages.

Incidence Rates

Cumulative Incidence Rates or Proportions

If we have a defined population and follow these persons for a period of time, we can count all new incident cases and divide these by the number of persons in the population. The result is the cumulative incidence, a dimensionless proportion. To interpret cumulative incidence correctly, we need some information about the time period over which the cases were counted. It would be misleading to compare the cumulative incidence of homicides in Baltimore in 1 month with the cumulative incidence of homicides in New York in 1 year, without knowledge of the time intervals used to collect the data.

Cumulative incidence is commonly used when the entire population from which the incident cases arise can be counted and followed to the conclusion of the observation period. Dire et al. (1992) treated patients for dog bite injuries at a military hospital in Fort Hood, Texas. Among 89 patients randomly assigned to receive antibiotics to prevent wound infection, only one became infected; cumulative incidence 0.011. Among 96 who were given no antibiotic, five became infected: cumulative incidence 0.052. Information about the time over which infection outcomes were collected is not critical here, as we can assume the interval was just a week or so. Case-fatality rates are a common example of cumulative incidence proportions.

As cumulative incidence is a proportion, binomial methods should be used for estimating confidence intervals, as described above.

Incidence Rates

When counts of incident cases are divided by the person-time from which the counts arose, the result is an incidence rate with units that are the inverse of a unit of time. We may express the results as incidence per person-day, person-year, or person-century. Mortality data are commonly presented per 100,000 person-years; this usually results in rounded numbers ranging from 0.0 to 999.9, which are easy to present in tables. Murray and Lopez (1996) estimated that there were 51,000 new or incident cases of spinal cord injury due to motor-vehicle crashes in the established market economies in 1990: incidence rate 6.4 per 100,000 person-years. The incidence in India was 4.2 per 100,000 person-years.

Incidence rates are ratios of counts to a measure of at-risk experience. The rate estimate is C/T, where T is a measure of person-time, or some other measure that expresses the amount of at-risk exposure that people or planes or trains had to the risk of some injury outcome, such as a broken leg or a crash event. Rates calculated from miles of travel are treated like person-time rates; they are not proportions and have units. Precision is commonly measured using Poisson methods for count data (Fisher and van Belle, 1993, pp. 214–17; Armitage and Berry, 1994, pp. 141–4; Rosner, 1995, pp. 179–80). An early example of Poisson methods was a study by von Bortkiewicz, published in 1898, of cavalrymen killed by a kick from a horse (Fisher and van Belle, 1993, p. 213). The Poisson distribution assumes that the mean count is the same as its variance, so an approximate 95% confidence interval for an incidence rate is $(C \pm 1.96 \times \sqrt{C})/T$. Note that precision depends entirely on the size of the count. This formula is adequate if the count is greater than 100. Exact methods are available in the cited textbooks and many statistical packages.

Proportional Incidence

Sometimes it is convenient to count incident cases, categorize them according to some characteristic, and present the proportion of cases in each category. For example, a regional trauma center may be unable to define the population from which its cases arise, and therefore cannot estimate incidence rates for admissions. However, if the hospital admitted 4000 male and 1000 female trauma patients in a year, they might report that men accounted for 0.8 of all admissions. This proportional incidence, leads to the inference that men are more prone to serious trauma then women; we can infer this because the number of men and women are roughly equal in most populations.

Proportional incidence or proportional mortality is sometimes used when an accurate denominator is not available. Often it is reported because investigators do not realize that they could report counts and incidence rates, which are usually more informative.

An example of proportional incidence is the annual estimate of the proportion of traffic crash fatalities in the United States that involved alcohol; this proportion decreased from 57.3% in 1982 to 38.6% in 1997 (National Highway Traffic Safety Administration, 1998, p. 32). If all we had were incidence proportions, we would not know if the proportions changed because crash deaths involving alcohol decreased, because deaths not involving alcohol increased, or a combination of these reasons. Fortunately, the published data includes counts and denominators for both person-years and vehicle-miles, so incidence rates can be estimated. As fatalities due to crashes are decreasing, and the proportion that involve alcohol is decreasing, we suspect that driver-miles generated by drinking drivers are decreasing.

Interval estimation for these proportions is based on binomial methods, described above.

Statistical Comparisons of Rates
Rates that are Actually Proportions

Between Populations

A more formal statistical test of a difference in two proportions is the chi-squared test; large sample and exact methods are available in virtually any statistical package. Subtracting one proportion from the other produces a risk difference, and dividing one by the other produces a risk ratio or relative risk. Large sample interval estimates may be generated for either of these (Fisher and van Belle, 1993, pp. 185–99; Rosner, 1995, pp. 362–4), and are available in software packages. If $C \times (1 - (C/N)) < 5$, exact methods should be used for interval estimates.

Trends Over Time

To determine whether there is a trend over time in the proportions, one can use a chi-squared test for trend, which will simply yield a p-value. Or logistic regression can be used, treating time as a linear predictor variable (Breslow and Day, 1980; Hosmer and Lemeshow, 1989; Kleinbaum, 1992).

Rates that are Ratios – Person-time or Other Denominators

Between Populations

Subtracting one proportion from the other produces a rate difference and dividing one by the other produces a rate ratio. A rate difference still has the units of the original rates, such as person-years, whereas a rate ratio has no units.

In generating interval estimates, rates that are ratios, with person-time or vehicle-miles in the denominator, should not be treated as if they were proportions. To generate an interval estimate, methods appropriate for person-time data should be used, such as maximum-likelihood Poisson methods (Agresti, 1996; Long, 1997; Rothman and Greenland, 1998, pp. 267–70). Suitable methods are now available in many statistical packages.

Trends Over Time

In examining trends over time, a first-step is to plot the rates. If the number of outcome events is large, and the confidence limits for each time interval narrow, this may be sufficient; sometimes the trend will be so smooth that a clear picture emerges, which need not be embellished by further tests. The investigator may simply comment, for example, that mortality decreased by 41% over a 17-year interval, and let the graphic show what happened.

For rates derived from smaller population groups, or for rare outcomes, there may be considerable annual variation in rates and one may be uncertain about the significance of any trend without the assistance of a statistical test. Furthermore, one may wish to test formally any change in rates, say before and after a new speed limit law was adopted. Constructing a rate-ratio, say, for just the first and last year of the data is an arbitrary choice and discards all the data for intervening years. We suggest that regression methods should be used.

In the past, least squares linear regression was often used to model rates. Now that software is more widely available with regression tools that are appropriate for count data, such as Poisson and negative binomial regression, we hope that the use of linear regression for incidence rates will fade away. In Poisson regression (Breslow and Day, 1987; Long, 1997), which has been used for several studies of injuries (Frome, 1983; Frome and Checkoway, 1985; Roberts and Power, 1996; Bailer et al., 1997), the outcome is the natural logarithm of the predicted count. The natural logarithm of the denominator for the rate, person-time, or vehicle-miles, is entered into the model as an "offset" term: that is a predictor variable with an assumed regression coefficient of one. Poisson methods assume that the mean count and its variance are equal. However, the observed variance might be greater; two methods allow for this possibility, adjustment of the Poisson variances, or negative binomial regression, which allows for extra-Poisson variation (McCullagh and Nelder, 1989, pp. 198–9; Gardner et al., 1995; Glynn and Buring, 1996; Long, 1997). Negative binomial models can also allow for possible nonindependence of multiple events within subjects. For example, it is possible that some people may be more likely than others to sustain several injuries, for reasons that we are unable to account for with our data. These reasons might include their use of alcohol or their temperament or physical disabilities. Some studies have dealt with this problem by only analyzing data until the first injury event, but negative binomial regression allows us to utilize all of the events that occurred in the population (Glynn and Buring, 1996). Several injury studies have used negative binomial regression or modifications of Poisson regression (Brenner et al., 1994; Levy et al., 1995; Cummings et al., 1997, 1998).

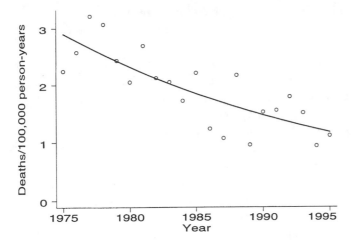

Figure 5.1. Annual incidence rates of drowning in King County, Washington, 1975–95. Circles are the actual rates. The line is the trend in rates estimated by negative binomial regression.

Cummings and Quan (1999) examined the trend in unintentional drownings in King County, Washington, a growing region with 1,507,319 residents in 1990. There were 539 drownings of county residents during 1975 through 1995. The annual rates showed considerable year-to-year variation (Figure 5.1). Negative binomial regression was used to estimate the change in mortality rates. The outcome was the log of the count of deaths in each year. The log of person-years for each year was entered as an offset predictor variable and the year was entered as a continuous linear variable. The overall change in mortality rates, from 1975 to 1995, was −59% (95% confidence interval, −70% to −46%).

Rate Adjustment

To compare the rates of injury in two or more regions, or between time periods, it is sometimes desirable to adjust for other factors, which may confound the comparison.

Adjustment Using Standard Population Weights – Direct Standardization

First we pick some standard population which will supply us with a distribution of person-time. Next we create subgroup-specific incidence rates for the study population; for example, rates within each five-year age group, or rates for men and women. To generate a standardized or adjusted rate, we take a weighted average of these subgroup-specific incidence rates, with the weights derived from the distribution of person-time in subgroups of the standard population:

standardized rate = sum($\text{rate}_i \times \text{weight}_i$)/sum($\text{weight}_i$), where the subscript i indicates each subgroup or stratum. The weights are the number of person-years in each stratum of the standard population, or the person-years divided by some scale factor: for example, dividing by the total person-years results in weights that conveniently sum to one. This method of standardization is sometimes called the direct method.

Adjustment can be made for age, sex, or any other characteristics or group of characteristics which are known for the incident cases, the population under study, and the standard population. Age-adjusted mortality rates are a familiar example of this method. Standardized rates are easy to present in tables and they allow for comparisons that account for differences between populations in regard to the variables used for adjustment. We can compare the rates of many populations, as long as they are adjusted to the same standard population.

One should bear in mind that standardized rates, while useful for comparisons, describe a hypothetical rate: what the crude rate would have been if the study population had the subgroup-specific incidence rates that were actually measured, but a stratified distribution of person-years which was that of the standard population.

Adjustment Using Study Population Weights – Indirect Standardization

Another common method of adjustment, sometimes called the indirect method, takes the standardization weights from the study population. First we calculate the observed crude incidence rate for the study population. Then we use the person-time of the study population to generate stratum-specific weights; these are total person-time in each stratum, or a scaled version of this person-time. Now we turn to the standard population (which is sometimes the entire population of a country) and, using information known about this population, we calculate rates for the same strata. We can now calculate an expected rate $= \text{sum}(\text{rate}_i \times \text{weight}_i)/\text{sum}(\text{weight}_i)$, where the rates come from the standard population, and the weights come from the study population. Finally, we compare the observed and expected rates; the ratio of observed to expected is called the standardized morbidity ratio or standardized mortality ratio.

Both of these adjustment methods, the first based on the distribution of the possible confounder in the standard population, the second based on the distribution in the study population, are valid methods. But there is an important difference. Suppose that we wish to compare the rates of fall-related mortality between Denmark, Australia, and China. If we arbitrarily select Denmark as the standard population and compute standardized mortality rates for Australia and China, we cannot only compare Australia and China to Denmark, but we can validly compare the standardized rates of Australia and China to each other. If, however, we again pick Denmark as the standard population, and compute crude rates, expected rates, and standardized mortality ratios for Australia and China, we cannot use these to compare mortality between Australia and China; such a comparison would only be valid if the standardization weights, the distribution of person-time by age in Australia and China, were fortuitously the same. Descriptions of these methods, with worked examples and formulas for interval estimation, can be found in several textbooks (Rothman, 1986, pp. 41–9; Fisher and van Belle, 1993, pp. 765–72).

Other Techniques

Investigators may wish to make use of stratified (Clayton and Hills, 1993) or regression methods that are suitable for counts. Poisson or negative binomial regression can produce incidence rate ratios, suitable for comparisons of incidence rates, and these can be easily adjusted for any known confounder.

Conclusions

We reiterate a few key points: (1) different rate denominators can address different questions; (2) rates that are proportions should be distinguished from rates that are ratios; (3) stratified and regression methods suitable for the analysis and comparison of incidence rates should be used more widely.

References

Agresti A (1996) An Introduction to Categorical Data Analysis. New York: John Wiley.

Armitage P and Berry G (1994) Statistical Methods in Medical Research, 3rd edn. London: Blackwell Scientific Publications.

Bailer AJ, Reed LD, Stayner LT (1997) Modeling fatal injury rates using Poisson regression: a case study of workers in agriculture, forestry, and fishing. J Safety Res 28(3):177–86.

Brenner RA, Smith GS, Overpeck MD (1994) Divergent trends in childhood drowning rates, 1971 through 1988. JAMA 271:1606–08.

Breslow NE, Day NE (1980) Statistical Methods in Cancer Research, Vol. I – The Analysis of Case–Control Studies. Lyon, France: International Agency for Research on Cancer.

(1987) Statistical Methods in Cancer Research, Vol. II – The Design and Analysis of Cohort Studies. Lyon, France: International Agency for Research on Cancer.

Clayton D, Hills M (1993) Statistical Methods in Epidemiology. New York: Oxford University Press.

Cummings P, Quan L (1999) Trends in unintentional drowning: the role of alcohol and medical care. JAMA 281:2198–202.

Cummings P, Grossman DG, Rivara FP, Koepsell TD (1997) State gun safe storage laws and child mortality due to firearms. JAMA 278:1084–6.

Cummings P, LeMier M, Keck, D (1998) Trends in firearm-related injuries in Washington State 1989–1995. Ann Emerg Med 32:37–43.

Dire DJ, Hogan DE, Walker JS (1992) Prophylactic oral antibiotics for low-risk dog bite wounds. Pediatr Emerg Care 8(4):194–9.

Fisher LD, van Belle G (1993) Biostatistics: a Methodology for the Health Sciences. New York: John Wiley & Sons.

Frome EL (1983) The analysis of rates using Poisson regression models. Biometrics 39:665–74.

Frome EL, Checkoway H (1985) Use of Poisson regression models in estimating incidence rates and ratios. Am J Epidemiol 121:309–23.

Gardner W, Mulvey EP, Shaw EC (1995) Regression analyses of counts and rates: Poisson, overdispersed Poisson, and negative binomial models. Psychol Bull 118(3):392–404.

Glynn RJ, Buring JE (1996) Ways of measuring rates of recurrent events. BMJ 312:364–7.

Hosmer DW, Lemeshow S (1989) Applied Logistic Regression. New York: John Wiley & Sons.

Insurance Institute for Highway Safety (1992) Crashes, fatal crashes per mile. Status Rep 27(11):1–7.

Kleinbaum DG (1992) Logistic Regression: a Self-learning Text. New York: Springer-Verlag.

Levy DT, Vernick JS, Howard KA (1995) Relationships between driver's license renewal policies and fatal crashes involving drivers 70 years or older. JAMA 274(13):1026–30.

Long JS (1997) Regression Models for Categorical and Limited Dependent Variables. Thousand Oaks, CA: SAGE Publications.

McCullagh P, Nelder J (1989) Generalized Linear Models, 2nd edn. New York: Chapman & Hall.

Murray CJL, Lopez AD (eds) (1996) The Global Burden of Disease: a Compendium of Incidence, Prevalence and Mortality Estimates for Over 200 Conditions. Boston, MA: Harvard School of Public Health.

National Highway Traffic Safety Administration (1998) Traffic Safety Facts 1997: A Compilation of Motor Vehicle Crash Data from the Fatality Analysis Reporting System and the General Estimates System. Washington, DC: US Department of Transportation.

Roberts I, Power C (1996) Does the decline in child injury mortality vary by social class? A comparison of class specific mortality in 1981 and 1991. BMJ 313:784–6.

Rosner B (1995) Fundamentals of Biostatistics, 4th edn. Belmont, CA: Duxbury Press.

Rothman KJ (1986) Modern Epidemiology, 1st edn. Boston: Little, Brown and Company.

Rothman KJ, Greenland S (1998) Modern Epidemiology, 2nd edn. Philadelphia: Lippincott-Raven.

6

Data Collection Methods

Carol W. Runyan and J. Michael Bowling

Introduction

Injury research employs a wide array of approaches including descriptive epidemiology, analytic epidemiology, behavioral research, policy analysis, and program evaluation. For each approach, alternative methods are available to collect information about exposures, outcomes, or both. No method is ideal for all situations, but certain principles apply across studies. The study question, logistical, sampling, and budget issues determine the data collection method. In this chapter, we consider the suitability of various methods for different research questions. We address issues of feasibility, logistics of instrument design, and methods to enhance response rates and data quality.

Sampling

Collecting information from everyone in a large population can be prohibitively expensive. For this reason, investigators will often sample the members of a study population.

The sample should represent the population to which the results are to be generalized and each person in the population of interest should have a calculable, nonzero probability of being selected. Achieving high response rates is important because of concerns regarding nonresponse bias (Lessler and Kalsbeek, 1992; Groves and Couper, 1998). Researchers often adjust or weight data so that the percent distribution of certain attributes of subjects (e.g., age, race, and sex) is equivalent to that in the population. This will reduce nonresponse bias to the degree that respondents within age–race–sex groups answer similarly to their nonrespondent counterparts.

Simple random sampling from a population has several advantages. First, the sample is easy to select when a list of all population members is available. Second, with simple survey designs, the statistical methods for data analysis are very straightforward. More complicated surveys conducted in multiple stages are more difficult to analyze appropriately and often require the assistance of a trained survey sampling researcher and use of specialized statistical programs.

One common method of selecting a random sample of people in a population is through the telephone. Because so many home phone numbers are unlisted and so many new listings are not yet in printed directories, telephone directories do not adequately reflect the entire population. For these reasons, investigators commonly resort to random digit dialing (Hartge et al., 1984; Groves et al., 1988; Lavrakas, 1993; Potthoff, 1994).

National survey research organizations can provide sample lists with names and addresses, but this sampling methodology should be scrutinized carefully. Lists derived from magazine subscriptions, club memberships, or other selective mechanisms can result in serious discrepancies between target and survey populations.

Random digit dialing (RDD) uses a random number generator to create telephone numbers. Telephone numbers in the United States consist of three distinct parts – a three-digit area code (specifies a regional calling area), a three-digit prefix (specifies a regional sub-unit), and a four-digit suffix. Simple RDD designs create a sample of telephone numbers to dial by attaching randomly generated suffixes to randomly selected area code/prefix combinations.

Other systems have been developed that begin with this process, and use a second stage of sampling to greatly increase the efficiency of telephone dialing (Mitofsky, 1970; Waksberg, 1978). Considerable cost is devoted to screening nonworking numbers using these approaches. Commercial vendors have recently begun to market lists of telephone numbers purged of many nonworking and commercial numbers. This allows researchers with smaller budgets to conduct telephone surveys with similar levels of efficiency to those of professional survey research units.

In order to achieve a population-based sample of individuals in a telephone survey, an eligible household member must be randomly selected from all those residents eligible for the study. Otherwise, samples would be disproportionately weighted towards those who are available at the time. In a general population survey women and older adults would predominate (Salmon and Nichols, 1983). Multiple telephone numbers to the same household also must be taken into consideration in a population-based design so that those households with multiple telephone lines are not over-represented.

In devising a sampling scheme, the investigator may have goals that take precedence over accurately estimating certain characteristics of all people in a defined population. Many observational studies are designed primarily to compare behaviors at different points in time (e.g., before vs. after legislation is enacted) and therefore seek to apply the same procedures over time rather than precisely estimating population parameters. For example, Coté et al. (1992) compared helmet use in three Baltimore counties with different approaches to bike helmet promotion. Forty observation sites were selected in each county to represent different socioeconomic strata with equal numbers of sites located around schools or recreation centers, county routes, residential streets, and parks or bike paths. Observations were held on two Saturdays, one in July (baseline) and one in May (follow-up) for a 45-minute duration with data collected on any bicyclist coming within an observer's field of vision.

Becker et al. (1996) compared two approaches to site selection for bike helmet observational studies designed to identify sites that yield a large number of bicyclists. One approach used the recommendations of local bicycle club members along with examination of maps to locate likely bike routes. The other method relied upon community informants to identify locations frequented by young bicyclists. Results indicated that knowledge about the community provided researchers with a more efficient and cost-effective method of identifying young bicyclists.

Choosing a Data Collection Method

Key issues related to the collection of data are the identification of an informant, and the method by which the informant interacts with the study staff. Informants can be the subject of interest or a proxy of the subject (e.g., parent or guardian). Methods to access the subjects or their proxies include telephone or mail surveys, in-person interviews, and behavioral observations.

Normally, data are collected directly from subjects. However, proxy respondents will be necessary if the subjects are very young, mentally compromised (e.g., severely brain injured), or deceased. For example, proxy respondents were necessary in a case–control study of homicide and firearms in the home as many questions related to the behavior of the decedent (Kellermann et al., 1993).

In mail, telephone, and in-person interviews, subjects usually report events or behavior. The validity of self-reported data may be threatened if the behavior is sensitive or illegal. For example, the validity of self-reported seat belt use has been examined by comparing observed use with self-reported use from the same area. Studies conducted in DeKalb County, Georgia and Madrid, Spain yielded telephone survey results that were nearly twice those estimated via observations (CDC, 1987, 1995). Nelson (1996), however, found less discrepancy between self-reported belt use and observational data. He concluded that the validity of self-reported behaviors will likely be higher when the actual prevalence of the behavior is high, but lower when the behavior is less common.

Customarily, information is gathered about the subject from a single source. However, using more than one source of data can be particularly useful in certain types of studies. In a case–control study of risk factors for fire death, data were collected from medical examiners, fire officials, and survivors (Runyan et al., 1992; Marshall et al., 1998). Similarly, a case–control study of adolescent suicide sought details about psychiatric diagnoses that may have been present before death. This required extensive interviewing with surviving family, other adults, and teachers (Shaffer et al., 1996). The process of collecting and interpreting data from more than one source or informant is often referred to as triangulation.

Instrument Development

The design and use of data collection instruments are central activities in quantitative studies. In some cases it is possible to use standardized instruments [e.g., the Functional Independence Measure^{TM} (FIM) for measuring functional outcomes; or the Things I have Seen and Heard Scale or the Women's Experiences with

Battering (WEB) scale] for studies of domestic violence. Individual items from other surveys (e.g., Health Interview Survey or the Behavioral Risk Factor Survey) can also be extracted and used in customized instruments. Comparisons are more easily made between studies if similar instruments or items are used.

Data collection instruments can be fully structured or semistructured. Semistructured instruments allow both quantitative and qualitative analysis. Quantitative data are much easier to analyze, but do not often provide the contextual depth of qualitative data (see chapter on Qualitative methods in injury research).

Selection of Instrument Items

Questionnaire items can be either open or close ended. Open-ended items invite respondents to use their own words to answer. For example, one item might read: What hazards have you encountered while working as a farm hand? This type of item would be particularly helpful if answers do not correspond to a list of hazards that the researcher could generate. A close-ended question might be structured to read: "Which of these hazards have you encountered while working as a farm hand? (a) tractor without rollover protection; (b) power take-off devices with shields removed; (c) heights above 15 feet; (d) working alone in a grain silo; (e) applying pesticides without a mask." Open-ended questions can add substantially to the time of survey administration and the time required for analyzing the results. Consequently, open-ended questions are used sparingly in quantitative studies. However, they can be useful if the goal is to obtain information about beliefs or attitudes which have not been identified in prior studies.

Items should be clear and should avoid being double-barreled or loaded. Double-barreled questions attempt to measure more than one construct at a time. For example, a question in a study of workplace safety should not ask: How often do you wear protective gloves or goggles? Rather, it would be better to construct questions that ask, How often do you wear protective gloves? followed by another item that asks: How often do you wear goggles? A question is considered loaded if it steers the respondent to a socially desirable response. An example of a loaded question would be: Do you always abide by the child safety seat law? A better question might read: How often do you use the child safety seat when transporting your child?

Questions about simple facts (e.g., Have you ever fallen off a horse? or Have you ever been the driver in a car crash?) can be asked in a straightforward manner without much preparation. Other questions, which require more difficult recall or reporting of sensitive information, require special attention to phrasing. For events difficult to recall, it is often helpful to restrict the time period of recall (e.g., During the past school year, did you ever ride your bicycle to school? or Since Christmas, have you worked the evening shift at your job? or During the time you were in college, were you ever threatened with a gun?). Alternatively, the questionnaire might gradually lead up to the desired type of response: Have you *ever* ridden your bicycle to school? followed by During the past school year, have you ridden your bicycle to school?

Questionnaires designed to elicit information that is personally sensitive may require lead-ins that give the respondent permission to report illegal or socially sanctioned behaviors. For example, a question designed to inquire about carrying concealed weapons might begin with: Some people carry concealed guns often when they go out in public, while others never carry them. Would you say that you usually, often, sometimes, rarely or never carry a concealed gun with you when you go out in your community?

The choice of response options is equally important to how questions are asked. The structure of the question and the response options must be appropriate to the question. For example, it would be inappropriate to ask the yes/no question: "Do you, as a pedestrian, ever cross the street in midblock? and include response options of often, sometimes, rarely, or never. Also, an investigator needs to be careful in choosing response options that are realistic. Very fine discriminations, while desirable, may simply not be possible for respondents to make. For example, a respondent being asked to indicate how many days of work he or she missed as a result of injuries may have a hard time providing the exact number. Rather, it may be more appropriate to provide meaningful groupings of days: none, less than a week, one week, more than a week but less than a month, a month or more. In other situations, it may be better to ask for a specific response, then group into categories later (e.g., age).

Process of Questionnaire Construction

Sufficient time should be allotted to the time-consuming task of developing a good data collection instrument. Sometimes it is helpful to use focus groups to learn the salient issues, the types of language used, and the constructs of interest (see chapter on Qualitative research methods). Constructing the instrument usually requires multiple drafts, with careful review of each draft by several persons having expertise in questionnaire design and the subject matter.

Once researchers develop a questionnaire to address all the variables of interest using language appropriate to the audience, the instrument is ready for pretesting. Dillman (1978) recommends that researchers pretest instruments with three separate groups – colleagues, potential users of the data, and people drawn from the population to be surveyed. This latter pretest often entails the selection of 20–50 respondents and can be used to evaluate questionnaire items, the quality of interviews, likelihood of controversy resulting from the survey, the likely non-response rate, and the cost and length of the interview (Warwick and Lininger, 1975). Researchers often debrief pilot test respondents after completing the interview in order to identify difficulties encountered in interpreting the meaning of the items or the response options. This also allows respondents to discuss issues associated with the sensitivity of questions or the interview administration. The information obtained from this kind of debriefing process is invaluable to permit revisions in the questionnaire or administration procedures.

Data Collection Methods

Three major categories of data collection are discussed: self-administered surveys; in-person interviews; and direct observation. Table 6.1 summarizes advantages and disadvantages of each method.

Self-administered Surveys

Self-administered surveys are used in injury research to obtain information about self-reported risk or protective behaviors, attitudes, and beliefs about proposed or implemented interventions, or to learn about injury experiences. They may be mailed or administered in a setting where subjects gather (e.g., clinic or school) and require that the respondent be able to read at the appropriate grade level. The method may be used to obtain information from an at-risk population (e.g., teenage workers reporting about hazards at the workplace; Schulman et al., 1997; Dunn et al., 1998), or about injured persons (e.g., survey of emergency department patients to learn about domestic violence experience; Waller et al., 1996).

Mail Surveys

Mail surveys are feasible when lists of names and addresses are available from administrative units such as employers, health care providers, clubs, or schools. Studies have shown consistently that the single most important technique to obtaining high response rates in mail surveys is to send out reminders (Dillman et al., 1974; Kanuk and Berenson, 1975; Yammarino et al., 1991; Mangione, 1995). Dillman (1978) has outlined a detailed plan of respondent reminders. Though not all steps are used in every study, the approach recommends, in addition to the initial mailing, a follow-up postcard reminder sent to everyone after one week has elapsed, a letter and questionnaire sent to nonresponders three weeks after the initial mailing, and a final mailing of a letter and questionnaire sent by certified mail. Telephone follow-up can also be used if appropriate.

Other techniques used to increase response rates are: (1) including a one-page introduction letter from an influential person on professionally produced letterhead; (2) providing a self-addressed envelope with return postage (preferably with a regular stamp); (3) keeping the questionnaire short; (4) making the questionnaire simple, easy to read and follow; and (5) emphasizing prestigious sponsorship such as a university, the federal government, or a professional organization (Fox et al., 1988; Mangione, 1995). In a meta-analysis of various methods identified to increase response rates of mail survey designs, Fox et al. (1988) found that university sponsorship, pre-notification by letter, and stamped return reply verses business reply yielded the largest increases in response. Postcard follow-up, first-class outgoing postage, green questionnaire versus white, and enclosing a small cash incentive also yielded significant improvements to response. Promised monetary awards as well as nonmonetary incentives such as pens and pencils have been found to increase response, but by less than enclosed monetary incentives (Hansen, 1980;

Table 6.1 Features of data collection methods

Method	Pros	Cons
Self-administered surveys		
Mailed survey	can be used with a widely dispersed geographic sample sampling frame obtainable from address-based list relatively inexpensive respondents have more time to think about answers privacy in responding respondents can visualize response options requires fewer personnel to administer appropriate for sensitive/threatening question	harder to use open-ended questions requires shorter instrument response rates lower than interviews requires addresses no opportunity to develop rapport with study subject difficult to maintain anonymity and conduct follow-up
Interviews		
Personal interview	highest response rates allows for complex questionnaire design nonverbal and verbal queues to respondent confusion easier to develop rapport combines well with observational methods respondents willing to take longer to answer questions than self-administered surveys or telephone interviews	risks to interviewers in dangerous neighborhoods may be less desirable for sensitive material precision of estimates reduced by design effects expensive difficult if study population geographically dispersed
Telephone interview	less expensive than personal interviews can be easier to preserve confidentiality (with random dialing) can complete survey relatively quickly verbal queues only to respondent confusion	less ability to develop rapport than in-person interview frame limited to individuals with telephones respondent cannot visualize lists response rates
Observational studies	can directly observe behavior or hazard, rather than relying on self-report more valid than self-reported information when actual behaviors are socially unacceptable	not feasible for measuring psychological variables (e.g., attitudes, beliefs) development of appropriate sampling design can be costly

Nederhof, 1983). Incentives should be meaningful to the respondent but not so large that it is coercive, an issue that human subjects boards will consider when reviewing a study protocol. In general, response rates to mail surveys range from 60% to 75% or lower (Marcus and Crane, 1986). Dillman (1978) claimed response rates of 85% using his Total Design Method approach.

Respondent anonymity is possible with mail questionnaires but studies have not clearly shown the advantage of anonymity over simple assurances of confidentiality (Futrell and Swan, 1977; Wildman, 1977; Mangione, 1995). Dillman (1978) recommends placing an identification number prominently on the first page of the questionnaire, emphasizing that all information will be treated confidentially, and acknowledging the purpose of identification to facilitate follow-up. If researchers conclude that anonymity is essential to the success of the survey, follow-ups should be sent to all participants. However, this does carry the risk that a respondent will return two questionnaires. An alternative is to provide each respondent with a postcard with identifying information that can be mailed simultaneously but separately from the questionnaires. Respondents are instructed to indicate on the postcard that either the questionnaire has been returned or that the respondent refuses to participate. This method permits researchers to track nonrespondents while keeping the returned questionnaires anonymous by virtue of their separation from identifying information (Mangione, 1995).

Computerized Self-administered Questionnaire

The computerized self-administered questionnaire (CSAQ) or audio computer-assisted self-interviewing (audio-CASI) approach to data collection has recently been developed to facilitate the private collection of sensitive data by allowing respondents to interact with a computer rather than an interviewer (Aday, 1989; Wright et al., 1997; Beebe et al., 1998; Turner et al., 1998). Computer-generated approaches to data collection have also become popular in surveying subjects with Internet access. The audio-CASI program leads respondents through written and audio electronic questionnaires and provides respondents with low literacy opportunities to complete self-administered questionnaires. Picture and video capabilities can also be programmed into the computer-generated interview. When used in an in-home survey, the computer-assisted approaches have been shown to increase the likelihood that respondents report sensitive information such as adolescent homosexual contact and drug use (Wright et al., 1997; Turner et al., 1998). In an in-school comparison of a CSAQ with a paper and pencil instrument, however, the computer-assisted mode was shown to identify fewer sensitive adolescent behaviors than the paper and pencil version (Beebe et al., 1998).

Personal Interviews

Choosing between a personal interview or telephone interview requires several considerations. The subject matter, the type of data required, and the accessibility of subjects may all influence this determination. Telephone interviews may be necessary if the subjects are dispersed over a large geographic area. Costs of conducting personal interviews are higher than telephone interviews. Personal interviews can also be used in conjunction with observational methods; for example, making direct observations of living conditions (e.g., presence of throw rugs, stairs, or bath rails) or personal behaviors (e.g., gait, shoe type).

Response rates to personal interview surveys exceed other data collection methods. In a side by side comparison of personal versus telephone designs, one study found that telephone administration of the National Health Interview Survey led to a 16% point drop in the response rate (96–80%) (National Center for Health Statistics, 1987). The response rates of well-designed population-based personal interview studies tend to exceed 80% (Siemiatycki, 1979; Aday, 1989). Estimates of costs, however, vary considerably across personal interview studies, but on the whole, exceed those of telephone surveys by a factor of two or three.

Another consideration is the safety of the interviewer and the respondent. For example, interviewing abused women at home may put them at increased risk if the batterer becomes suspicious that the interview will reveal his abusive behavior. Abused women may be unable or unwilling to give honest answers in a home interview for fear of personal safety. Enrollment of subjects in high crime areas may impose unacceptable risks on solitary interviewers. Though sending more than one member of a study team into a home may alleviate concerns about safety, it is costly, and may also be intimidating for respondents.

Traditionally, personal interviewers have relied on paper and pencil questionnaires, although it has become increasingly popular to use laptop computers for survey administration and data entry. Interviewers read questions and enter responses, eliminating the need for the time-consuming process of hard copy editing and data entry. The National Center for Health Statistics (NCHS) uses this technology for the administration of the National Health Interview Survey (National Center for Health Statistics and U.S. Bureau of the Census, 1988; National Center for Health Statistics, 1999).

Telephone Interviews

The use of the telephone to conduct interviews has grown in popularity over the past two decades (Frankel and Frankel, 1987; Frey, 1989). The training of interviewers and preparation of data collection instruments must be structured specifically for telephone use. The telephone interviewer must develop the ability to judge auditory cues signaling the degree of trust between respondent and interviewer, levels of uncertainty about question clarity or response choices, discomfort with certain topics, or background distractions (e.g., tending a child, cooking a meal, or watching television) or what may be a threatening situation (e.g., presence of an abusive partner listening to responses to a survey about violence).

Multiple attempts will be needed to reach selected households or specific respondents (Traugott, 1987). Most investigators use different protocols for call-backs, but typically six attempts at different times of the day and different days of the week are sufficient to reach the great majority of the sample in a general population survey (Frey, 1989).

Response rates to telephone surveys usually exceed rates from mail surveys, but are often lower than for personal interviews. They tend to be in the range of 70–85%, but are likely to vary considerably depending upon the subject matter and target population (Groves and Kahn, 1979; Aday, 1989; Frey, 1989). Response rates reflect the success of a researcher in contacting and completing an interview with eligible respondents. The basic calculation is:

$$\text{Response rate} = \frac{\text{completed interviews}}{\text{eligible respondents}}$$

Eligibility, however, is often not obtainable for those telephone numbers that are dropped from dialing because of no answers after a prearranged number of attempts. This complicates the calculation of response rates in telephone survey designs with higher rates calculated if all numbers with unknown eligibility are excluded from consideration and lower rates calculated if unknowns are all considered eligible (Frey, 1989). A reasonable compromise to this conundrum was advanced by the Council of American Survey Research Organizations (CASRO) that assigned the proportion eligible in the known cases to those that are unknown (CASRO, 1982).

Computer-assisted telephone interviewing systems (CATI) are also available to improve the efficiency of data collection tasks (Frey, 1989; Lavrakas, 1993). In this case, the questions are programmed into a computer so that the interviewer reads them on a screen and records the answers directly on to the computer. Computerization reduces errors associated with data entry and makes it easier for the interviewer to follow skip patterns designed so that different questions are asked depending on answers given by the respondent.

Examples of large-scale telephone interview studies used by injury researchers are the National Crime Victimization Survey (Bachman and Saltzman, 1995), the Health Interview Survey (NCHS, 1988), the Behavioral Risk Factor Survey (BRFS) (CDC, 1999), and the Injury Control and Risk Survey (ICARUS) developed at the National Center for Injury Prevention and Control (Sacks et al., 1996). Other studies have used telephone interviewing to obtain information about teen work experiences (Schulman et al., 1997; Dunn et al., 1998), gun storage and use practices (Hemenway et al., 1995), and the occurrence of injuries to children in child care (Kotch et al., 1997).

Observational Methods

Observational approaches to data collection involve the visual identification and codification of particular situations, events, or occurrences by trained observers. These methods differ by the level of involvement of observers (participant vs. nonparticipant) and the degree of structure in the data collection protocol.

Most uses of the observational approach in injury research have involved nonparticipant structured designs in which behaviors or hazards are observed and coded by trained observers. Among the issues to consider are the selection of observational sites, how the site or behavior in question is observed and recorded, and procedures for interobserver reliability.

Some observational studies of seat belt use have collected data from moving vehicles rather than from a stationary site. For example, a driver and accompanying observer made observations over a predetermined route on roadways primarily in downtown or commercial areas that had at least two lanes in the direction that the observers were traveling. Driving in the right lane at less than the posted speed, observers coded seat belt use within the vehicles that passed on the left or stopped abreast at stop signs or stoplights (Williams et al., 1987a). A study of seat belt use in four states with seat belt laws used a similar approach (Williams et al., 1987b). These approaches, however, were not population-based and may not have yielded representative samples of drivers during the time periods for which observations were made.

Many states have used a multistaged probability sampling technique designed to yield precise estimates of seat belt use. In North Carolina the methodology calls for the collection of observational data from a subset of the most populous 48 of 100 counties. The selection process specifies a first-stage random sample of counties, a second-stage random sample of road segments from within counties, reflecting different types of roads and use patterns, and a third-stage selection, which determines the stop-light controlled intersection where the observations are made.

In a non-traffic example, Sacks used observational methods to assess the presence of hazards on playgrounds in Atlanta before and after an intervention (Sacks et al., 1989, 1990, 1992). He trained observers to use standardized measures derived from the Consumer Product Safety Commission guidelines for safe playgrounds, to assess equipment height, distances between equipment, and the fall zone around equipment, pinching hazards, and surface depth.

In any observational study, observers must be given very clear guidelines for what is to be counted and how to make assessments (e.g., what constitutes a passenger in a vehicle, how to estimate age of a passenger, how to measure the depth of surface material under playground equipment, slipperiness of floors in nursing homes, or noise in an industrial worksite). Often more than one observer is used to make assessments, with comparisons done in both the training and data collection process to assure high interobserver reliability.

Conclusions

Each strategy of data collection has different strengths, depending on the study question and setting. Regardless of the method chosen, care must be exercised in sampling, developing, and pretesting appropriate instruments, and in training data collectors to ensure the collection of valid and reliable information.

References

Aday LA (1989) Designing and conducting health surveys: A comprehensive guide. San Francisco, CA: Jossey-Bass Publishers.

Bachman R, Saltzman LE (1995) Violence against women: Estimates from the redesigned survey. NCJ-154348. Washington, DC: Bureau of Justice Statistics.

Beebe TJ, Harrison PA, McRae JA, Anderson RE, Fulkerson JA (1998) An evaluation of computer-assisted self-interviews in a school setting. Public Opin Q 62:623–32.

Becker LR, Mandell MB, Wood K, Schmidt ER, O'Hara F (1996) A community based approach to bicycle helmet use counts. Injury Prev 2:283–5.

Centers for Disease Control (1999) Behavioral risk factor surveillance system. Available from URL: http://www.cdc.gov/nccdphp/brfss/about.htm

   (1987) Use of seat belts – Madrid, Spain, 1994. MMWR 44:150–3.

   (1995) Use of safety belts – DeKalb County, Georgia, 1986. MMWR 36:433–7.

Coté TR, Sacks JJ, Lambert-Huber DA, Dannenberg MD, Kresnow M, Lipsitz CM, Schmidt ER (1992) Bicycle helmet use among Maryland children: Effect of legislation and education. Pediatrics 89:1216–20.

Council of American Survey Research Organizations (1982) On the definition of response rates. A Special Report of the CASRO Task Force on Completion Rates, Council of American Survey Research Organizations.

Dillman DA (1978) Mail and telephone surveys: The total design method. New York: John Wiley.

Dillman D, Carpenter E, Christenson J, Brooks R (1974) Increasing mail questionnaire response: A four state comparison. Am Sociol Review 39:744–56.

Dunn KA, Runyan CW, Cohen LR, Schulman MD (1998) Teens at work: A statewide study of jobs, hazards, and injuries. J Adolesc Health 22:19–25.

Fox RJ, Crask MR, Jonghoon K (1988) A meta-analysis of selected techniques for inducing response. Public Opin Q 52:467–91.

Frey JH (1989) Survey research by telephone, 2nd edn. Beverly Hills, CA: Sage Publications.

Frankel MR, Frankel LR (1987) Fifty years of survey sampling in the United States. Public Opin Q 51:127–38.

Futrell CM, Swan JE (1977) Anonymity and response by salespeople to a mail questionnaire. J Marketing Res 14:611–16.

Groves RM, Couper MP (1998) Nonresponse in household interview surveys. New York: Wiley.

Groves RM, Kahn RL (1979) Surveys by telephone: A national comparison with personal interviews. New York: Academic Press.

Groves RM, Biermer PP, Lyberg LE, Massey JT, Nicholls WL, Waskberg J (1988) Telephone survey methodology. New York: John Wiley and Sons.

Hansen RA (1980) A self-perception interpretation of the effect of monetary and nonmonetary incentives on mail survey respondent behavior. J Marketing Res 17:77–83.

Hartge P, Brinton LA, Rosenthal JF, Cahill JI, Hoover RN, Waksberg J (1984) Random digit dialing in selecting a population based group. Am J Epidemiol 120: 825–33.

Hemenway D, Solnick SJ, Azrael DR (1995) Firearm training and storage. JAMA 273:46–50.

Kanuk L, Berenson C (1975) Mail surveys and response rates: A literature review. J Marketing Res 12:440–53.

Kellermann AL, Rivara FP, Rushforth NB, Banton JG, Reay DT, Francisco JT, Locci AB, Prodzinski J, Hackman BB, Somes G (1993) Gun ownership as a risk factor for homicide in the home. N Engl J Med 329:1084–91.

Kotch JB, Dufort VM, Sieberg SJ, McMurray M, OBrien S, Ngui EM, Brennan M (1997) Injuries among children in home and out-of-home care. Injury Prev 3:267–71.

Lavrakas PJ (1993) Telephone survey methods: Sampling, selection, and supervision, 2nd edn. Applied Social Research Methods Series, Vol. 7. Newbury Park, NY: Sage Publications, Inc.

Lessler JT, Kalsbeek WD (1992) Nonsampling Error in Surveys. New York, NY: Wiley.

Mangione TW (1995) Mail surveys: Improving the quality. Applied Social Research Methods Series, Vol. 40. Newbury Park, NY: Sage Publications.

Marcus AC, Crane LA (1986) Telephone surveys in public health research. Med Care 24:97–112.

Marshall SW, Runyan CW, Bangdiwala SI, Linzer MA, Sacks JJ, Butts JD (1998) Fatal residential fires: Who dies and who survives? JAMA 279:1633–7.

Mitofsky WJ (1970) Sampling of telephone households [Mimeo]. New York: CBS News.

National Center for Health Statistics and US Bureau of the Census (1988) Report of the 1987 Automated National Health Interview Survey Feasibility Study: An Investigation of Computer-Assisted Personal Interviews. Hyattsville, MD: National Center for Health Statistics.

National Center for Health Statistics (1987) An experimental comparison of telephone personal health interview surveys. DHHS Publication no. (PHS) 87–1380. Vital and Health Statistics Series 2, no. 106. Washington, DC: US Government Printing Office.

(1999) National health interview survey flow. Available from URL: http://www.cdc.gov/nchswww/about/major/nhis/nhisflow.htm

Nederhof AJ (1983) The effects of material incentives in mail surveys: Two studies. Public Opin Q 47:107–11.

Nelson DE (1996) Validity of self reported data on injury prevention behavior: Lessons from observational and self reported surveys of safety belt use in the US. Injury Prev 2: 67–9.

Potthoff RF (1994) Telephone sampling in epidemiologic research: To reap the benefits, avoid the pitfalls. Am J Epidemiol 139:967–78.

Runyan CW, Bangdiwala SI, Linzer MA, Sacks JJ, Butts JD (1992) Risk factors for fatal residential fires. N Engl J Med 327:859–63.

Sacks JJ, Brantley MD, Holmgreen P, Rochat RW (1992) Evaluation of an intervention to reduce playground hazards in Atlanta child-care centers. Am J Public Health 82:429–31.

Sacks JJ, Holt KW, Holmgreen P, Colwell LS, Brown JM (1990) Playground hazards in Atlanta child-care centers, Am J Public Health 80:986–8.

Sacks JJ, Smith JD, Kaplan KM, Lambert DA, Sattin RW, Sikes KS (1989) The epidemiology of injuries in Atlanta day-care centers. JAMA 262:1641–5.

Sacks JJ, Kresnow M, Houston B (1996) Dog bites: How big a problem? Injury Prev 2:52–4.

Salmon CT, Nichols JS (1983) The next-birthday method for respondent selection. Public Opin Q 47: 210–76.

Schulman MD, Evenson CT, Runyan CW, Cohen LR, Dunn KA (1997) Farm work is dangerous for teens: Agricultural hazards and injuries. J Rural Health 13:295–305.

Siemiatycki J (1979) A comparison of mail, telephone, and home interview strategies for household health surveys. Am J Public Health 69:3238–45.

Shaffer D, Gould MS, Fisher P, Tautman P, Moreau D, Kleinman M, Flory M (1996) Psychiatric diagnosis in child and adolescent psychiatry. Arch Gen Psychiatry 53: 339–48.

Traugott MR (1987) The importance of persistence in respondent selection for preelection surveys. Public Opin Q 51:48–57.

Turner CF, Ku L, Rogers SM, Lindberg LD, Pleck JH, Sonenstein FL (1998) Adolescent sexual behavior, drug use, and violence: Increased reporting with computer survey technology. Science 280:867–73.

Waksberg J (1978) Sampling methods for random digit dialing. J Am Stat Assoc 73:40–6.

Waller AE, Hohenhaus SM, Shah PJ, Stern EA (1996) Development and validation of emergency department screening and referral protocol of victims of domestic violence. Ann Emerg Med 27:6.

Warwick DP, Lininger CA (1975) The sample survey: Theory and practice. New York: McGraw-Hill.

Wildman RC (1977) Effects of anonymity and social setting on survey responses. Public Opin Q 41:74–9.

Williams AF, Lund AK, Preusser DF, Blomberg RD (1987a) Results of a seat belt use law enforcement and publicity campaign in Elmira, New York. Accid Anal Prev 19:243–9.

Williams AF, Wells JK, Lund AK (1987b) Shoulder belt use in four states with belt use laws. Accid Anal and Prev 19:251–60.

Wright DL, Aquiline WS, Supple AJ (1997) A comparison of computer-assisted and paper and pencil self-administered questionnaires in a survey of smoking, alcohol, and drug use. Public Opin Q 62:331–53.

Yammarino FJ, Skinner SJ, Childers TL (1991) Understanding mail survey response behavior. Public Opin Q 55:613–39.

7

Selecting a Study Design for Injury Research

Thomas D. Koepsell

Introduction

The first step in conducting an injury-related research project is to specify the research question. The second step is to choose a study design.

What exactly is meant by a study design? In broad terms, it is a plan for identifying study subjects and for obtaining data on them. The study subjects are often people, but they can be other kinds of observation units, including social groups, physical settings, time periods, devices, published articles, and so on. Data on study subjects can come from pre-existing sources or can be gathered anew by a wide variety of methods ranging from ethnographic observation to questionnaires to specialized physiologic measurements. Many study designs involve comparing data between groups of study subjects or on the same subjects monitored over time.

The number of different study designs is potentially infinite, and they can be classified in many ways. The organizing scheme used here, shown in Figure 7.1, draws its terminology from epidemiology, biomedical research, and the social sciences. However, the underlying ideas are quite general, and this scheme can be usefully applied to a wide range of injury research. This chapter seeks to provide an overview of the major study designs, to highlight factors that guide the investigator to an appropriate design choice, and to illustrate the application of several commonly used study designs to injury research through examples.

Questions to Consider in Choosing a Design
Does the Primary Research Aim Involve Description or Hypothesis Testing?

Some research merely seeks to characterize a prevailing state of affairs, without any advance prediction or expectation about what might be found. For example: What are the most common clinical presentations among persons injured in a motorcycle collision? How common are burns and scalds among preschool children? This kind of research question is typically best addressed with a descriptive study.

In contrast, other studies seek explicitly or implicitly to test a specific hypothesis. For example: Does a program to prevent falls in the elderly significantly reduce the incidence of falls? Do bicycle helmets protect wearers against head injury in a bicycle crash? This kind of research question is usually best addressed with an

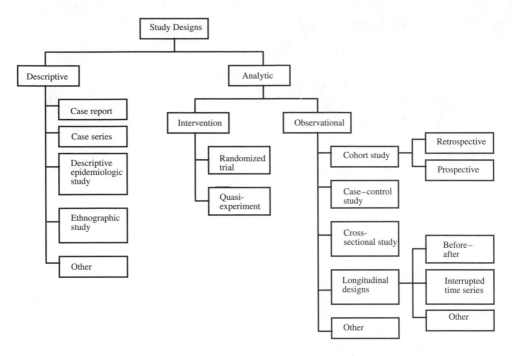

Figure 7.1 Tree diagram of study design types.

analytic study design. Often the research question for an analytic study is whether a certain cause (which may be an intervention) leads to a certain effect.

Can a Subject's Exposure to a Potential Causal or Protective Factor be Manipulated by the Investigator?

Among analytic study designs, a key distinction is between intervention studies and observational studies. In intervention studies, the investigator can manipulate the exposure of subjects to a factor that is thought to be related to injury occurrence or another injury-related outcome. For example, alternative clinical treatments for trauma patients can sometimes be compared by applying one treatment to some patients and another to other patients, in order to determine which form of treatment is more effective. Likewise, intervention programs aimed at injury prevention can often be implemented in such a way that part of the potential target population is exposed to the intervention, leaving others as an unexposed control group.

In observational studies, the investigator plays a more passive part, lacking the ability to dictate which study subjects are exposed to a factor of interest and which are not. Exposures that must typically be studied with observational study designs include lifestyle choices (such as driving while intoxicated), public policies (such as laws requiring all new automobiles to be equipped with passenger-side air bags), or clinical features of injury presentation that may affect prognosis (such as closed vs. penetrating head injury).

How Often and How Soon do We Expect to
Observe the Outcome of Interest?

As discussed below, some analytic study designs are inefficient for rare or delayed outcome events. For example, fatal episodes of child abuse are (fortunately) quite rare in most settings, making it difficult to study their causes prospectively by following a cohort of children, particularly if primary data collection is needed. Other study designs – especially the case–control study design – excel for study of rare outcomes and may offer dramatic savings in money and time.

Sometimes a long time may need to pass between a cause and a hypothesized effect, as in studying childhood characteristics or experiences as predictors of adult violent behavior. A prospective cohort study on this topic could be very expensive and time-consuming. However, if good historical data were available, a retrospective cohort study could be much cheaper and quicker.

Are there Important Local Opportunities or Barriers?

Sometimes unusual circumstances in a particular population, setting, or time period can strongly affect the feasibility of a particular study design, either positively or negatively, and trump scientific considerations that would otherwise prevail. For example, one research study can often provide a springboard for other related studies. Once a special surveillance system has been set up to obtain valid and reliable statistics on the incidence of domestic violence episodes, such a system may provide an easy way to identify cases for a case–control study of risk factors for domestic violence. Similarly, access to diagnostic data from hospital admissions and clinic visits in a Health Maintenance Organization may make it possible to study injury occurrence relatively cheaply in a large cohort of people.

In other situations, local history or other idiosyncrasies can create barriers for a study plan that might otherwise work well scientifically. For example, conducting a school survey to characterize the injury risk behavior of children may be very difficult if local schools have recently been bombarded with requests from other organizations to permit their students to be surveyed.

Descriptive Study Designs
Case Report

Perhaps the simplest descriptive study design is a narrative account of a specific clinical injury case. A case report describes some newsworthy clinical occurrence, such as an unusual type of injury event, use of an unusual treatment, or a treatment error with a lesson. The report may stimulate other clinicians to be on the lookout for such cases, and it may lead to more formal attempts to quantify the magnitude of the problem. Results are generally reported simply as a clinical narrative. The story of the case may generate hypotheses that can be followed up more formally in analytic studies. For example, Chin and Berns (1995) described a 23-month-old girl who was nearly strangulated while playing with a popular toy necklace – a previously unrecognized hazard of such toys.

Case Series

A case report shows that something can happen once; a case series shows that it can happen repeatedly. It also provides an opportunity to identify common features among multiple cases and to describe patterns of variability. Results are usually reported using simple descriptive statistics, such as means, ranges, standard deviations, and percentages. Internal comparisons may also be made within the case series. For example, Rabban et al. (1997) described a series of 16 cases of electrical injury from contact with subway third rails, pointing out that the seven episodes involving subway workers tended to be less severe, nonfatal injuries, compared with the nine occurring among nonoccupational victims.

Cummings and Weiss (1998) noted that a case series can sometimes also be viewed as a primitive relative of a case–control study. In a case series, one often looks for unexpected features in the background of cases. Expectations are implicitly based on what one judges would be found in a comparable series of non-cases, even though no such non-cases are actually studied. These authors also point out that a so-called "exposure series" may serve a similar purpose, reporting on the fate of a series of persons who shared exposure to some factor or experience. The observed outcomes would be interpreted in relation to outcomes expected in a set of otherwise comparable unexposed persons.

Case series that include all eligible cases in a defined population can be of special value, because they avoid selection biases due to referral of certain kinds of patients to a particular clinical center. For example, Orsay et al. (1995) summarized the characteristics of 1231 motorcycle crash victims treated in all 73 Level I or II trauma centers throughout Illinois in order to estimate the burden of motorcycle trauma in the state. While generalization from one setting to another always requires caution, we can at least be more confident that the cases in a population-based case series are representative of the setting from which the cases were drawn.

Descriptive Epidemiologic Study

A descriptive epidemiologic study combines data on a population-based set of cases with denominator data. This research approach is often used when little is known about the frequency and risk factors for injury of a certain type. It serves to quantify the burden of the injury on a population in terms of standard measures of disease frequency, including incidence, prevalence, or mortality rates. Descriptive epidemiologic studies can be a rich source of hypotheses that can be followed up in analytic studies.

Most descriptive epidemiologic studies rely on data from existing sources, such as death certificates or an area-wide trauma registry. Primary data collection is necessary if no such data sources exist. The time-honored conceptual framework of descriptive epidemiology is person, place, and time. Injury frequency is compared across subpopulations defined on the basis of personal characteristics such as age, sex, race, income, or other sociodemographic factors; among geographic areas or between urban and rural settings; or over time, considered in terms of long-term secular trends in injury occurrence and cyclic variation in relation to time of day, day of week, month of year, or season.

The *Injury Fact Book* by Baker et al. (1992), exemplifies descriptive epidemiologic research based chiefly on injury mortality data for the United States. It provides a wealth of data that highlight the significance of injury as a public-health problem and that identify high-risk subpopulations. Schwarz et al. (1994) carried out a careful descriptive epidemiologic study of injuries in a predominantly African-American part of Philadelphia. To study both fatal and non-fatal injuries, they set up their own injury-surveillance system through multiple hospital emergency departments in order to capture nearly all medically treated injuries among residents of the study area. Population denominator data came from the U.S. census. The findings called attention to the high incidence of intentional interpersonal injury in the inner city and the high risk of recurrent interpersonal injury among persons with an initial injury.

Ethnography

Ethnographic research is particularly valuable for enriching our understanding of the cultural antecedents and consequences of injury (see chapter 8). Classically, ethnography involves participant observation and in-depth interviews of key informants by a trained cultural anthropologist, seeking to uncover the meaning behind what people do and say. Lundsgaarde's book *Murder in Space City* (1977) described an ethnographic study of all homicides in Houston, Texas that occurred during one year. The study involved the anthropologist-author's review of police files; interviews with police detectives, lawyers, and forensic pathologists; and observation of homicide investigations, including interrogation of killers and witnesses. Among many findings, the study revealed the close social similarity between most killers and their victims; the frequency with which fatal violence stemmed from apparently trivial disagreements; and the strong association between severity of punishment for homicide and the nature of the killer–victim relationship, with more severe penalties for those who killed a stranger than for those who killed an acquaintance or family member.

Analytic Study Designs

An analytic study focuses on one or more hypotheses to be tested. Often the main hypothesis is that some factor increases or decreases the risk of some outcome. The (possibly) causal factor is commonly termed an exposure. In studies of injury causation or prevention, the outcome is occurrence of the kind of injury of interest, while in studies of injury treatment or prognosis, the outcome may be death, occurrence of complications, or some other adverse effect of sustaining an injury.

The unit of study is not always a person. Some injury research involves studying groups of persons en bloc. Using groups as units of analysis is suitable when the relevant exposure is a policy or program that applies to everyone in the group, as with a state law. In other situations, the individual-level relationship between exposure and outcome is of interest, but only group-level data are available and are therefore used by necessity. Studies using group-level data are often termed ecologic studies, which are discussed by Hingson et al. (chapter 12).

Intervention Studies

In an intervention study, the investigator can manipulate the exposure status of study subjects. Often this capability is used to arrange groups of exposed and nonexposed subjects so as to maximize the validity of comparisons.

Randomized Trials

The randomized trial is the king of study designs: all else being equal, it is more likely than any other study design to give the correct answer about whether the exposure is causally related to the outcome. The reason for this is that random assignment of subjects to different exposure groups tends, on average, to balance the groups on other factors that could influence the outcome. This feature of randomization works well even for factors that may be hard to measure or that may not be known to the investigator. Thus, an observed difference in outcomes between groups at the end of the study can be ascribed with high confidence to the difference in exposure that the study was designed to investigate.

A simple two-group randomized trial design is shown in Figure 7.2. Potential study subjects are screened for eligibility, and those found eligible are asked to give their informed consent to participate. These eligible and willing subjects are then assigned at random to one of two groups, here called Treatment A and Treatment B. Often one treatment is experimental; the other may be no treatment, a specific alternative treatment, or usual care. In any case, both groups are then followed prospectively, and the incidence of good and bad outcomes is measured and compared.

Brochgrevink et al. (1998) randomly assigned 201 patients with whiplash injury after a car crash to receive either (1) a soft collar to immobilize the neck for 14 days and time off from work; or (2) encouragement to resume normal daily activities. Six months later, 54% of the immobilized group reported no neck stiffness, compared with 69% of those in the act-as-usual group ($p < 0.04$). The act-as-usual group also fared significantly better on several other head and neck symptoms.

As the design of choice among intervention studies, the randomized trial should usually be the first study design option considered for treatment and program evaluations, resorting to other less rigorous designs only if there are major obstacles to a randomized trial. Even when a nonrandomized design must be used, its protocol can often be guided by considering how the corresponding randomized trial would be conducted. In addition to the parallel-groups design portrayed in

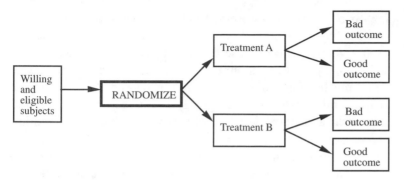

Figure 7.2 Randomized trial.

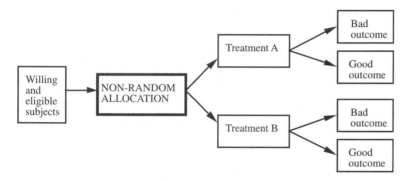

Figure 7.3 Quasi-experimental trial.

Figure 7.2, there are many useful variations of the randomized trial design, as described by Koepsell (chapter 9). These include designs that permit concurrent study of two or more interventions (factorial designs), designs that are well-suited to interventions aimed at pre-existing social groups (group-randomized designs), and designs that enhance statistical power and validity by exposing each participant to two intervention conditions at different times (crossover studies).

Like prospective cohort studies and quasi-experiments (next section), randomized trials may be too expensive or infeasible if the primary outcome of interest is rare, or if long periods of follow-up would be required before any intervention effects appear. Randomization may also sometimes be politically unacceptable to collaborating organizations or participants.

Quasi-experiments

An intervention study that does not involve random assignment of subjects to comparison groups is sometimes termed a quasi-experiment (Cook and Campbell, 1979). This label derives from the fact that a randomized trial is sometimes called a true experiment. This design is diagrammed in Figure 7.3. For example, DiGuiseppi et al. (1989) evaluated a multifaceted bicycle helmet wearing campaign in Seattle, Washington by comparing observed helmet-wearing behavior in the intervention area with helmet-wearing in Portland, Oregon, a control site. Seattle was chosen as the intervention site because the investigators were based there, making it easier and less expensive to mount the intervention program. Bicycle riders obviously could not be assigned at random to one city or the other, so the investigators measured and controlled in the analysis for factors that differed between cities and that were associated with helmet-wearing, such as rider's gender, race, and bicycle type.

Although a quasi-experiment is an intervention study, in one important way it is more like an observational study than like a randomized trial. One cannot depend on the intervention and control groups being similar with regard to other determinants of outcome. Hence the burden is on the investigator to assess and control such confounding factors in the design and analysis of a quasi-experiment.

Observational Studies

In an observational study, the investigator has no control over which study subjects are exposed and which are not. Instead, a subject's exposure status may be determined by the subject (such as deciding whether or not to wear a seat belt), by a health-care provider (such as deciding whether to prescribe psychotropic medication for a certain patient), or by other forces beyond the control of any of the parties involved (such as the presence or absence of comorbid conditions in an elderly person at risk for falls). An important methodological issue in all observational studies is confounding, which is discussed before describing several specific study designs.

Confounding

Confounding is a very important issue in judging whether an exposure–outcome association in an observational study truly represents cause and effect. The central problem is that people who are exposed to the factor of primary interest may differ systematically in other ways from persons not so exposed. Moreover, some of those other differences may affect the likelihood of experiencing the outcome of interest. For example, suppose that the incidence of injury is found to be lower for children who are up to date on immunizations than for children who are behind on immunizations in a certain health insurance plan. Although this comparison focuses on immunization history as the exposure, being current on immunizations may merely reflect parental education or prevention awareness rather than any biological effect of immunization on injury risk.

Fortunately, several tools are available to remove bias due to confounding in observational studies. While a full discussion of all of them is beyond the scope of this chapter, details can be found in several standard references and texts (Anderson et al., 1980; Kleinbaum et al., 1982; Kelsey et al., 1996; Rothman and Greenland, 1998).

Some methods to control confounding can be used in the design phase. As noted earlier, randomization is the most powerful method because it controls, on average, both known and unknown confounding factors. However, it is not available for use in observational studies. Restriction involves confining all study subjects to one category of a confounding factor: for example, studying only males removes any possibility that gender could be a confounding factor. Matching involves pairing each individual in one group to a similar individual in the other group, with "similarity" referring to the confounding factor(s) of concern. For example, in a study of falls in relation to use of psychotropic medication, each person who took such a drug might be matched to a person of similar age and gender who did not take the drug, comparing fall incidence between these two matched cohorts. Matching can also be used in case–control studies. In general, a matched analysis must be conducted if a matched study design is used.

Other methods to control confounding can be applied in data analysis. Restriction or matching can be carried out after data collection is complete, but in practice this is rarely done because it wastes data already collected. Stratification on the confounding factor(s) is often employed, however, and involves comparing like with like. To control for age by stratification, for example, the investigator subdivides study subjects according to age category, then examines exposure–outcome associations within each age category. If similar associations are found, the results can be statistically combined across age groups to summarize the effect of exposure on outcome. Finally, multivariate analysis can be employed. The outcome variable is modeled statistically as a function of several predictor variables, one predictor being the exposure of main interest and others being confounding factors. These multivariate methods can isolate the effect of the exposure on the outcome, even if exposure is correlated with other measured characteristics.

Cohort Studies

A cohort is a group of people who have some common characteristic or experience and who are followed together over time. In a cohort study, this shared characteristic is degree of exposure to the risk factor of interest. The first step is thus to assemble at least two cohorts, one exposed and one non-exposed. The second step is to follow these cohorts concurrently over time, measuring and comparing the incidence of good and bad outcomes in them.

There are two main kinds of cohort studies, prospective and retrospective, as shown in Figures 7.4a and b. In a prospective cohort study, both of the steps described above are carried out in real time once the study has been conceived and initiated. At the beginning of the study, none of the outcomes of interest have occurred yet. In contrast, a retrospective cohort study involves reconstructing from historical data a cohort study that has already taken place. The investigator first goes back in time to identify an exposed and a nonexposed group at some time in the past, usually relying on an existing data source to do so. The follow-up period extends from that past time of exposure toward the present. Thus, the

(a)

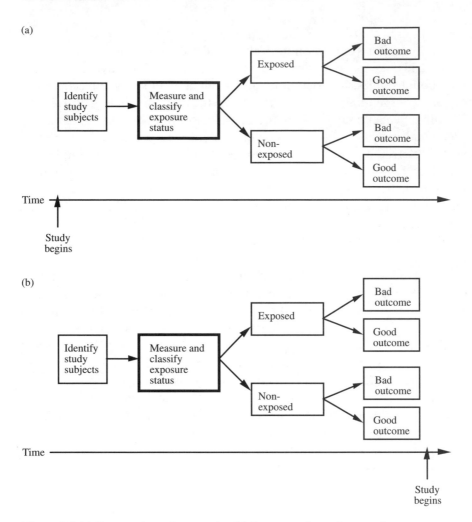

(b)

Figure 7.4 (a) Prospective cohort study; (b) Retrospective cohort study.

cohorts existed before the investigator identified them for research purposes, and the outcome events of interest have already taken place by the time the study is initiated.

As an example of a prospective cohort study, Tinetti et al. (1995) investigated risk factors for falls among 1103 community-dwelling adults aged 72 years or older. All participants underwent a baseline examination to measure the presence or absence of several potential risk factors. They were then followed for 1 year, measuring the incidence of falls by mailed-back monthly postcards indicating days on which a fall occurred, telephone follow-up if an expected postcard was not received, and surveillance through emergency rooms and hospital admission logs. Among the cohort of 131 subjects who were taking a psychotropic medication at baseline, 66% experienced a fall during the year; in contrast, among the cohort of 972 subjects not taking a psychotropic drug at baseline, 47% experienced a fall during the year.

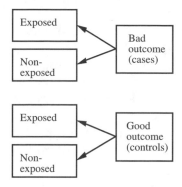

Figure 7.5 Case–control study.

As an example of a retrospective cohort study, Ray et al. (1992) investigated the incidence of injurious motor-vehicle crashes among older drivers in relation to exposure to psychoactive drugs. They linked enrollment and health-care utilization data from the Tennessee Medicaid program with Tennessee drivers-license data and police reports of injurious crashes for the years 1984–88. During 21,578 person-years in which no psychoactive drug was taken, the incidence of injurious crashes was 11.3 per 1000 person-years. During 5530 person-years in which an older driver was currently taking a psychoactive drug, the incidence of injurious crashes was 17.2 per 1000 person-years, or 1.5-fold higher than during nonexposed time at risk. Note that the study was not begun until after 1988, by which time the crashes of interest had already occurred.

A prospective study is a good choice when the outcome of interest is common and the follow-up period needed to measure its incidence is not too long. The Tinetti study of falls exploited these characteristics of falls in the elderly: they are common – some 49% of study participants experienced a fall during follow-up – and any effect of psychoactive drug use on their incidence would occur almost immediately. The cohort study design is also useful for studying rare exposures, such as an unusual occupation or pastime. All available exposed individuals can then form one cohort, and a sample of the many nonexposed individuals can form a comparison cohort. Cohort studies also yield information about absolute level of risk (i.e., incidence estimates) for exposed and nonexposed persons.

As the Ray et al. (1992) study illustrates, a retrospective cohort study can sometimes avoid what would otherwise be limitations of a cohort study design. Although motor-vehicle collision injuries were relatively rare, the investigators were able to use a large pre-existing population of elderly Medicaid enrollees and a 5-year surveillance period without adding greatly to the cost and duration of their study. However, such a study was possible only because detailed archival data existed that allowed retrospective identification of exposed persons and injuries. In general, the feasibility of a retrospective cohort study depends heavily on the existence of historical data with details on subjects' exposure status at some time in the past, and on having comparable follow-up data on exposed and nonexposed subjects.

Case–Control Studies

At first blush, a case–control study seems to approach testing a causal hypothesis backwards by proceeding from effect to cause. As shown in Figure 7.5, the investigator begins by identifying (1) a group of persons known to have sustained an adverse outcome of interest, such as occurrence of a certain kind of injury – the cases; and (2) a group of individuals known not to have experienced the adverse outcome – the controls. The next step is to gather data about the frequency of past exposure to the risk factor of interest in the case and control groups. Only exposure that preceded the outcome in cases (or a comparable "reference time" in controls) is considered. As described in chapter 11), the resulting data can be analyzed to estimate the strength and statistical significance of the association between exposure and outcome. The cases in a case–control study may already have occurred when the study begins, or they may be new cases that occur as the study proceeds. Thus, like cohort studies, case–control studies may be either retrospective or prospective.

Leveille et al. (1994) investigated the association between use of psychoactive drugs and risk of injury in a motor-vehicle collision among older drivers, using a case–control study design. During 1987–88, 234 older drivers who belonged to a large prepaid health plan and were injured in a crash while driving became the cases. For comparison, 447 controls who had sustained no such injury were identified from health plan enrollment files and were matched to the cases on age, sex, and county of residence. Exposure to psychoactive drugs on the date of the crash, or on an assigned reference date for controls, was ascertained from computerized pharmacy data files obtained from the health plan. The results showed that, compared with nonusers, older drivers who had used one psychoactive drug within the previous 60 days had a 1.3-fold increased risk of crash injury, and those who had used two or more psychoactive drugs had a 2.0-fold increased risk.

A major advantage of the case–control study design is that it is efficient for study of rare outcomes. All available cases of the outcome can be identified to form the case group, and a representative sample of the many noncases can be identified to form the control group. In general, studying more than three or four times as many controls as cases yields only a negligible increase in statistical power, so the total number of subjects needed under the case–control design can be much smaller than would be needed for a cohort study of the same hypothesis. Case–control studies are also easily extended to studying multiple risk factors for the same outcome: once the case and control groups are formed, there is little additional work involved in adding another item to an exposure data-collection form. A disadvantage, however, is that case–control studies do not directly yield information about absolute risk, only relative risk.

Cross-sectional Studies

In a cross-sectional study, each study subject's status on both outcome and exposure is ascertained as of the same time point or time period. Thus, one cannot tell from the data which came first, and because of this limitation, a cross-sectional study is rarely the preferred design for testing a cause–effect hypothesis. However, a cross-sectional study may nonetheless reveal useful associations even if they are not necessarily causal. For example, Sosin et al. (1995) used data from a national survey of adolescents to investigate associations between several problem behaviors, including fighting. Those reporting a fight in the previous 30 days were much more likely than nonfighters to report carrying firearms, using cocaine, drunk driving, and other risky behaviors, suggesting that a health-care encounter for treatment of a fight-related injury may provide an opportunity for detection and intervention aimed at these other problems.

Longitudinal Studies

In contrast to the above study designs, which usually involve measurement of the outcome for each study subject only once, longitudinal studies involve repeated assessments at the individual or group level over time. Changes in outcomes are then examined in relation to known changes in exposures.

A before–after study compares the frequency of an outcome in a single group on two occasions, before and after the occurrence of some exposure. For example, Erdmann et al. (1991) showed that the proportion of Seattle-area homes with tap water temperatures over 54°C. fell significantly after passage of a state law requiring newly installed water heaters to be preset at 49°C.

A limitation of the before–after design is that any differences observed may just represent continuation of a pre-existing secular trend. Some protection against this misinterpretation is offered by the interrupted time-series design, which involves taking multiple measurements of outcome frequency over time, both before and after a new program or policy begins. An effect of a new program or policy may appear as a sudden reduction in outcome frequency just when the program or policy begins, or as a change in slope of the time trend. For example, Loftin et al. (1991) noted an abrupt reduction in firearm homicides in Washington, DC soon after the adoption of a gun-licensing law, with no similar decline in violent deaths by other mechanisms.

More elaborate longitudinal study designs can involve concurrent monitoring of two or more groups with different exposure experience over time, in order to control for secular trends. For example, Wagenaar et al. (1990) studied the effects of raising the speed limit on certain highways in Michigan by comparing temporal trends in crash, injury, and death rates between roads with raised speed limits versus roads with unchanged speed limits, finding a 19% increase in fatalities associated with raised limits.

Other Designs

A variety of other analytic study designs are available for injury research. Most were developed for specialized research purposes and hence are less commonly used. Two will be mentioned briefly here. The case–crossover design, first described by Maclure (1991), is useful for investigating the incidence of an acute event in relation to a factor to which people are exposed intermittently, and which may confer a temporary increase or decrease in risk. The general approach is to determine whether exposure at the time an event occurs is more or less common than would be expected from the historical pattern of exposure in cases before the event. For example, this design has been used to study whether the risk of a motor-vehicle crash increases while the driver is using a cellular telephone (Redelmeier and Tibshirani, 1997).

The regression-discontinuity design (Trochim, 1990) can be useful for evaluating the effect of a program or policy that is applied only to persons who, at baseline, score above or below some cutoff value on a scale that predicts later outcomes. For example, Johnston et al. (1995) describe a hypothetical study in which a rehabilitation program is applied only for patients who score poorly on a baseline measure of function. Later, function is measured again on everyone, regardless of program participation. Benefit from the program is inferred if the follow-up level of function among those treated is significantly better than would be predicted from the regression of follow-up function scores against baseline scores on everyone.

Conclusions

In order to emphasize "the big picture," this chapter has omitted most details about how the study designs described are actually implemented. In addition, research projects often have two or more objectives, and the best design to meet one objective may not be optimal for another. Thus, the process of choosing a research design often involves priority-setting among the objectives and iterative refinement of the research questions. The principles outlined here can help direct the injury research-er's attention to a few of the most suitable design options, including some that might not otherwise have been considered. Once a tentative design choice has been made, Chapters 8–13 can be consulted for more details about it.

References

Anderson S, Auquier A, Hauck WW, Oakes D, Vandaele W, Weisberg HI (1980) Statistical Methods for Comparative Studies. Techniques for Bias Reduction. New York: Wiley and Sons.

Baker SP, O'Neill B, Ginsburg MJ, Li G (1992) The Injury Fact Book, 2nd edn. New York: Oxford University Press.

Brochgrevink GE, Kaasa A, McDonagh D, Stiles TC, Haraldseth O, Lereim I (1998) Acute treatment of whiplash neck sprain injuries. A randomized trial of treatment during the first 14 days after a car accident. Spine 23:25–31.

Chin N, Berns SD (1995) Near-hanging caused by a toy necklace. Ann Emerg Med 26:522–5.

Cook TD, Campbell DT (1979) Quasi-experimentation: design and analysis issues for field settings. Boston: Houghton Mifflin.

Cummings P, Weiss NS (1998) Case series and exposure series: the role of studies without controls in providing information about the etiology of injury or disease. Injury Prev 4:54–7.

DiGuiseppi CG, Rivara FP, Koepsell TD, Polissar L (1989) Bicycle helmet use by children. Evaluation of a community-wide helmet campaign. JAMA 262:2256–61.

Erdmann TC, Feldman KW, Rivara FP, Heimbach DM, Wall HA (1991) Tap water burn prevention: the effect of legislation. Pediatrics 88:572–7.

Johnston MV, Ottenbacher KJ, Reichardt CS (1995) Strong quasi-experimental designs for research on the effectiveness of rehabilitation. Am J Phys Med Rehab 74:383–92.

Kelsey JL, Whittemore AS, Evans AS, Thompson WD (1996) Methods in Observational Epidemiology, 2nd edn. New York: Oxford University Press.

Kleinbaum DG, Kupper LL, Morgenstern H (1982) Epidemiologic research: principles and quantitative methods. New York: Van Nostrand Reinhold.

Leveille SG, Buchner DM, Koepsell TD, McCloskey LW, Wolf ME, Wagner EH (1994) Psychoactive medications and injurious motor vehicle collisions involving older drivers. Epidemiology 5:591–8.

Loftin C, McDowall D, Wiersema B, Cottey TJ (1991) Effects of restrictive licensing of handguns on homicide and suicide in the District of Columbia. N Engl J Med 325:1615–20.

Lundsgaarde HP (1977) Murder in Space City: A Cultural Analysis of Houston Homicide Patterns. New York: Oxford University Press.

Maclure M (1991) The case–crossover design: a method for studying transient effects on the risk of acute events. Am J Epidemiol 133:144–53.

Orsay E, Holden JA, Williams J, Lumpkin JR (1995) Motorcycle trauma in the state of Illinois: analysis of the Illinois Department of Public Health Trauma Registry. Ann Emerg Med 26:455–60.

Rabban J, Adler J, Rosen C, Blair J, Sheridan R (1997) Electrical injury from subway third rails: serious injury associated with intermediate voltage contact. Burns 23:515–18.

Ray WA, Fought RL, Decker MD (1992) Psychoactive drugs and the risk of injurious motor vehicle crashes in elderly drivers. Am J Epidemiol 136:873–83.

Redelmeier DA, Tibshirani RJ (1997) Association between cellular-telephone calls and motor vehicle collisions. N Engl J Med 336:453–8.

Rothman KJ, Greenland S (1998) Modern epidemiology, 2nd edn. Philadelphia: Lippincott-Raven.

Schwarz DF, Grisso JA, Miles CG, Holmes JH, Wishner AR, Sutton RL (1994) A longitudinal study of injury morbidity in an African-American population. JAMA 271:755–60.

Sosin DM, Koepsell TD, Rivara FP, Mercy JA (1995) Fighting as a marker for multiple problem behaviors in adolescents. J Adolesc Health 16:209–15.

Tinetti ME, Doucette J, Claus E, Marottoli R (1995) Risk factors for serious injury during falls by older persons in the community. J Am Geriatr Soc 43:1214–21.

Trochim WMK (1990) The regression–discontinuity design. In: Sechrest L, Perrin E, Bunker J (eds), Research Methodology: strengthening causal interpretations of nonexperimental data. Washington, DC: US Department of Health and Human Services Publication No. 90-3454.

Wagenaar AC, Streff FM, Schultz RH (1990) Effects of the 65 mph speed limit on injury morbidity and mortality. Accid Anal Prev 22:571–85.

8

Qualitative Methods in Injury Research

David C. Grossman and Lorna Rhodes

Overview

Much of the content of this book is devoted to research methods that are anchored in the collection, analysis, and interpretation of numerical data. This is often referred to as quantitative research. All disciplines involved in the field of injury control predominantly make use of quantitative techniques in the conduct of research. Another domain of research methodology relies largely on the use of nonquantitative data and is broadly referred to as qualitative research.

This chapter will concentrate on the potential roles of qualitative research in the conduct of injury research investigations. An overview of methodologic issues in qualitative research will also be presented with reference to three major qualitative research traditions: ethnography (and ethnographic interviewing), participant observation, and focus groups. Sampling, data collection, and measures to ensure reliability and validity of qualitative studies are discussed.

Definition of Qualitative Research

Qualitative research is a broad term designating a family of diverse research traditions that share some common features. One key shared feature is the use of non-numerical data. Instead of collecting and analyzing numbers, most qualitative methods focus on the collection and analysis of narrative data. The family of qualitative traditions includes ethnography, focus group methodology, grounded theory, case studies, participant observation, phenomenology, and others.

Qualitative research methods are, in some respects, fundamentally different from traditional quantitative methods used in epidemiology, biostatistics, and health services research. The qualitative and quantitative paradigms are complementary approaches associated with different strengths and weaknesses. The challenge for the researcher is to recognize method most suitable for the type of question being addressed (Berkwits and Aronowitz, 1995).

One of the greatest strengths of qualitative methodology is its greater potential to develop explanatory models and theories regarding injury related human behavior (Roberts, 1997). For example, quantitative approaches can be useful to analyze specific risk factors for lack of seat belt use among adults, such as alcohol use, male sex, and age. Risk factors derived from epidemiology can be used to locate target groups for intervention, but the development of interventions will likely require a greater understanding of why these groups are at high risk. Qualitative research methods can extend such research in two ways. First, these methods may help to identify new risk factors not yet examined in epidemiologic studies. Second, they can provide contextual depth to the superficial labels often attached to subjects, for example, yes/no, male/female, young/old. Qualitative methods suggest how these characteristics can be combined into a richer model that addresses seat belt nonuse, and address why these risk groups do not use belts.

Etiologic studies using epidemiologic methods are inferential and use hypothetico-deductive reasoning to reach conclusions regarding associations of outcomes and risk factors. Although epidemiological activity does not usually include the development of theoretical models, it certainly does include the testing of theory. Epidemiological studies are often categorized in a hierarchy of design rigor, with randomized controlled trials classified as the most rigorous, and case reports being the weakest (Sackett et al., 1985). However, the evolution of quasi-experimental and experimental studies in medicine not infrequently arises from initial case studies and case series that point to novel observations or challenge conventional thinking (Hunter, 1991).

Qualitative investigations are not hypothesis driven but, instead, rely on inductive reasoning (Cook and Reichart, 1979). Honing research questions into a concise, narrow framework is strongly discouraged in qualitative research as the question is progressively defined only through initial interaction with the subjects under study. For example, one study that was initially designed to explore the meaning of adolescent suicide in an American Indian community changed its focus, once underway, to the meaning of premature death. Exploratory interviews with key informants revealed that few of the deaths initially classified by the investigators as suicides were viewed as such by the subjects. Though subjects clearly recognized the impact of early mortality, they did not think of these as intentional injury deaths (Grossman et al., 1993).

There are few research questions for which qualitative and quantitative methods would be interchangeable. Many investigators choose to take advantage of the unique, complementary strengths of qualitative and quantitative approaches and employ both in serial fashion (Stange et al., 1994). For example, an investigator may choose to develop a structured closed-ended questionnaire about why children choose to wear bicycle helmets in order to develop a better understanding of the underpinnings of this behavior. But, prior to the development of the individual instrument items, this investigator may choose to hold several focus groups with children to determine the general domains of attitudes and beliefs that belong in the questionnaire. During the focus group, the investigator may learn that there are seasonal changes in behavior among some subjects in the focus groups and that these changes are attributable to an association between higher temperatures and decreased helmet wearing. Unless the investigator had learned this information from another study, or from personal experience, it might not have emerged as an item to ask in the survey. Qualitative strategies, such as these focus groups, allowed this investigator to explore, in open-ended fashion without hypotheses, assumptions, or narrowly defined questions, about what children thought concerning the use of bicycle helmets.

In general, qualitative techniques are most likely to reveal new information in injury related studies when employed in studies of attitudes and perceptions of injuries, risks and preventive measures, and in studies of functional outcomes and rehabilitation of injuries. Qualitative methods have had a limited role in the study of acute care, except in the area of performance improvement and patient satisfaction (see chapter by Maier and Rhodes, this volume). Qualitative methods can also be extremely useful in cross-cultural studies (with "cross-cultural" broadly defined such as studies of different ethnic, professional, or linguistic groups) of injury risk and may yield insights as to why certain groups are at higher risk for particular injuries. (The term "culture" is not a simple or unitary concept. See Clifford and Marcus (1986) for further discussion.) For example, a number of qualitative and mixed-method studies have sought to determine the perception of injury risks and intervention strategies from the subject's point of view (Haught et al., 1995; Aminzadeh and Edwards, 1998; Green and Hart, 1998; Zakocs et al., 1998).

Despite their potential usefulness in some areas of investigation, qualitative methods have rarely been used in injury research. A literature search of the MEDLINE (1966–98), PSYCHINFO (1967–98), SOCIOFILE (1963–98), and HEALTHSTAR (1981–98) databases by the authors revealed a total of only 65 journal references that included mention of using a qualitative technique in a study regarding some aspect of injury control. Of these, 27 were related to prevention, 19 to rehabilitation care, and 10 to acute care of injuries. Ten articles focused on occupational health. Of the studies, 26 used focus group methodology, 33 used ethnographic techniques, 10 used participant observation, and 7 used mixed qualitative and quantitative methods. Clearly, many more opportunities exist to employ these relatively unknown methods in injury control (Roberts, 1997).

Table 8.1 lists some research areas for each of the phases of injury control (acute care, prevention, and rehabilitation) in which qualitative or combined qualitative/quantitative research approaches have been used or might be used in the future.

Methods of Qualitative Data Collection and Analysis
Research Traditions in Qualitative Research

There is great diversity in qualitative approaches to research. Despite some semantic variations, most of these methods draw on common characteristics of ethnography. Most methods termed "qualitative," however, have their origin in ethnographic approaches that have developed within anthropology and sociology over the past 100 years.

Ethnography is the work of describing one or more aspects of a culture (Spradley, 1980), whether it be a culture of physicians and attitudes toward domestic violence (Sugg and Inui, 1992), the culture of child cyclists, or the culture of a Native American tribe. For brevity, this chapter will primarily discuss three common ethnographic research traditions: participant observation, ethnographic interviewing, and focus groups.

Table 8.1 Potential injury control topics for qualitative investigation

Acute care

    Ethical issues in acute care management of trauma victims
    Patient centered outcomes of acute care (patient satisfaction, quality of life)
    Cultural differences in attitudes toward care
    Physician attitudes toward care of injured patients
    Ethnographic analysis of the process of care
    Experience of patients in the health-care system
    Preferences for care

Prevention

    Cross-cultural aspects of risk perceptions
    Attitudes toward participation in specific prevention strategies
    Barriers and enabling factors for prevention
    Attitudes and opinions regarding environmental factors raising risk

Rehabilitation

    Narratives of patient healing and coping
    Perceptions of quality of care
    Impact of injuries on functional status
    Ethnography of rehabilitation hospital culture
    Preferences for care
    Ethical issues in care

Participant observation is commonly used by anthropologists to study a culture in depth. Researchers immerse themselves in a culture and make longitudinal observations over time. Data consist of observations of behavior, and subject narrative collected by notes or audiotape. These methods have been used, for example, to develop an in-depth understanding of such subcultures as alcohol abusers (Spradley, 1970) or drug abusers (Agar and Stephens, 1975). Participant observation requires extensive time of an investigator and the development of trust of a social group. There are very few examples of participant observation in injury control. One year-long investigation sought to study parent's actions and remediative responses to children following actual injuries (Peterson et al., 1995). The investigators were interested in exploring actual, observed responses to injury, rather than subjective parent views of their responses.

Ethnographic interviewing is a method derived from ethnography that uses in-depth interviewing to pursue a general topic of interest to the investigator. This is also known as focused ethnographic interviewing or focused ethnography. Ethnographic interviews usually focus on a specific area of interest but are held one-on-one with the investigator (Spradley, 1980). This method is also suitable for investigations about personal beliefs and attitudes about risk and prevention. Compared with focus groups, ethnographic interviewing takes considerable time, with interviews often lasting between 60 and 90 minutes, depending on the subject matter. However, these interviews, because of their depth, often yield much richer and coherent data. Ethnographic interviews can also be nested in participant observation activities but are always conducted in the subject's community setting. Ethnographic investigations in the field of injury control have included inquiries into the impact of traumatic brain injury (Crisp, 1993), hip fractures (Borkan et al., 1991), and childhood burns (Mason, 1993) on patients and their families, as well as the community effects of land mines in four war zones (Andersson et al., 1995).

Focus groups provide a much narrower view of cultural beliefs by conducting a targeted collective discussion on a particular topic among members of the culture under study (Basch, 1987; Kitzinger, 1996). These moderated discussions provide a relatively rapid method for gleaning information about a specific area of interest. Focus groups were largely developed by businesses interested in doing marketing research about potential products and thus do not have the same grounding in social science as ethnographic interviewing or participant observation. Unlike most other qualitative methods, focus groups are usually convened in the investigator's, rather than the subject's, environment.

Focus groups provide a relatively efficient method to elicit beliefs and attitude from multiple individuals simultaneously. Members of the group may elicit reactions and comments from other participants but, unlike ethnographic interviews, investigators can rarely gain in-depth information because group interactions make it difficult for a moderator to pursue new information with a single informant. Focus groups may not be appropriate when the subject matter is personally sensitive, such as in discussions about illegal or sanctioned behavior, although some researchers believe that some sensitive topics will receive greater discussion in a group (Folch-Lyon and Trost, 1981). Focus groups have been used to explore injury topics such as firearm counseling in primary care (Haught et al., 1995), views of hazards in the workplace environment for adolescents (Zakocs et al., 1998) and firefighters (Conrad et al., 1994), adolescent views regarding suicide prevention (Coggan and Patterson, 1998), and elders' views about external hip protectors (Cameron and Quine, 1994).

The investigator needs to decide on a method best suited for the goals of the project. If the purpose of a study is to gain a greater appreciation about the diversity of attitudes, knowledge, and beliefs of a target group, then either focus groups or ethnographic interviews may be appropriate methods. If an investigator wishes to develop an in-depth understanding of the behavior and interaction of community members, then participant observation would be preferred.

Sampling

In contrast to quantitative approaches, in which the sampling of subjects is designed to make the overall sample representative of the broader population under study, qualitative studies are focused on capturing the full thematic range of beliefs in a relatively small sample size (Mays and Pope, 1995). Because of the lack of randomness in sample selection, qualitative studies cannot be used to estimate the prevalence of specific health attitudes or behaviors in a population but they can be used to elicit the full spectrum of health beliefs that may be prevalent in the general population (Glaser and Strauss, 1967).

Sampling strategies depend on the goal of the study and the culture under study, but many studies employ one of several strategies or a combination. Two common strategies are key informant sampling, and snowball sampling. The key informant approach uses a method of referral in which the investigator is introduced to subjects by one of more key informants. Key informants are usually members of the community under study who provide access to the community for the investigator and also can assist the investigator with the identification of potential subjects with wide-ranging beliefs on the topic of interest (Gilchrist, 1992). An investigator may choose to employ more than one key informant to maximize the opportunities to enroll a diverse sample. The snowball technique of sampling relies on subjects themselves for referral of other subjects to the study. For example, the investigator may ask the subject at the conclusion of an in-depth interview to select another community member who may or may not share the informant's point of view (Kuzel, 1992). This process of purposive sampling depends on whether the investigator is deliberately seeking disconfirming evidence or developing a new understanding of a network of shared belief systems (Good, 1977; Kleinman, 1980). Key informants, especially if recognized to have broad access to community members, may facilitate the snowball referral process by serving as a conduit between investigators and subjects.

The number of subjects needed in a qualitative study is usually not known at the outset because the investigator cannot usually predict in advance the number of different belief patterns that might be encountered. Sample size is usually considered adequate when the investigator reaches a state of theoretical saturation, in which no new themes emerge from the latter interviews, despite vigorous efforts to sample divergent beliefs (Glaser and Strauss, 1967). The investigator recognizes this milestone when he or she stops hearing new information from subjects on the subject of interest. In practice, studies in public health that employ ethnographic interviewing often have between 20 and 50 subjects.

Sample size for focus groups is a practical matter as each group can have between 5 and 10 individuals. Multiple focus groups may need to be held with membership determined by an important characteristic. For example, one study of children's views of injury risks and prevention used 16 focus groups organized by age group, residential location (rural/urban), and gender (Green and Hart, 1998). In general, the composition of focus groups is not intended to sample for diversity, but rather to facilitate interaction among a relatively homogenous group.

Data Collection

Another distinguishing feature of qualitative research is its reliance on narrative and direct observation, rather than on numerical data. Media to collect these data include notetaking, audiotape with transcriptions, and videotape. Fieldnotes are a method long used by anthropologists to develop complete ethnographies of other cultures (Spradley, 1980). The advantage of using paper notebooks is the portability of the method, the lack of reliance on technology and transcription, and the relative efficiency of using human judgment to record only salient narrative and observations. Many investigators using the short-term qualitative methods discussed here now prefer to tape interviews and interactions so that the data will not be subject to undue filtering by the interviewer (Mays and Pope, 1995). However, audiotape and videotape are both mildly intrusive and may alter the respondent's narrative if he/she is uncomfortable speaking on tape. In these situations, one may have to resort to fieldnote methods to record data. Institutional review boards may also request separate signed consent from subjects for recording interviews on tape.

One of the most foreign concepts to quantitative researchers unfamiliar with qualitative methodology is the relative lack of structure in the data collection phase. Unlike descriptive ethnographies, ethnographic interviews and focus groups usually revolve around a central thematic question of interest. For example, several qualitative studies have attempted to use focus groups and ethnographic interviewing to determine potential barriers to the identification and treatment of family violence (Sugg, 1992; Cohen et al., 1997).

The interviewer generally prepares a set of probe questions that help to guide the interview to some required domains of inquiry (Britten, 1995). These questions are broad, open-ended, and do not take the iterative form of most clinical interviews, in which initial hypotheses are formed, and then tested (Sackett et al., 1985). The questions can be presented in any order and are usually used as a guide to assure the completion of a minimum data set. Open-ended ethnographic interviews frequently lead to subject matter that was not anticipated by the interviewer (Glaser and Strauss, 1967; Mishler, 1986). For example, in a focus group of parents of low-income pediatric patients about gun safety counseling, the investigators were surprised to learn that parents expressed reluctance to admit gun ownership because of fear that social service agencies (e.g. child protective services) would be contacted (Haught et al., 1995). Morse and Field (1995, p. 98) outline an excellent review of potential pitfalls to avoid during interviews.

Interviewers are encouraged to use open-ended questions to pursue these "leads." Complete transcripts of tapes that include the voice of the interviewer allow reviewers to judge whether subjects were improperly asked leading questions. Finally, as in survey research, many investigators choose to reimburse subjects with a small stipend, in exchange for their time spent on the lengthy interview.

Data Management

After completion of interviews, audiotapes are often transcribed into a word processing software program and then imported into a qualitative software program that facilitates coding and organization of narrative text. Like relational database software, these qualitative analysis programs can assist the investigator with the organization of data, but they cannot be used for analysis or tests (Weitzman and Miles, 1995). Two examples of commonly used qualitative software programs are QSR NUD*IST (Qualitative Solutions & Research Pty Ltd, Melbourne, Australia) and The Ethnograph (Qualis Research Associates, Salt Lake City, UT, USA). The U.S. Centers for Disease Control and Prevention also recently introduced text analysis software (CDC EZ-Text) for analysis of narrative data (Centers for Disease Control; Carey et al., 1996). (A useful source of information on computer aided analysis of qualitative data can be found on the internet at http://www.quarc.de/english.html)

The task of qualitative analysis is to reduce voluminous data to key themes and meanings derived from the text. Narrative data are coded on the software using thematic codes that capture the meaning of individual words, sentences, or paragraphs. The unit of coding depends on many factors and can consist of one or more sentences or paragraphs of narrative (Reid, 1992). For example, a 40-page transcript from an interview with a parent about car seat use may have 10 separate references made by the subject in the interview about how the subject traveled in cars when she was a toddler. These repeated references to the subject's own early childhood would probably be coded together using a code such as childhood. Narrative data chunks can be coded with more than one code if multiple concepts and ideas emerge in a segment of text. Similarly, not all narrative must be coded. An initial unsorted group of coded text components is further organized into a taxonomy consisting of domains that best describe this group of components. For example, an example of a possible taxonomy of themes and domains related to car seat use are shown in Table 8.2.

The analysis of narrative or observational data relies on an iterative process in which each subject's data helps to shape the investigator's interpretation of the data. The exposure of the interviewer to open-ended interviews results in early impressions, hypotheses, and ideas that are usually recorded in a notebook for later reference.

Trustworthiness

Validity and reliability are issues of concern in the conduct of qualitative research (Kirk and Miller, 1986). Medical qualitative researchers have placed an increasing emphasis on having more than one investigator code the same set of narrative data. The purpose of dual coding is to enhance the reliability of the data interpretation, and decrease the opportunity for selective interpretations by single investigators (Inui and Frankel, 1991; Mays and Pope, 1995; Greenhalgh and Taylor, 1997).

Qualitative research is thought by many to have strong validity as the researcher's framework is defined by the community. However, some measures can still be taken to enhance the validity of the findings. Triangulation refers to an approach in which additional, independent sources of evidence are sought to confirm or enhance the validity of findings. Conclusions can be supported by relying on data from more than one source or type. For example, one participant observation study of homicide in Houston (Lundsgaarde, 1977) combined data from direct observations of homicide detectives, police reports, and interview data to reach conclusions about the subculture of homicide perpetrators and victims.

The validity of findings can also be enhanced when the researcher shares the interpretation of data with subjects from the study. This process, often referred to as member checks, can occur by either having subjects individually review the domain analysis or by having the investigator share these concepts with a group of subjects.

Table 8.2 Hypothetical domain analysis of ethnographic interviews related to lack of booster car seat use by toddlers. Interviews conducted with parents known not to use booster seats

Domains	Components
Child characteristics	weight, height, head size, position of leg on seat
Car seat characteristics	seat height, cost, design, quality, effectiveness
Car characteristics	car age, seat belt types, number of seat belts
Reinforcements for use	fear of police, parent belt use, coupons, public health nurse visits, knowing a victim
Ease of use	installation manual, installation time, compatibility between cars, personal instruction,
Parental risk perceptions	fear of entrapment, fear of crash fire, risk of crash, risk of seatbelt injury
Distractions related to modern life	Trying to feed restless infant while driving

One can use a focus group format, in which the participants are allowed to comment, in open-ended fashion, on the analysis. This form of subject verification is widely thought to strengthen the validity of the data interpretation as it provides subjects a further opportunity to clarify their thinking and for the investigator to refine the analysis of the meaning of the narrative. Ideally, this session, too, should be recorded and transcribed for other investigators to review.

Potential Uses of Qualitative Research in Future Injury Research

Several factors may account for the finding that qualitative methods have been used only infrequently in injury research. First, the field of injury control is still in its relative infancy. Much effort has been expended on defining the epidemiology of injury, both descriptively and analytically. While many strides have been made in the definition of descriptive epidemiology, the science of injury prevention, particularly interventions focused on behavior, appears to lag behind.

The second reason for the relative dearth of qualitative research probably is associated with the strong emphasis by injury control researchers on controlling the environment. Though there is ample reason to justify this approach, evaluations of environmental or passive intervention do not often converge with the strengths of qualitative techniques. Nonetheless, the design of legislative interventions may be better informed by investigating the acceptability and enforcement potential of new laws, both among citizens and law enforcement officers. Failure of certain population subgroups to comply with laws may also represent another opportunity for qualitative investigations.

Passive solutions may induce behavioral responses and lead to qualitative investigations. The study of the effectiveness of purely passive interventions, in which human behavior is largely irrelevant, does not revolve around human choice, and thus is much better suited for quantitative methods. In the field of prevention, qualitative research may be best suited to facilitate the design, implementation, and even evaluation, of prevention programs that involve some degree of active behavior. For example, the implementation of air bags in passenger vehicles was a purely passive prevention measure that represented a combination of engineering (for design and evaluation) and epidemiology (for evaluation). After air bags were associated with deaths among children and adults, the public took a much harder look at air bags and their potential risks. What once seemed to be the perfectly passive solution to occupant injuries led to active behavior by the public and legislators to request modifications in the design of air bags and the installation of cutoff switches. Subsequent efforts to move children to rear seats represented new efforts to induce active behavior on the part of parents. Qualitative efforts could be very useful to understand the motivations and barriers of parents to place their children in rear seats in air bag equipped cars.

As the field of medicine becomes more sensitive to the needs and preferences of its patients, there will be an increased need for qualitative research to examine the subjective experience and outcomes of patients after injury. Clinical investigators may be in an excellent position to conduct these types of studies because of their intimate involvement with care. Several qualitative investigations have resulted in better understanding of patient preferences (Singer et al., 1999) and the importance of improvement in physician-patient communication (Levinson et al., 1997; Suchman et al., 1997).

Summary

Three main qualitative research strategies have been used to a limited extent in previous injury investigations: participant observation, ethnographic interviews, and focus groups. Though few researchers have employed these techniques in research related to injury control, they hold particular promise in study questions revolving around human behavior and perceptions, ethics, and cross-cultural studies. Qualitative research methods can also be effectively combined with quantitative methods to both derive and test hypotheses regarding human aspects of injury control.

References

Agar MH, Stephens RC (1975) The methadone street scene: the addict's view. Psychiatry 38(4):381–7.

Aminzadeh F, Edwards N (1998) Exploring seniors' views on the use of assistive devices in fall prevention. Public Health Nurs 15:297–304.

Andersson N, da Sousa CP, Paredes S (1995) Social cost of land mines in four countries: Afghanistan, Bosnia, Cambodia, and Mozambique. Br Med J 311:718–21.

Basch CE (1987) Focus group interview: an underutilized research technique for improving theory and practice in health education. Health Education Quarterly 14:411–48.

Berkwits M, Aronowitz R (1995) Different questions beg different methods. J Gen Intern Med 10:409–10.

Borkan JM, Quirk M, Sullivan M (1991) Finding meaning after the fall: injury narratives from elderly hip fracture patients. Soc Sci Med 33:947–57.

Britten N (1995) Qualitative interviews in medical research. Br Med J 3111:251–3.

Cameron ID, Quine S (1994) External hip protectors: likely non-compliance among high risk elderly people living in the community. Arch Gerontol Geriatr 19:273–81.

Carey JW, Wenzel PH, Reilly C, Sheridan J, Steinberg JM (1996) CDC EZ-Text: software for management and analysis of semistructured qualitative data sets. Cultural Anthropol Methods 10:14–20.

Centers for Disease Control and Prevention. CDC EZ-Text; Internet address: *http:// www.cdc.gov/nchstp/hiv_aids/software/ez-text.htm*

Coggan C, Patterson P (1998) Focus groups with youth to enhance knowledge of ways to address youth suicide. In: Kosky RJ, Eshkevari HS (eds), Suicide Prevention; the Global Context, pp. 259–268. New York: Plenum Press.

Cohen S, De Vos E, Newberger E (1997) Barriers to physician identification and treatment of family violence: lessons from five communities. Acad Med 72(Suppl. 1):S19–25.

Conrad KM, Balch GI, Reichelt PA, Muran S, Oh K (1994) Musculoskeletal injuries in the fire service; views from a focus group study. AAOHN J 42:572–81.

Cook TD, Reichart CS (eds) (1979) Qualitative and Quantitative Methods in Evaluation Research. Beverly Hills, CA: Sage Publications.

Clifford J, Marcus GE (eds) (1986) Writing Culture: the poetics and politics of ethnography. Berkeley: University of California Press.

Crisp R (1993) Personal responses to traumatic brain injury: a qualitative study. Disab Handicap Soc 8:393–404.

Folch-Lyon E, Trost J (1981) Conducting focus group sessions. Stud Fam Plann 12:443–9.

Gilchrist V (1992) Key Informant Interviews. In: Crabtree BF, Miller WL (eds), Doing Qualitative Research, p. 74. Newbury Park, CA: Sage Publications.

Glaser BG, Strauss AS (1967) The Discovery of Grounded Theory, p. 45. Chicago, IL: Aldine Publishing.

Good BJ (1977) The heart of what's the matter. The semantics of illness in Iran. Cult Med Psychiatry 1(1):25–58.

Green J, Hart L (1998) Children's views of accident risks and prevention: a qualitative study. Injury Prev 4:14–21.

Greenhalgh T, Taylor R (1997) How to read a paper: papers that go beyond numbers (qualitative research). Br Med J 315:740–3.

Grossman DC, Putsch R, Inui TS (1993) The meaning of death to adolescents in an American Indian community. Family Med 25:593–7.

Haught K, Grossman DC, Connell F (1995) Parents' attitudes toward firearm injury prevention counseling in urban pediatric clinics. Pediatrics 96:649–53.

Hunter KM (1991) Doctor's Stories: the Narrative Structure of Medical Knowledge. Princeton: Princeton University Press.

Inui TS, Frankel R (1991) Evaluating the quality of qualitative research: a proposal pro tem. J Gen Intern Med 6:485–6.

Kirk J, Miller ML (1986) Reliability and Validity in Qualitative Research. Beverly Hills: Sage Publications.

Kleinman A (1980) Patients and Healers in the Context of Culture; an exploration of the borderland of Anthropology, Medicine and Psychiatry. Berkeley, CA: University of California Press.

Kitzinger J (1996) Introducing focus groups In: Mays N, Pope C (eds), Qualitative Research in Health Care. London: BMJ Publishing Group.

Kuzel AJ (1992) Sampling in qualitative research. In: Crabtree BF, Miller WL (eds), Doing Qualitative Research, p. 40. Newbury Park, CA: Sage Publications.

Levinson W, Roter DL, Mullooly JP, Dull VT, Frankel R (1997) Physician-patient communication; the relationship with malpractice claims among primary care physicians and surgeons. JAMA 277:553–9.

Lundsgaarde H (1977) Murder in Space City: a cultural analysis of Houston homicide patterns. New York: Oxford University Press.

Mason SA (1993) Young, scarred children and their mothers – a short term investigation into the practical, psychological and social implications of thermal injury to the preschool child; Part I: Implications for the mother. Burns 19:495–500.

Mays N, Pope C (1995) Rigour and qualitative research. Br Med J 311:109–13.

Mishler E (1986) Research Interviewing: context and narrative. Cambridge, MA: Harvard University Press.

Morse JM, Field PA (1995) Qualitative Research Methods for Health Professionals, p. 31. Thousand Oaks, CA: Sage.

Peterson L, Bartelstone J, Kern T, Gillies R (1995) Parent's socialization of children's injury prevention: description and some initial parameters. Child Dev 66:224–35.

Reid AO (1992) Computer management strategies for text data. In: Crabtree BF, Miller WL (eds), Doing Qualitative Research. Newbury Park, CA: Sage Publications.

Roberts H (1997) Qualitative research methods in interventions in injury. Arch Dis Child 76:487–9.

Sackett DL, Haynes RB, Tugwell P (1985) Clinical Epidemiology; a Basic Science for Clinical Medicine, p. 3. Toronto: Little Brown.

Singer PA, Martin DK, Kelner M (1999) Quality end-of-life care: patients' perspectives. JAMA 281:163–8.

Spradley JP (1970) You Owe Yourself a Drunk: an Ethnography of Urban Nomads. Boston: Little, Brown.

(1980) Participant Observation, p. 63. New York: Holt Rinehart, Winston.

Stange KC, Miller WL, Crabtree BF, O'Connor PJ, Zyanski SJ (1994) Multimethod research: approaches for integrating qualitative and quantitative methods. J Gen Intern Med 9:278–82.

Suchman AL, Markakis K, Beckman HB, Frankel R (1997) A model of empathic communication in the medical interview. JAMA 277:678–82.

Sugg NK, Inui T (1992) Primary care physicians' response to domestic violence. Opening Pandora's box. JAMA 267(23):3157–60.

Weitzman E, Miles MB (1995) Computer Programs for Qualitative Analysis. Thousand Oaks, CA: Sage Publications.

Zakocs RC, Runyan CW, Schulman MD, Dunn KA, Evensen CT (1998) Improving safety for teens working in the retail trade sector: opportunities and obstacles. Am J Ind Med 34:342–50.

9

Randomized Trials

Thomas D. Koepsell

Introduction

A randomized trial is a comparative study in which subjects are assigned among alternative intervention strategies according to random chance. It is a relatively new tool in health research. The first clinical trial involving randomization of individual patients, reported in 1948, compared streptomycin with bed rest for pulmonary tuberculosis (Medical Research Council, 1948). Since then, it is estimated that over 300,000 randomized trials have been conducted (Randal, 1999).

This chapter seeks to orient the injury researcher to important methodologic issues in applying the randomized trial design, to illustrate how the design has been applied in injury research, and to provide entry points into the literature on randomized trial methodology. More information can be found in several good books (Pocock, 1983; Meinert, 1986; Chow and Liu, 1998; Friedman et al., 1998).

Prototype Design

The term randomized trial encompasses a family of designs. Probably the simplest version is a two-arm, parallel-groups randomized trial, shown in Figure 9.1. Potential study subjects are identified from a source, such as patients receiving care from a certain provider or hospital. Those who satisfy criteria for eligibility are informed about the trial and invited to participate. Consenting subjects are assigned at random to one of two intervention strategies (arms), and are monitored over time to measure the incidence of good and bad outcomes.

An example of this study design was the Prevention of Falls in the Elderly Trial (PROFET), conducted by Close et al. (1999). Over a 7-month period, 1031 elderly Londoners who visited an accident and emergency department after having fallen were screened for eligibility. Patients who were institutionalized, had dementia, did not speak English, could not be re-contacted, or declined consent were excluded. Of the remaining 397 fallers, 184 were randomly assigned to an intervention involving assessment and treatment of medical risk factors for falls plus an occupational-therapy evaluation that included a home visit to remedy environmental hazards. The other 213 patients received no special program. A year later, 77% of subjects in each arm remained in the study. The odds of falling was significantly reduced in the intervention group (odds ratio = 0.39, 95% CI = 0.23–0.66).

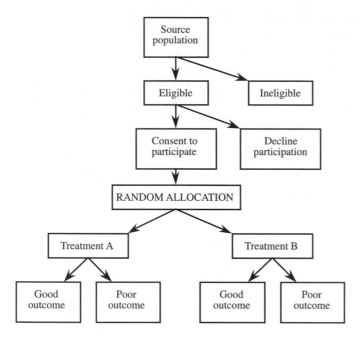

Figure 9.1 Basic randomized trial design.

Special Strengths of Randomized Trials

Randomized trials offer two main advantages over other designs. First, randomization forms comparison groups that are generally similar on factors that may affect the likelihood of a good or bad outcome, even if those factors are difficult to measure or are unknown to the investigator. In the PROFET study, the two study groups proved to be similar at baseline on age, gender, history of falls, index fall circumstances, and other characteristics. They are also likely to have been similar on other unmeasured risk factors.

Second, common tests of statistical significance assume independent random samples from the same underlying population (Armitage and Berry, 1994). In non-randomized studies, this assumption is known a priori to be false, but in a randomized trial, it actually is satisfied, leading to more trustworthy p-values.

Applicability of Randomized Trials

With rare exceptions, randomized trials require that the researcher be able to control which intervention a subject receives. In injury research, the main opportunities for randomized trials include evaluating a preventive intervention or assessing clinical practices for the care of injured patients. Randomized trials generally cannot be used to study exposures over which researchers have no control, such as patients' genetic background or past experiences. For ethical reasons, there must also be sufficient uncertainty about the relative superiority of the intervention strategies being compared to justify assigning subjects between them at random.

Randomized trials are facilitated if the outcome event is reasonably common. The PROFET study was feasible in part because falls are common in elderly adults. For rare outcomes, a randomized trial with adequate statistical power may require too many subjects or too long an observation period to be feasible.

Unusual opportunities do arise: Hearst et al. (1986) studied injury mortality among young U.S. males after a draft lottery during the Vietnam-War years. Although the investigators had no control over the lottery, it randomized men into two groups that would be expected to have similar injury mortality in the absence of an effect of military service. Men whose draft-lottery numbers made them eligible for the draft proved to have significantly higher mortality from suicide and vehicular trauma, suggesting long-term effects of such service on risk of death from certain injuries.

Interventions
Experimental Arm

The idea for a randomized trial usually originates from interest in the effects of a particular intervention, which becomes one arm of the trial. Within this framework, trials range from explanatory to pragmatic (Schwarz and Lellouch, 1967; Charlton, 1994). An explanatory trial tests a scientific theory, focusing on the efficacy of an experimental intervention under tightly controlled conditions. For example, Gentilello et al. (1997) tested the theory that prolonged hypothermia is an independent determinant of outcome in victims of major trauma. In the experimental arm, hypothermic patients' body temperatures were rapidly raised using continuous arteriovenous rewarming, while those in the control arm received standard rewarming. Experimental-group patients required significantly less fluid during treatment to achieve similar hemodynamic status, and fewer died. Although continuous arteriovenous rewarming is currently feasible only in specialized centers, the findings confirmed that prolonged hypothermia in such patients has a net deleterious effect.

In contrast, a pragmatic trial seeks to evaluate whether an intervention with potentially broad applicability is beneficial in typical settings and with relatively unselected target populations. Its focus is on determining effectiveness of the intervention in the "real world." For example, Clamp and Kendrick (1998) conducted a randomized trial of providing safety advice and low-cost safety equipment during well-child or acute-care visits for families with children under 5 years of age. The study enrolled 98% of such families in a general practice in Nottingham, England. The results showed significantly lower prevalence of several child safety hazards in the intervention arm, suggesting that this low-cost, practical intervention may make homes safer. Whether injury incidence itself would be reduced remains unknown.

Control Arm

Although the experimental intervention may follow automatically from the trial's original scientific motivation, it may not be obvious what should happen in the comparison arm. The answer often depends on the current state of knowledge. One possibility, particularly in explanatory trials, may be a placebo – something that outwardly resembles the experimental intervention but that lacks a true biological effect. A placebo is useful and justified when no alternative to the experimental treatment has been proven effective and when measured outcomes may be influenced by non-specific features of the intervention. In drug trials, the placebo is a pill or injection like the test drug but containing only biologically inert ingredients. For example, Madsen et al. (1996) randomized patients with open hand or foot wounds involving the bone, tendon, or joint to one of three treatment arms. Group A received an injection of penicillin and placebo pills for 6 days, group B received a placebo injection and oral penicillin pills, and group C received a placebo injection and placebo pills. The incidence of wound infection was significantly lower in group A than in group C, while other pairwise comparisons showed no significant differences. For other kinds of interventions, such as educational programs aimed at injury prevention, a placebo program aimed at some non-injury behavior might be offered in the control arm in order to equalize the amount of special attention given to study subjects.

When an effective intervention is already available, it would be improper to offer only a placebo to subjects in the control arm. Instead, control subjects may receive the best current alternative to the experimental intervention.

Lastly, the experimental intervention may be compared to usual care – a less well-defined alternative that is minimally disruptive to normal clinical operations and that is often used in pragmatic trials. This option was employed in the PROFET fall-prevention trial and in the Clamp and Kendrick study of home safety hazards.

Subject Recruitment

A randomized trial needs explicit eligibility criteria, to clarify the target population to whom the results can be applied. Patients for whom either intervention arm would pose unreasonable risk – such as patients with known allergy to a drug they might receive – are excluded. Some eligibility criteria may safeguard the trial's internal validity – its likelihood of yielding the correct conclusion for persons actually enrolled. Patients with known dementia were excluded from the PROFET study because self-reported data on subsequent falls might be inaccurate. Other criteria may affect the external validity, or generalizability, of the trial. The Clamp and Kendrick study of home safety advice used deliberately broad inclusion criteria, enrolling nearly all families with young children in the study's general-practice setting so that the results would apply to such families in other similar practices. Lastly, some eligibility requirements can simplify study logistics or contain costs. Patients who do not speak the investigators' native language are often excluded because of the difficulty of translating instructions and data-collection instruments adequately into other languages.

How many study subjects are needed? For the two-arm randomized trial shown in Figure 9.1, with a binary outcome variable, the following formula applies:

$$n = \frac{2(Z_\alpha + Z_\beta)^2 \cdot \bar{p}(1 - \bar{p})}{(p_1 - p_0)^2}$$

Here, n is the required number of subjects in each study arm. Z_α is a standard normal deviate corresponding to the threshold for statistical significance (α) and whether a one- or two-tailed significance test is used. For a two-tailed test at $\alpha = 0.05$, $Z_\alpha = 1.96$. Z_β is a one-tailed standard normal deviate corresponding to the highest tolerable probability (β) of accepting the null hypothesis when, in fact, a specified alternative hypothesis is true. For $\beta = 0.10$, $Z_\beta = 1.28$. The projected overall incidence of the outcome event across both study arms is $\bar{p}$. Under equal allocation, $\bar{p} = (p_1 + p_0)/2$, where p_1 is the projected incidence in one arm and p_0 is the projected incidence in the other arm. Note that the investigator must estimate p_0 and p_1 in advance. A p_0 estimate may be available from other studies of similar populations or from pilot data. The $p_1 - p_0$ in the denominator represents the hypothesized difference in cumulative incidence between arms – ideally, the smallest such difference that would be theoretically or practically important. Examples of sample-size and power calculations appear in Hulley and Cummings (1988). Techniques for more complex designs and for outcomes measured on other scales appear in Lachin (1981), Donner (1984), Friedman et al. (1998). Several computer programs are available to assist with the calculations.

With rare exceptions, study subjects must give their informed consent to participate. In the United States, federal regulations mandate that subjects be told the purpose of the research, procedures involved, risks and benefits of interventions to which they might be exposed, arrangements for handling adverse effects, the voluntary nature of their participation and their right to withdraw, who will have access to data about them and how long the data will be retained, and whom they can contact with questions (Friedman et al., 1998). The project protocol and proposed consent form must be approved by an Institutional Review Board, whose composition and procedures are designed to safeguard subject welfare. Many research organizations require that such review and consent procedures be followed regardless of funding source.

Unexpectedly low rates of subject accrual are a common problem. Estimates of the number of potential subjects available and their willingness to participate are often too optimistic. Pilot studies can be very valuable for working out study logistics and for developing realistic estimates of subject availability. Hunninghake et al. (1987) review ways of enhancing subject recruitment and retention.

Randomization

Random allocation, the feature that distinguishes a randomized trial from other study designs, is responsible for the substantial advantages of this design. If randomization is worth doing, it is worth doing right. Various forms of systematic allocation – such as assigning subjects alternately between arms, or based on day of the week, or on subjects' birthdays, or on medical record number – appear occasionally in injury research, but they are not truly random and should be avoided. An investigator may be tempted to regard these methods as effectively random, being unable to think of how they could be biased. But evidence suggests that proceeding on this assumption is a risky and unnecessary gamble. In one review by Chalmers et al. (1983) of 145 trials, the frequency of significant differences between study arms on variables measured at baseline was more than twice as common when true random assignment had not been used.

Two issues are at stake. One is whether the assignment sequence that specifies which subject goes to which intervention arm is truly random. The other is allocation concealment – whether the intervention assignment of a subject is adequately hidden from persons involved in deciding whether and when the subject enters the trial. Flaws in either process can lead to bias. Fortunately, it is quite easy to do both properly.

Generating the Assignment Sequence

Most standard biostatistics texts include a table of random numbers that can be used to create an assignment sequence by hand. Nowadays, it is easier and arguably better to use a computer, in order to minimize mistakes and to allow the assignment process to be audited if necessary. The necessary steps can be carried out with most standard statistical packages (Le and Lindgren, 1988), or even with a spreadsheet program (see next section).

All Subjects Known at Beginning of Trial

Sometimes all study subjects can be identified at the outset. For example, in the Clamp and Kendrick (1998) study of home safety advice, all families with a preschool child who were registered in a certain primary care practice were deemed eligible. The task is to divide such a list at random into sublists, one for each study arm. A simple method is shown in Table 9.1 for eight hypothetical subjects.

In panel 1, subjects have been listed in a spreadsheet – here, alphabetically, but the ordering is immaterial. In panel 2, a computer-generated random number in the range 0–1 has been added to each row. The specific way to do this depends on the software. In panel 3, the rows have been sorted by column B. The top half of the list was assigned to intervention group 1 and the bottom half to group 2.

This approach assures that the sizes of the two intervention groups will be equal or nearly equal. It can also be extended to guarantee balance on one or more baseline factors. For example, to assure gender balance, the method could be carried out separately for males and females – a process termed stratified randomization (Kernan et al., 1999). To balance two or more factors simultaneously, a separate list would be created for each unique combination of values on the stratification factors and randomization performed within each list. In multicenter studies, center is usually one stratification factor. Each additional factor creates smaller strata, however, and eventually stratification becomes self-defeating: strata with, say, one, three, or five subjects cannot be divided equally between intervention groups, and there may be many such strata. Friedman et al. (1998) advise that the number of stratification factors, if any, be kept small, and they should generally be factors known to be strongly associated with the main outcome.

Table 9.1 Randomizing a predefined list of study subjects

(1) Initial listing

A
Name
Adams
Brown
Chester
Davis
Edwards
Fulton
Graham
Harris

(2) After adding a computer-generated
     random number to each row

A	B
Name	*Computer-generated random no.*
Adams	0.81422
Brown	0.90634
Chester	0.32979
Davis	0.05449
Edwards	0.32959
Fulton	0.06776
Graham	0.72420
Harris	0.55622

(3) After sorting by column B and then assigning individuals to
     interventions based on list position

A	B	C
Name	*Computer-generated random no.*	*Intervention group assignment*
Davis	0.05449	1
Fulton	0.06776	1
Edwards	0.32959	1
Chester	0.32979	1
Harris	0.55622	2
Graham	0.72420	2
Adams	0.81422	2
Brown	0.90634	2

Subjects Identified Sequentially

In other situations, subjects are recruited as the trial progresses and must be randomized on the fly. The assignment sequence itself can still be created in advance. Simple randomization is tantamount to flipping a coin for each subject.

In practice, the investigator could create a long list of random numbers like those in column B of Table 9.1, then map each random number less than 0.5 to group 1 and the rest to group 2. A disadvantage of simple randomization is that the resulting groups may not be equal in size, which can lead to a loss of statistical power for a given trial size.

To avoid this problem, blocked randomization is often used. Positions on the assignment list are pre-grouped into small sets or blocks, with the size of each block being a small multiple of the number of study arms. For a two-arm trial, block 1 may be the first four positions, block 2 may be the next four, and so on. Within each block, the method of Table 9.1 is then used to determine at random which two block members go to intervention group 1, with the other two going to group 2. Intervention group sizes will automatically be equal at the end of each block. As noted below, it is important that the assignment sequence be hidden and unpredictable: an observer should not be able to look ahead or to examine the pattern of past assignments and determine easily what the next assignment will be. Hence block sizes of two are best avoided: once the assignment for the first subject in each pair is known, the next assignment is obvious. Block sizes of four, six, or eight make the pattern harder to decipher. Even better, block sizes can be varied within the sequence.

To prevent imbalance on an important characteristic, blocking and stratification can be combined. For example, there may be separate lists, each organized in blocks, for males and females. A new subject would then be logged into the next opening on the appropriate gender-specific list.

Concealing the Assignment Sequence

Bias can occur if decisions about whether subjects enter the trial, or the order in which they enter, are influenced by the assignments they would receive (Schulz, 1995). Schulz et al. (1995) found that apparent treatment effects were systematically larger in trial reports that suggested inadequately concealed methods of randomization. Under such conditions, someone's preference for one intervention over the other, rather than random chance, could determine membership of the intervention groups. Comparability can no longer be assumed, and the damage may be impossible to repair. Prevention of the problem is usually easy. Assignment of subjects is best done by trained study staff whose primary job is faithful implementation of the study protocol. When possible, it is best that control over subject registration and assignment remain in a central study office, which is contacted whenever a new subject is identified. If logistics require randomization in the field, the sequence of individual assignments can be put into numbered, opaque, sealed envelopes. Each new subject is first logged in on a list showing the envelope number, and only then is the envelope opened to reveal the group assignment.

Data Collection

Issues to consider in designing and applying good data-collection methods are covered in the chapter by Runyan and Bowling (this volume). Good advice can also be found in Meinert (1986), Friedman et al. (1998), Hulley and Cummings (1988), and McFadden (1998).

Baseline data serve in part to verify trial eligibility. Characteristics that are likely to influence outcomes above and beyond the intervention received are typically measured at baseline, in order to assess the similarity of intervention groups. Some of these factors may later be used in the analysis to adjust for any imbalances, to improve study power, or to define subgroups that may respond differently to the interventions being compared.

As the trial proceeds, it is useful to monitor whether interventions are actually implemented as intended, including subject compliance. This information can later aid interpretation of results, especially if the trial finds no statistically significant differences in outcome between treatment arms. In the PROFET study to prevent falls, the investigators reported the number of patients in the intervention arm who received the medical and occupational-therapy assessments as intended (Close et al., 1999). In the study of antibiotic propylaxis against hand and foot wound infections, the investigators counted remaining pills at follow-up, reporting high compliance across intervention groups (Madsen et al., 1996).

When outcome measurements involve perception or judgment by subjects or study staff, blinding is highly desirable. A trial is double blind if both subjects and investigators responsible for outcome measurements are unaware of which inter- vention group the subject is in. A trial is single blind if one of these two parties knows the subject's group assignment but the other does not. The system of placebos in the Madsen et al. (1996) study of wound infection prophylaxis enabled that study to be double blinded. To assess the success of attempted blinding, participants can be asked at the end of the trial to guess which group they were in. Blinding is not always possible: in the Clamp and Kendrick (1998) study of home safety advice to prevent child injury, each family should clearly have known whether they received such advice or not.

Data Analysis

The first step in analysis is usually to compare the intervention groups on baseline characteristics. These results are often summarized in Table 1 of the published report, which characterizes the study population, helps readers judge similarity to their own settings, and identifies prognostically important factors that were unbalanced between groups despite randomization.

The main analysis compares outcomes between intervention groups. It should follow the intent-to-treat principle: each subject remains in the group to which he or she was randomly assigned, even if later events created a discrepancy between the intervention intended and that actually received. The reason is that the major benefits of randomization obtain only if the groups formed by random assignment are kept intact. Departures from the intended regimen will tend to reduce differ- ences between comparison groups in an intent-to-treat analysis – a conservative bias. The injury trial examples cited above followed this widely accepted principle. Sometimes a secondary analysis by treatment actually received can also be informative, particularly if an intent-to-treat analysis is negative and many subjects received an intervention other than intended. However, the onus is then on the investigator to identify and control for differences between groups. Such a comparison converts a randomized trial into an observational study.

Sequential analysis (Friedman et al., 1998) involves monitoring outcomes periodically or even continuously as the trial proceeds, so that a superior treatment can be identified early. Braakman et al. (1983) randomized severely head-injured patients to receive either high-dose corticosteroids or placebo. One-month survival was monitored throughout the trial so that the experiment could be terminated promptly if early data indicated clear superiority of one regimen. In this instance, no significant differences were observed in 161 patients, after which the trial was stopped. Because sequential analysis involves repeated looks at the results and thus multiple statistical tests, special statistical methods are required to avoid falsely rejecting the null hypothesis (Whitehead, 1997).

Subgroup analyses may identify a subpopulation for whom the experimental intervention was especially effective. Ray et al. (1997) reported a randomized trial of a fall-prevention consultation service in Tennessee nursing homes. During follow-up, 13.7 injurious falls occurred per 100 patient-years in intervention-group sites, compared with 19.9 falls per 100 patient-years in control sites ($p = 0.22$). However, nearly all of the difference observed stemmed from a 49% reduction in fall rate among patients who had had three or more falls in the previous year ($p = 0.06$); little effect was seen in other patients. Subgroup analyses should be approached with caution, however. There are many ways to divide participants into subgroups, and performing many significance tests will inevitably lead to some apparently significant p-values by chance (Yusuf et al., 1991; Oxman and Guyatt, 1992).

An international consortium of trialists and journal editors (Begg et al., 1996) has proposed that reporting of randomized trials follow a set of guidelines designed to maximize readers' ability to understand and to judge the quality of a study. These guidelines may also facilitate future meta-analysis.

Design Variations

Several other randomized-trial designs can be useful in injury research. In a factorial trial, two or more interventions are studied simultaneously (Stampfer et al., 1985). A separate group is formed for each possible combination of interventions: for example, in a study of interventions A and B, group 1 would receive both, group 2 A only, group 3 B only, and group 4 neither. If one intervention magnifies or inhibits the other's effects, a factorial design can detect the interaction. In the absence of interaction, the design offers efficiency by addressing two research questions for little more than the price of one.

In a crossover trial, each subject is exposed to each intervention at different time periods. The design applies when each intervention has only short-term effects that subside when the intervention is stopped. Because each person is exposed to each intervention, within-person comparisons of efficacy can be made, which can reduce sample-size requirements. Robbins and Waked (1997) reported a randomized crossover study involving four shoe-sole materials suitable for use in athletic footwear. They found that vertical impact and balance problems, both thought to be related to sports injuries, were inversely associated with sole and surface material hardness.

Finally, group-randomized trials involve allocation of pre-existing clusters of individuals en bloc to different interventions (Murray, 1998). The clusters may be families, physicians' practices, classrooms, workplaces, or entire communities. This design is appropriate when an intervention would apply nonselectively to an entire group of people, as would a mass-media campaign. It can also be useful when communication between people could create unacceptable contamination of control subjects if randomized individually. Grossman et al. (1997) evaluated a school-based violence-prevention program by randomizing six pairs of elementary schools to receive or not receive an experimental curriculum. Several special methodological challenges arise in conducting group-randomized studies (Koepsell, 1998; Murray, 1998), including increased sample-size requirements, increased likelihood of unbalanced intervention groups, and the need for special forms of analysis to obtain valid significance tests.

Conclusion

Randomized trials have important scientific advantages over other study designs, and injury researchers should be alert for opportunities to reap those benefits. Influential organizations such as the US Preventive Services Task Force (1996), the Evidence-Based Medicine Working Group (Guyatt et al., 1993), and the Cochrane Collaboration (Chalmers, 1993) place randomized trials at the top of the evidence hierarchy. Thus, findings from well-conducted randomized trials are likely to be recognized and to have an impact.

References

Armitage P, Berry G (1994) Statistical Methods in Medical Research, 3rd edn. London: Blackwell Science.
Begg C, Cho M, Eastwood S, Horton R, Moher D, Olkin I, Pitkin R, Rennie D, Schulz KF, Simel D, Stroup DF (1996) Improving the quality of reporting of randomized controlled trials. The CONSORT statement. JAMA 276:637–9.
Braakman R, Schouten HJ, Blaauw-van Dishoeck M, Minderhoud JM (1983) Megadose steroids in severe head injury. Results of a prospective double-blind clinical trial. J Neurosurg 58:326–30.
Chalmers I (1993) The Cochrane Collaboration: preparing, maintaining, and disseminating systematic reviews of the effects of health care. Ann NY Acad Sci 703:156–63.
Chalmers T, Celano P, Sacks HS, Smith H Jr (1983) Bias in treatment assignment in controlled clinical trials. N Engl J Med 309:1358–61.
Charlton BG (1994) Understanding randomized controlled trials: Explanatory or pragmatic? Fam Pract 11:243–4.
Chow S-C, Liu J-P (1998) Design and Analysis of Clinical Trials: Concepts and Methodologies. New York: John Wiley & Sons.
Close J, Ellis M, Hooper R, Glucksman E, Jackson S, Swift C (1999) Prevention of falls in the elderly trial (PROFET): a randomized controlled trial. Lancet 353:93–7.

Clamp M, Kendrick D (1998) A randomized controlled trial of general practitioner safety advice for families with children under 5 years. Br Med J 316:1576–9.

Donner A (1984) Approaches to sample size estimation in the design of clinical trials – a review. Stat Med 3:199–214.

Gentilello LM, Jurkovich GJ, Stark MS, Hassantash SA, O'Keefe GE (1997) Is hypothermia in the victim of major trauma protective or harmful? A randomized, prospective study. Ann Surg 226:439–47.

Grossman DC, Neckerman HJ, Koepsell TD et al. (1997) Effectiveness of a violence prevention curriculum among children in elementary school: a randomized controlled trial. JAMA 277:1605–11.

Guyatt GH, Sackett DL, Cook DJ (1993) Users' guides to the medical literature. II. How to use an article about therapy or prevention. A. Are the results of the study valid? Evidence-Based Medicine Working Group. JAMA 270:2598–601.

Friedman LM, Furberg CD, DeMets DL (1998) Fundamentals of Clinical Trials, 3rd edn. New York: Springer-Verlag.

Hearst N, Newman TB, Hulley SB (1988) Delayed effects of the military draft on mortality: A randomized natural experiment. N Engl J Med 314:620–4.

Hulley SB, Cummings S (1988) Designing Clinical Research. Baltimore: Williams and Wilkins.

Hunninghake DB, Darby CA, Probstfield JL (1987) Recruitment experience in clinical trials: literature summary and annotated bibliography. Controlled Clin Trials 8(Suppl 4):6S–30S.

Kernan WN, Viscoli CM, Makuch RW, Brass LM, Horwitz RI (1999) Stratified randomization for clinical trials. J Clin Epidemiol 52:19–26.

Koepsell TD (1998) Epidemiologic issues in the design of community trials. In: Brownson R, Petitti DB (eds), Applied Epidemiology. New York: Oxford University Press.

Lachin JM (1981) Introduction to sample size determination and power analysis for clinical trials. Controlled Clin Trials 2:93–133.

Le CT, Lindgren BR (1988) Randomization using packaged programs. Comput Biomed Res 21:593–6.

Madsen MS, Neumann L, Andersen JA (1996) Penicillin prophylaxis in complicated wounds of hands and feet: a randomized, double-blind trial. Injury 27:275–8.

McFadden E (1998) Management of Data in Clinical Trials. New York: John Wiley & Sons.

Medical Research Council (1948) Streptomycin treatment of pulmonary tuberculosis. Br Med J 2:769–82.

Meinert CL (1986) Clinical Trials: Design, Conduct, and Analysis. New York: Oxford University Press.

Murray DM (1998) Design and Analysis of Group-Randomized Trials. New York: Oxford University Press.

Oxman AD, Guyatt GH (1992) A consumer's guide to subgroup analyses. Ann Intern Med 116:78–84.

Pocock SJ (1983) Clinical Trials: A Practical Approach. New York: Wiley & Sons.

Randal J (1999) Randomized controlled trials mark a golden anniversary. J Natl Cancer Inst 91:10–12.

Ray WA, Taylor JA, Meador KG et al. (1997) A randomized trial of a consultation service to reduce falls in nursing homes. JAMA 278:557–62.

Robbins S, Waked E (1997) Balance and vertical impact in sports: role of shoe sole materials. Arch Phys Med Rehabil 78:463–7.

Schulz KF (1995) Subverting randomization in controlled trials. JAMA 274:1456–8.

Schulz KF, Chalmers I, Hayes RJ, Altman DG (1995) Empirical evidence of bias. Dimensions of methodological quality associated with estimates of treatment effects in controlled trials. JAMA 273:408–12.

Schwarz D, Lellouch J (1967) Explanatory and pragmatic attitudes in therapeutic trials. J Chron Dis 20:637–48.

Stampfer MJ, Buring JE, Willett W, Rosner B, Eberlein K, Hennekens CH (1985) The 2×2 factorial design: its application to a randomized trial of aspirin and carotene in U.S. physicians. Stat Med 4:111–16.

US Preventive Services Task Force (1996) Guide to Clinical Preventive Services, 2nd edn. Alexandria, VA: International Medical Publishing.

Whitehead J (1997) The Design and Analysis of Sequential Clinical Trials, 2nd edn. New York: John Wiley & Sons.

Yusuf S, Wittes J, Probstfield J, Tyroler HA (1991) Analysis and interpretation of treatment effects in subgroups of patients in randomized clinical trials. JAMA 266:93–8.

10

Cohort Studies in Injury Research

Jess F. Kraus

Definition of a Cohort Study

Cohort studies have been used extensively in past decades to describe and identify risk factors for human afflictions or to test specific hypotheses aimed at determining causal relationships between risk factors and outcomes. The definition of a cohort study varies, but most references include a study method in which a designated group of people are defined, some are exposed and some not exposed (or there is variation in degree of exposure) to a factor of interest, and they are followed over a period of time during which observations are made, according to exposure categories, of outcomes such as death or incidence of new affliction (Last, 1995). The key elements in the definition of cohort studies are the designation of a population in which exposure status is determined, then a period of time elapses, and one or more outcomes are observed. The term exposure means any factor which the investigator wishes to study for its possible promotion of or prevention of the study outcomes.

There are a number of merits in cohort studies. Prospective cohort studies may more accurately measure prognostic or risk factors than other study designs as information about the risk factors is generally obtained prior to the onset of outcomes. When a substantial period of time elapses between exposure and outcome, prospective cohort studies, which can measure many explanatory factors long before the outcomes, may have an advantage over case–control studies, which must reconstruct the past exposure history after the outcome events have occurred. Furthermore, a cohort study can measure incidence rates among those exposed and unexposed to the factor(s) of interest (see the chapter by Cummings, Norton, and Koepsell, this volume). There are several drawbacks to cohort studies, however. They can be expensive and time-consuming and large numbers of subjects or lengthy follow-up are required to study rare outcomes.

There are two general types of cohort studies, prospective and retrospective. In the prospective form the investigator identifies the study population and assesses current risk factors, and then monitors occurrence of outcomes into the future. The planned duration of follow-up may be based on the level of anticipated incidence of outcomes, if reasonable estimates are known. The prospective form has advantages, including the ability to control for many extraneous and confounding factors, and to assess accurately exposure status and outcome events under the watchful eye of the investigator. There are disadvantages as well, including cost, time, and loss of persons to follow-up because of migration or failure to properly monitor.

The retrospective cohort design relies on past records to identify a study group and, at the same time, to identify within those records the nature and amount of exposure. Follow-up for outcome events occurs from the date of historical group identification and proceeds to a specific date in the recent past or even into the future. The advantage of this design is that all or much of the study period has already occurred, and therefore the investigator may proceed rapidly to analyzing the results. However, the assessment of risk factors is beyond the investigator's control, and little can be done to remedy any inadequacy or incompleteness in these measurements.

Analytic Methods

Analytic methods for cohort studies have been reviewed in a journal volume edited by Samet and Munoz (1998) and are described in many textbooks (Breslow and Day, 1987; Rothman and Greenland, 1998). In the next sections are discussed a number of potentially useful measures with application to cohort studies of injuries.

For illustration purposes, data from a report by Felson and associates (1989) on the Framingham Study Cohort are used to show the effect of impaired vision on hip fracture in older adults. In 1973–75, members of the cohort underwent a thorough eye examination and were grossly classified as good vision in both eyes or any impaired vision in either eye. All those examined were followed for 10 years. The findings from this cohort study are shown in Table 10.1.

Crude Estimates of Risk and Relative Risk

Two forms of incidence may be calculated, cumulative and the incidence (density) rate (see chapter by Cummings, Norton, and Koepsell, this volume).

$$\text{cumulative incidence} = \frac{\text{number of new events over time}}{\text{number of persons at risk}} = I_c$$

$$\text{incidence (density) rate} = \frac{\text{number of new events over time}}{\text{person-time of exposure}} = I_d$$

From our example, the cumulative incidence was 3.0 per 100 persons per 10 years with good vision and 9.4 per 100 persons per 10 years with impaired vision. If we assume all persons were followed for the full 10-year period, the incidence density rates using person-years of follow-up can be derived: 3.0 and 9.4 per 1000 person-year, respectively.

From these rates, the most common measure of effect, the risk ratio, can be derived. It is the ratio of the incidence in those exposed to the risk factor, impaired vision (I_E), relative to the incidence in those unexposed to the risk factor (I_U); that is, $I_E \div I_U = 9.4 \div 3.0 = 3.1$.

Table 10.1 Data from the Framingham Study cohort, comparing those with good vision with those with impaired vision, in regard to the subsequent cumulative incidence of hip fracture

Risk factor	Population at risk	No. with hip fracture	Cumulative incidence per 100 persons per 10 years	Symbol
Impaired vision	502	47	9.4	I_E
Good vision	2131	63	3.0	I_U
Total cohort	2633	110	4.2	I_P

The risk ratio answers the question of how many times greater (or smaller) is the risk of outcome in people exposed compared with those unexposed to the factor of interest. In our example, persons with impaired vision have about three times the risk of hip fracture compared with persons whose vision is unimpaired.

Risk Difference or Attributable Risk

Risk difference (RD) is calculated by subtracting the incidence rate in the unexposed from the incidence rate in the exposed. The resulting unit is a rate; $I_E - I_U = RD$. From our example, $9.4 - 3.0 = 6.4$ per 1000 person-years. This measures the amount of absolute risk (the incidence rate) that can be attributed to a specific risk factor or exposure. The risk difference addresses two important questions, namely, how much of the incidence rate in the exposed is due to the exposure itself (6.4 per 1000 person-years), and second, if the risk factor or the exposure could be eliminated, what level of the incidence rate would be eliminated in the exposed population (6.4 per 1000 person-years).

Etiologic Fraction Percent (EF%), or Attributable Fraction Percent

This measure is calculated by subtracting the incidence rate in the unexposed from the incidence in the exposed, and then dividing the result by the incidence in the exposed population, times 100: $[(I_E - I_U) \div I_E] \times 100 = EF\%$ or $[(9.4 - 3.0) \div 9.4] \times 100$ or 68%. This measures the percent of the outcomes among the exposed that can be attributed to the exposure. In our example, if the exposure were eliminated (i.e., impaired vision) we would expect that the incidence of outcomes (hip fracture) would decrease by 68% among the exposed.

Multivariate Techniques

The measures of effect summarized above are crude measures, unadjusted for possible confounding factors. In a cohort study, those who are exposed and unexposed may differ in regard to factors other than their level of exposure. Confounding is present if the crude relative risk estimates do not accurately reflect the underlying association between exposure and outcome due to failure to account for the effects of additional factors. In order to control for possible confounding factors in an analysis, we can either use stratified methods, such as Mantel–Haenszel estimators, or regression methods, such as Poisson regression or Cox proportional hazard models. These techniques are discussed in the citations given previously.

Injury Cohort Studies
A Classification Scheme

For the purposes of this chapter, I have classified cohort studies used in injury research into three groups, based on the criteria for assembling the cohort: (1) cohorts based on broad inclusion criteria that do not require an illness or injury (the cohort may represent persons in a defined population); (2) cohorts formed from persons with a non-injury illness; and (3) cohorts which include only persons who have been injured.

Population-based Cohort Studies

The Prototype Design

The first major group includes population-based studies, in which an entire population, or a sample from a population, is characterized on certain attributes and then followed for the occurrence of injury. An example of this general type of population-based cohort was described by Fujiwara and associates (1991) and involved the original Adult Health Study Cohort of about 20,000 residents of Hiroshima and Nagasaki identified in 1950. This cohort was divided on the basis of distance from the hypocenter of the bomb blast (the risk factor) and by gender and age at time of exposure; incidence of thoracic vertebral fractures was obtained from 1958 to 1986. The investigators found no relationship between radiation exposure and risk of later vertebral fracture.

Cohort Studies of Entire Populations or Subsets of a Population

Examples of these studies can include birth cohorts such as the prospective Dunedin Birth Cohort Study, initiated in 1972–73 in New Zealand (Silva, 1990). Other retrospective birth cohort studies have been reported from Montreal, Canada (Larson and Pless, 1988), the United Kingdom (Pless et al., 1989), and Tennessee (Scholer et al., 1997). Some prospective cohort studies enrolled subsets of large adult populations, for example the Framingham Study Cohort (Felson et al., 1989). The Finnish twin cohort study (Romanov et al., 1994) involved a retrospective approach. Some population-based retrospective cohort studies were formed on the basis of exposure to a single catastrophic event such as the Hiroshima and Nagasaki survivors (Fujiwara et al., 1991). Some retrospective cohort studies were formed on the basis of membership in health maintenance organizations (HMOs), for example, the Kaiser Permanente Medical Care Program (Braun et al., 1998) or the members of the Group Health Cooperative of Puget Sound (Thompson et al., 1993).

The exposures or risk factors that were studied vary across these cohort studies. In the Framingham Study Cohort, visual acuity was the exposure of interest (Felson et al., 1989). In the Finnish male cohort (Pekkanen et al., 1989), serum cholesterol was the risk factor on which the cohort was classified. In the Finnish twin cohort (Romanov et al., 1994), hostility, derived from self-report, was the basis for determining cohort exposure status. The cohort formed from the Kaiser Permanente Medical Group (Braun et al., 1998) used self-reported marijuana and alcohol use as the basis for cohort exposure classification.

Some form of injury, such as traffic crash injuries (Thompson et al., 1993), was the outcome of interest in these examples. Several studies either linked national records systems for entire countries, such as Finland (Pekkanen et al., 1989) and Sweden (Mallmin et al., 1993), or linked data found in existing health care records, as located in an HMO (Thompson et al., 1993). These records were then used as the basis for exposure delineation and additional records (e.g., death certificates) were used for outcome assessment. The investigators thus made use of existing data to form their cohorts and conduct their analyses.

Cohort Studies Defined by Work or Employment

There are studies where the cohort of interest was defined on the basis of a specific occupation or type of work. A variety of study populations have been used, including fishermen (Tomaszuna et al., 1988), postal workers (Zwerling et al., 1993), veterinarians (Wilkins et al., 1997), and military cadets (Bijur et al., 1997). These cohorts used a variety of exposures including type of work, category of occupation, and employee use of substances (caffeine, alcohol, or controlled substances). A number of methods were incorporated in these studies including the use of rates (Driscoll and Hanson, 1997) and regression analysis (Zwerling et al., 1993) to adjust for covariates.

Cohort Studies of Sport or Recreational Groups

Sports and recreational groups are commonly used to define cohorts; then outcomes are assessed following exposure to play or sporting activity. Haddon and associates (1962) conducted a study in Mount Snow, Vermont, which identified a prospective cohort of skiers. They used a sampling method that has been repeated on several subsequent occasions; they randomly selected persons waiting to use the ski lifts. The outcomes were reported as incidence rates by level of experience, gender, and age of skier. Exposure times were obtained from lift tickets and sample interviews. The investigators found injury rates per 1000 ski-person days significantly higher for women compared with men skiers and for skiers less than 20 years of age compared with older skiers. In 1969, Kraus and Gullen reported on the risks of injury during football games among college students. A variety of individual, game-related, and environmental factors were measured prior to the 8-week exposure period. Age-specific injury rates per 100 players were directly related to age, previous high school or college football injury history, or history of any prior high school disabling injury.

Schafle and associates (1990) and Bahr and Bahr (1997) conducted prospective cohort studies defined by membership on volleyball teams while Lee and associates (1997) and Gissane and associates (1998) defined cohorts of rugby team members. U.S. amateur boxers were the cohort studied by Stewart and associates in 1994. These studies used rates to measure outcomes and exposure periods were precisely recorded.

Cohort Studies of Persons with Pre-existing Noninjury Illnesses or Conditions

Cohorts may be defined on the basis of existing morbidity. Several recently published studies illustrate differences in the nature of eligibility for membership in this type of cohort design. In a report from Japan (Asada et al., 1996) two prospective cohorts were formed, one composed of medically diagnosed dementia patients and the other a comparison cohort. The exposure of interest was the presence or absence of dementia and information on confounders was also recorded. A logistic regression model was used to evaluate the risk for falls among those with strokes compared with others. The community-based assessment had well-defined end points and exposure definitions, although there were concerns of external validity. A fall in the year previous to the study was one of the major risk factors for a fall during the study period. A similar type of prospective study was reported in the Netherlands (Tutuarima et al., 1997) in which stroke patients in 23 Dutch hospitals were evaluated at baseline for a variety of medical conditions. The outcome of interest was falls and crude and adjusted relative risk estimates were calculated. Poisson regression was used to control for potential confounders. Those with heart disease, mental decline, and urinary incontinence were at highest risk of falling, compared with stroke victims without these conditions.

Cohort Studies with Injury as a Criteria for Inclusion in the Study

The third major group of cohort studies are those which require an injury for membership in the cohort. Individuals are usually identified from a medical facility and followed for some outcome. These studies of outcomes after injury are in essence studies of prognosis, but they do not differ in principle from cohort studies of the causes of injury.

Cohort Studies of Persons who Share a Common Mechanism of Injury

Many cohort studies are composed of injured persons involved in a motor vehicle crash. Wolf et al. (1993), assembled a cohort of pregnant women of greater than 19 weeks gestation who were drivers in a motor vehicle crash. The outcomes of low birth weight and fetal death were more common among women who were unrestrained in the crash, compared with those who used restraints. Braithwaite et al. (1998), studied the outcomes of persons with an Injury Severity Score of greater than 15 who were discharged alive from one of 16 hospitals in the United Kingdom;

about three-fourths of those with the highest Injury Severity Scores had persistent disability, compared with smaller proportions among those with lower scores.

Cohort Studies of Persons who Share a Common Anatomic Site of Injury

One of the early attempts to study traumatic brain injury using a cohort approach was reported by Kraus and associates (1984) using San Diego County residents as the population base. The exposure was traumatic brain injury stratified by severity. Outcomes were those defined by the Glasgow Outcome Scale (Jennett and Bond, 1975) and the case-fatality rate. The study identified all cases, including those who died, through a well-coordinated emergency medical services system. Williams and associates (1991) used the Mayo Clinic registry to identify individuals with traumatic brain injury and to follow them for a significant period of time to look for the onset of dementia and other degenerative diseases. Gender, severity of brain injury, and number of head trauma exposures were the main risk factors studied. Using an existing database, the investigators found no increased risk of neurologic diseases or disorders following a traumatic brain injury based on standardized mortality ratios or standardized incidence ratios (see chapter by Cummings, Norton, and Koepsell, this volume).

Cohort studies of patients with spinal cord injury are mostly of a retrospective design and date back over 3 decades. One of the largest, from the United States, was reported by DeVivo and associates (1993), who specified membership on the basis of survival following injury for at least 24 hours. Follow-up was through patient record monitoring and outcomes were compared with the U.S. population using standardized mortality ratios. The risk factors were age at time of injury and level and extent of injury. Fatal septicemia and pulmonary complications were more frequently observed than expected among those of younger age (less than 25 years) or with complete quadriplegia.

Cohort Studies among Persons in other Injury Categories

Hall and associates (1998) defined a cohort based on patients discharged from a hospital in Scotland after a suicide attempt. A sample in excess of 8300 patients was identified and the incidence of readmissions and death were measured. The major classification of the cohort was on gender with higher than expected occurrences of unintentional deaths among men and greater than expected homicide rates among women. This study design is possible when reporting of hospital admissions and other health events is available through existing health record monitoring systems. A report from Quebec, Canada (Abenhaim et al., 1995) illustrated the use of workers compensation data to identify persons with long-term chronic low back pain, with monitoring of outcomes following a low back injury claim over a period of several years. Risk of chronic back problems was associated with older age ($\geq$ 45 years) and amount of daily compensation.

Future Prospects of Injury Cohort Studies

Many cohorts are readily available for study with information on a number of potentially important factors already recorded, such as persons in health maintenance organizations or specific subsets of populations such as housing facilities for the elderly.

Cohorts with variations in risk factors (or levels of one risk factor) are continually being formed, such as runners in a marathon, bicyclists at a cycling event, or workers at a factory. With minimal resources and good public relations it may be possible to address questions of differential risk of injury within these groups by studying variations in exposure, such as using or not using a bicycle helmet or the type of helmet worn by motorcyclists.

In work settings, changes in work practices, environmental layouts or worker behavioral change requirements can sometimes be evaluated with respect to injury reductions. Although a randomized controlled trial is the benchmark of evidence-based prevention or treatment practice, real-world circumstances suggest that quasi-experimental approaches using cohorts can sometimes result in realistic appraisals of effectiveness. Although the investigator is restricted to observational data instead of experimental data, results may nonetheless be valid.

Follow-up of cohort members can be relatively easy in some groups identified by a common factor such as employment, specific locale, or common activity (i.e., sports team). Even so, long-term follow-up and monitoring for outcomes poses additional difficulties, namely loss of members of the group or lack of information on health status at the termination of the observation period. Short-term follow-up periods pose fewer problems but the size of the cohort must increase accordingly to ensure an outcome occurrence of sufficient size to meet the statistical needs of the study.

One of the major advances in recent years has been the ability to link databases for defined cohorts. National health care systems with common record linkage offer great advantages over systems that rely on information from a number of different sources with no common linkage capability. Exposure information, for example, may come from police reports and outcome data from death certificates or medical records. Often these may be linkable, although information on variables crucial to some analyses may be missing.

The examples cited in this chapter, although not intended as a complete listing of all possible cohort designs or their exposures and outcomes, are examples of the rich variety of approaches and results that have been undertaken with success in recent years. Cohort studies are practical and valid ways to extract useful information regarding differences in risk of an outcome according to levels of an exposure.

Acknowledgments

My thanks to David McArthur PhD for undertaking the article search, providing a critical reading and offering valuable editorial comments. Also my gratitude to

David Watson and Tad Stephen for word processing and careful reading of the chapter.

References

Abenhaim L, Rossignol M, Gobeille D, Bonvalot Y, Fines P, Scott S (1995) The prognostic consequences in the making of the initial medical diagnosis of work-related back injuries. Spine 20:791–5.

Asada T, Kariya T, Kinoshita T, Asaka A, Morikawa S, Yoshioka M, Kakuma T (1996) Predictors of fall-related injuries among community-dwelling elderly people with dementia. Age Ageing 25:22–8.

Bahr R, Bahr IA (1997) Incidence of acute volleyball injuries: a prospective cohort study of injury mechanisms and risk factors. Scand J Med Sci Sports 7:166–71.

Bijur PE, Horodyski M, Egerton W, Kurzon M, Lifrak S, Friedman S (1997) Comparison of injury during cadet basic training by gender. Ach Pediatr Adoles Med 151:456–61.

Braithwaite IJ, Boot DA, Patterson M, Robinson A (1998) Disability after severe injury: five year follow up of a large cohort. Injury 29:55–9.

Breslow NE, Day NE (1987) Statistical Methods in Cancer Research. Volume II. The design and analysis of cohort studies. Lyon, France: International Agency for Research on Cancer.

Braun BL, Tekawa IS, Gerberich SG, Sidney S (1998) Marijuana use and medically attended injury events. Ann Emerg Med 32:353–60.

DeVivo MJ, Black KJ, Stover SL (1993) Causes of death during the first 12 years after spinal cord injury. Arch Phys Med Rehab 74:248–54.

Driscoll T, Hanson M (1997) Work-related injuries in trade apprentices. Aust NZ J Public Health 21:767–72.

Felson DT, Anderson JJ, Hannan MT, Milton RC, Wilson PWF, Kiel DP (1989) Impaired vision and hip fracture. The Framingham Study. J Am Geriatr Soc 37:495–500.

Fujiwara S, Mizuno S, Ochi Y, Sasaki H, Kodama K, Russell WJ, Hosoda Y (1991) The incidence of thoracic vertebral fractures in a Japanese population, Hiroshima and Nagasaki, 1958–86. J Clin Epidemiol 44:1007–14.

Gissane C, Jennings D, White J, Cumine A (1998) Injury in summer rugby league football: the experiences of one club. Br J Sports Med 32:149–52.

Haddon W, Ellison AE, Carroll RE (1962) Skiing injuries. Public Health Rep 77:975–85.

Hall DJ, O'Brien F, Stark C, Pelosi A, Smith H (1998) Thirteen-year follow-up of deliberate self-harm, using linked data. Br J Psychiatry 172:239–42.

Jennett B, Bond M (1975) Assessment of outcome after severe brain injury. Lancet i:480–4.

Kraus JF, Gullen WH (1969) An epidemiologic investigation of predictor variables associated with intramural touch football injuries. Am J Public Health 59:2144–55.

Kraus JF, Black MA, Hessol N, Ley P, Rokaw W, Sullivan C, Bowers S, Knowlton S, Marshall L (1984) The incidence of acute brain injury and serious impairment in a defined population. Am J Epidemiol 119:189–201.

Last JM (ed.) (1995) A Dictionary of Epidemiology. New York: Oxford University Press.

Larson CP, Pless IB (1988) Risk factors for injury in a 3-year-old birth cohort. Am J Dis Child 142:1052–7.

Lee AJ, Myers JL, Garraway WM (1997) Influence of players' physique on rugby football injuries. Br J Sports Med 31:135–8.

Mallmin H, Ljunghall S, Persson I, Naessaen T, Krusemo UB, Bergstreom R (1993) Fracture of the distal forearm as a forecaster of subsequent hip fracture: A population-based cohort study with 24 years of follow-up. Calcified Tissue Int 52:269–72.

Pekkanen J, Nissinen A, Punsar S, Karvonen MJ (1989) Serum cholesterol and risk of accidental or violent death in a 25-year follow-up. The Finnish cohorts of the Seven Countries Study. Arch Intern Med 149:1589–91.

Pless IB, Peckham CS, Power C (1989) Predicting traffic injuries in childhood: A cohort analysis. J Pediatrics 115:932–8.

Rothman KJ, Greenland S (1998) Modern Epidemiology. Philadelphia: Lippincott-Raven.

Romanov K, Hatakka M, Keskinen E, Laaksonen H, Kaprio J, Rose RJ, Kosenvuo M (1994) Self-reported hostility and suicidal acts, accidents, and accidental deaths: A prospective study of 21,443 adults aged 25 to 59. Psychosom Med 56:328–36.

Samet JM, Munoz A (eds) (1998) Cohort studies. Epidemiol Rev 20:1–136.

Schafle MD, Requa RK, Patton WL, Garrick JG (1990) Injuries in the 1987 national amateur volleyball tournament. Am J Sports Med 6:624–31.

Scholer SJ, Mitchel EF Jr, Ray WA (1997) Predictors of injury mortality in early childhood. Pediatrics 100:342–7.

Silva PA (1990) The Dunedin multidisciplinary health and development study: A fifteen year longitudinal study. Perinat Paediatr Epidemiol 4:76–107.

Stewart WF, Gordon B, Selnes O, Bandeen-Roche K, Zeger S, Tusa RJ, Celentano DD, Shechter A, Liberman J, Hall C, Simon D, Lesser R, Randall RD (1994) Prospective study of central nervous system function in amateur boxers in the United States. Am J Epidemiol 139:573–88.

Thompson DC, Rivara FP, Thompson RS, Salzberg PM, Wolf ME, Pearson DC (1993) Use of behavioral risk factor surveys to predict alcohol-related motor vehicle events. Am J Prev Med 9:224–30.

Tomaszuna S, Weclawik Z, Lewiski M (1988) Morbidity, injuries and sick absence in fishermen and seafarers – a prospective study. Bull Inst Maritime Trop Med Gdynia 39:125–35.

Tutuarima JA, van der Meulen JH, de Haan RJ, van Straten A, Limburg M (1997) Risk factors for falls of hospitalized stroke patients. Stroke 28:297–301.

Wilkins JR, Bowman ME (1997) Needlestick injuries among female veterinarians: frequency, syringe contents and side-effects. Occup Med 47:451–7.

Williams DB, Annegers JF, Kokmen E, O'Brien PC, Kurland LT (1991) Brain injury and neurologic sequelae: a cohort study of dementia, parkinsonism, and amyotrophic lateral sclerosis. Neurology 41:1554–7.

Wolf ME, Alexander BH, Rivara FP, Hickok DE, Maier RV, Starzyk PM (1993) A retrospective cohort study of seatbelt use and pregnancy outcome after a motor vehicle crash. J Trauma 34:116–19.

Zwerling C, Sprince NL, Ryan J, Jones MP (1993) Occupational injuries: comparing the rates of male and female postal workers. Am J Epidemiol 138:46–55.

11

Case–Control Studies in Injury Research

Peter Cummings, Thomas D. Koepsell, and Ian Roberts

Introduction

In 1935, a research group in Evanston, Illinois, began measuring the alcohol content in urine from drivers who were hospitalized after a traffic crash. Over 3 years, they found that 47% of 268 injured drivers had been drinking, and 25% had measurements consistent with a blood alcohol level of 21.7 μmol/L or greater. The researchers reasoned that if alcohol use was a cause of traffic crashes, then the prevalence of alcohol in the blood of injured drivers should be greater than that in drivers who had not crashed. To test this hypothesis, they developed a machine which could measure alcohol in expired air. In April of 1938, they towed this machine to several sites in Evanston and measured alcohol levels in 1726 drivers at all hours of the day and night. They found that only 12% of drivers had alcohol in their breath, and only 2% had values consistent with a blood level of 21.7 μmol/L or more. When Holcomb (1938) published these findings, he made no mention of the case–control design, as this term had not yet been coined.

The case–control study design was more formally developed in the 1950s with a series of papers regarding the causes of cancer. The first statistical methods for analyzing these studies, still in use today, were formulated during the same era (Cornfield, 1951; Mantel and Haenszel, 1959). Had the Evanston researchers known these methods, they could have estimated that the crude relative risk of hospitalization due to a crash was 22 (95% confidence interval, 14–34) for drivers with blood alcohol levels of 21.7 μmol/L or greater compared with drivers with no alcohol in their blood. Formal case–control studies of injuries first appeared in 1961 and 1962; Haddon et al. (1961) reported an association between alcohol use by pedestrians and death from being struck by a vehicle, while McCarroll and Haddon (1962) reported a strong association between alcohol use by automobile drivers and driver death in a motor-vehicle crash. More recently, case–control methods have been applied to many types of injury, including pool drownings in Australia (Inter-Governmental Working Party on Swimming Pool Safety, 1988), suicides in Pennsylvania, Tennessee, and Washington (Brent et al., 1991; Kellermann et al., 1992), deaths in house fires in North Carolina (Runyan et al., 1992), and pediatric vehicular injuries in New Zealand driveways (Roberts et al., 1995b).

Why Use a Case–Control Design?

Many exposures that may cause or prevent injuries cannot be manipulated in randomized studies. For example, a randomized trial of the effect of alcohol use on the risk of a traffic crash will never be performed. To study exposures which cannot be randomly assigned, we usually turn to comparative observational study designs: either cohort or case–control studies. The case–control study is often preferred over a cohort design in three situations. First, when an outcome is rare, but the exposure common, the case–control study is relatively more efficient; the investigator can estimate the association of interest with less effort and expense. Second, in studies of injury, we are sometimes interested in a short-term exposure: was a person wearing a bicycle helmet when they crashed or intoxicated just before their car collided with a tree? A case–control study, which need only determine the exposure just before the outcome, may be more practical than a cohort design, which would have to repeatedly assess exposure every time the person engaged in an activity that could result in the injury outcome of interest. Finally, the investigator often faces practical problems in finding or assembling a cohort for which information on exposures and outcomes is or will become available. Series of cases, however, are relatively easy to collect in a health-care system or death records system, and the investigator can usually devise a method for finding suitable controls.

A Brief Review of Case–Control Study Design

The design and analysis of case–control studies have been well described in texts (Breslow and Day, 1980; Schlesselman, 1982; Rothman and Greenland, 1998) and reviews (Wacholder et al., 1992a; Armenian, 1994). Here we give a brief review of how this design estimates relative risks.

Although a case–control study does not directly yield information about absolute risk in persons with or without exposure to some factor, it does allow estimation of the risk of injury in persons with a given exposure relative to that of unexposed persons. As estimation of relative risks from case–control data may seem counterintuitive, we first describe an imaginary cohort study. We wish to know if wearing a life vest while boating is associated with the risk of death due to submersion. Our cohort consists of 1 million adult boaters who are all about the same age, have similar boats, and boat with equal frequency on the same body of water. One-fourth of these boaters wear life vests every time they go out, while the others never use a life vest. Over a year, we classify boaters according to outcome and use of life vests (Table 11.1). Using the cell labels in Table 11.1, the relative risk of drowning while boating with a life vest compared with boating without a vest is the ratio of the two outcome probabilities = probability of death if wearing a vest $\div$ probability of death if not wearing = $[A/(A + B)] \div [C/(C + D)] = (25/250000) \div (150/750000) = 0.50$ (95% confidence interval, 0.33–0.76).

Collecting information about 1 million boaters would be expensive. To save money, let's redesign our imaginary study as a case–control study. With the cooperation of area medical examiners, we get life vest information regarding

Table 11.1 Results of a hypothetical cohort study of boaters

Life vest use	Outcome after 1 year			
	Drowned		Survived	Total
Always	(A)	25	(B) 249,975	250,000
Never	(C)	150	(D) 749,850	750,000
Total		175	999,825	1,000,000

Table 11.2 Results of a hypothetical case–control study of boaters

Life vest use	Outcome during 1 year			
	Drowned		Controls	Total
Always	(A)	25	(B) 131	156
Never	(C)	150	(D) 394	544
Total		175	525	700

every boater who drowns in the study area; these are the cases. Using observers in boats, we assess the life vest use of a random sample of living boaters. If we sample all of the 175 cases and three control boaters for each case, our new data will contain the same information about fatalities, but information about only 525 control boaters. On average, subject to variation in sampling, the distribution of vest use among the controls will represent the distribution of vest use among all living boaters (Table 11.2).

Having collected the data, it occurs to us that the probabilities of death while wearing and not wearing a vest cannot be obtained from Table 11.2. How can we derive the relative risk estimate? In 1951, Cornfield (1951) pointed out that if the probability of the outcome is small in the study population, as it is in Table 11.1, then the risk $A/(A + B)$ may be approximated by A/B and the risk $C/(C + D)$ may be approximated by C/D. The relative risk of drowning associated with life vest use in Table 11.1 may then be estimated as $(A/B) \div (C/D) = (25/249,975) \div (150/749,850) = 0.50$. As A/B and C/D are the odds of drowning for each level of exposure, their ratio is called the odds ratio.

This odds ratio can also be expressed as the ratio of the odds of exposure, $(A/C) \div (B/D)$. If controls are sampled correctly, the ratio of B to D in Tables 11.1 and 11.2 will be, on average, the same; as cells A and C are the same in both Tables 11.1 and 11.2, we should be able to derive the same odds ratio from both tables. In Table 11.2, the odds ratio for drowning, if a boater wears a vest, is $(A/B) \div (C/D) = (25/131) \div (150/394) = 0.50$ (95% confidence interval, 0.32–0.80). Rounded to two decimals, this is the same as the risk ratio from Table 11.1; the confidence limits are only slightly wider.

The cost and effort involved in obtaining the data for this imaginary case–control study should be considerably less than for its sister cohort study. The case–control design required information about only 700 boaters, compared with information regarding 1 million boaters in the cohort study, and obtained the same result with only a small loss of precision, as measured by the confidence interval. In summary, as the outcome becomes rarer, the cost advantage of a case–control study over a cohort study will become relatively greater, and the case–control generated odds ratio will more closely approximate the relative risk.

The Study Population or Study Base

In planning a case–control study, it is helpful to think of the study as being set in a specific population or cohort, even though most members of that population will not participate in the study. The study population usually represents a sample of person-time, not actual persons. For example, if the study base were defined as the residents of an area or participants in a health plan, during the 4-year period of 1990 through 1993, some people might belong to the study population for only 9 months, before moving to another area, dying, or switching health plans. Others might be born into the population, or move to the area, or join the plan before the end of 1993, contributing person-time to the population from which both cases and controls are derived.

The cases would be newly injured persons who are members of the study population; they must be people who we could sample as controls. If injuries are plentiful, we may choose only a sample of the injured persons in the source population as cases. Conversely, the controls must also be members of the study base; people who we could ascertain and count as cases if they were injured. The function of the control group is to provide an estimate of exposure prevalence in the study base.

In studies of injury, we are sometimes interested only in person-time spent in certain activities (Roberts, 1995). In a study of alcohol use and traffic crashes, we are only interested in person-time spent as a driver of a vehicle. Persons who do not drive would not be part of the study base; they would not be eligible for selection as either cases or controls.

We distinguish between a study that is population-based and one that is not. If we are confident that all the injured persons within a region must come to a group of hospitals, and if we limit cases to residents of that region, then our study would be population-based in the sense that we could, in theory, list all the members of the population from which the cases are derived. It would be clear to us that controls should be sampled only from residents of the region. Sometimes, however, cases are selected from all persons who come to a group of hospitals, regardless of where they live or even where they were injured. We must now think of the source population in more hypothetical terms: all persons who would use these hospitals if they were similarly injured. Sampling controls from this source population would be difficult, because visitors to the local region, as well as some persons who live at considerable distance from the region, should be sampled. Hospital-based case–control studies try to obviate this difficulty by selecting controls referred to the same group of hospitals for conditions other than the outcome that defines the cases. Because referral and admission patterns might be very different for different conditions, it would be hard to be confident that any group of hospitalized patients could represent the exposure prevalence of the hypothetical controls.

It is important to define the source population for the cases as clearly as possible, in order to facilitate our ability to decide who should be selected or excluded as a potential control. In defining the source population, we should consider the manner in which we will select controls. If, for example, we plan to select controls by using random digit dialing (Hartge et al., 1984), then the source population should consist of persons who have residential telephones; cases without residential telephones should be excluded from the study, as they did not arise from the study population (Greenberg, 1990; Potthoff, 1994). Similarly, if information is to be collected through interviews, and if the interviewers speak only English, then the source population must be restricted to English-speaking persons. Restricting the source population may mean that the study results cannot be generalized to some groups of persons. This is a small price to pay, however, for decreasing the potential for bias in the study. Valid results describe associations in the study population and perhaps other populations; biased results do not describe associations in any population.

Selection of Cases

We are normally testing hypotheses about factors that may increase or decrease the incidence of injury, not the prevalence of persons with injury-related disabilities or a history of injury in the population. For injuries with long-term sequelae, such as head or spinal cord injuries, this can be an important distinction. Hence we normally prefer incident cases: persons with new injury during the defined study period. If prevalent cases are used, associations with exposure may merely reflect differences in the chronicity of, or survival with, the condition in relation to exposure.

The definition of a case depends on the question the investigators wish to answer. In studying head injuries incurred in bicycle crashes, it seems reasonable to include as cases persons with both fatal and nonfatal head injuries (Thompson et al., 1996). However, if we wish to study firearm ownership as a risk factor for suicide (Kellermann et al., 1992; Brent et al., 1993; Cummings and Koepsell, 1998), there are several reasons for not including suicide attempts in the study. Chief among these is that this outcome may be thought of as a success, a suicide effort that failed. If gun ownership truly increases the risk of death by suicide, this might occur because using a gun is a more lethal method than, say, taking pills. Because of this, gun owners might be more likely to complete a suicide compared with other persons. Including as cases persons who attempted suicide will not help us estimate any association between gun ownership and death by suicide.

In selecting cases, we should consider the step in the causal chain that we wish to study. For example, suppose we wish to study the properties of footwear that may be associated with hip fractures. If features of shoes are related to the risk of having a hip fracture, they probably do so by making it more or less likely that someone will fall. As falls are much more common than hip fractures, it may be perfectly reasonable to choose as cases people who fall, regardless of whether or not they break their hip. This would make it much easier for us to study shoe-related factors that contribute to the risk of falling, and by inference, to the risk of hip fracture. On the other hand, suppose that we wish to study the association between wearing padded clothing and the risk of hip fracture. Padding over the hip is probably unrelated to the risk of falling, but may exert an influence over whether or not the hip fractures when a fall occurs. Therefore, to study this exposure, we will want to choose as cases those persons with hip fractures.

It is not required that we study only one step in the causal chain of events. For example, in a study of fires, Runyan et al. (1992) chose as cases those households that experienced one or more fire-related deaths. Controls were sampled from other households that experienced a fire, but had no resulting death. The authors reported that a death was more likely in a residence without a smoke detector: risk ratio 3.4. This study examined only one step in the causal chain: given a fire, did a death result? In another study of fires, Ballard et al. (1992) chose as cases households which had a death or injury due to a fire. The controls were other households contacted by random digit dialing; these residences had had no fire. The authors reported that the risk of a household fire injury was greater in residences with someone who smoked compared with other homes: risk ratio 4.8. This study combined two steps of the causal chain in one study: first a fire had to occur, then an injury had to result.

Whether we study one or more steps in the chain of injury causation may often depend on practical considerations. For example, in the hypothetical study of life vests that we described earlier in the review of case–control study design, we might really wish to study the association of life vests with drowning given that a boater falls into the water. It seems likely that if life vests have any influence on the risk of drowning, this is confined to what happens after the boater is in the water. But finding controls who have fallen out of their boat into the water may be very difficult. We may decide, therefore, to measure life vest use among control boaters who are still in their boats, and then account for the confounding influence of weather, boater age, alcohol use, and other factors that might influence both the likelihood of falling out of a boat and the likelihood of drowning once the boater is in the water.

Cases need not be persons. In the fire-related examples above, cases were households, rather than individuals. One of us studied injuries to elderly pedestrians by defining a case as an intersection where an elderly pedestrian was struck by a vehicle. Other intersections were selected as controls. Characteristics of intersections were measured, such as the frequency with which they were traversed by both pedestrians and vehicles, the paint pattern of the cross-walks, and the timing of the traffic lights. Similarly, a study of drowning and pool fencing might define a case as a pool in which a child drowned.

Cases may be found from many sources, such as the office of the medical examiner or police crash reports. As persons who suffer a serious injury often present to an emergency department, this setting is an appealing one for collecting injury cases (Cummings et al., 1998). For economy, it is also attractive to collect controls from the same source. A few case–control studies of injury have drawn both cases and controls from emergency department patients. Five studies of the protective effect of bicycle helmets selected persons with head injuries sustained in bicycle crashes as cases, using other persons injured in bicycle crashes who did not sustain a head injury as controls (Thompson et al., 1996). Schieber et al. (1996) used a similar design to examine whether wrist guards prevented wrist injuries among persons who fell while in-line skating.

Whether cases can be adequately sampled from one or several emergency departments, however, may depend on the type of injury. In a study of hazards in day-care, investigators defined a case as a child who visited a health professional for an injury which occurred in day-care; only 42% of these children were taken to an emergency department (Cummings et al., 1996). Day-care injuries are frequently minor and therefore emergency departments alone are inadequate locations for ascertainment of many cases. Conversely, injured persons who die at the scene may be taken to the medical examiner, not an emergency department. In a study of gunshot injuries in Memphis, Seattle, and Galveston, 11% of 1915 wounded persons died at the scene (Kellermann et al., 1996). A case–control study might also seek cases brought to the coroner or medical examiner for a geographic region. In a study of bicycle-helmet effectiveness, 3849 injured bicyclists were identified in seven emergency departments and five additional cases were identified by the medical examiner's office (Thompson et al., 1996). If one is willing to limit cases to those with injuries severe enough to use an emergency department, and possibly supplement case-finding by seeking those who die at the scene, one or several emergency departments can be an excellent location for identifying persons with injuries.

Bias in case ascertainment can arise if the exposure of interest has an important effect on the likelihood that a case will be identified, independent of the exposure's effect on the occurrence of injury. This bias might arise, for example, if we decided to study whether intoxication with alcohol was associated with injuries due to assault. It is easy to imagine that alcohol might be associated with assault-related injury; persons who are intoxicated might be less able to defend themselves against assault and they might be more likely to provoke disputes. But aside from the injuries that a person might suffer in a beating, the person's use of alcohol might influence the decision to come to seek medical care. Friends or paramedics might fear that the victim's slurred speech could be due to brain injury, rather than alcohol, or they might insist on transport to the hospital because otherwise the beaten victim would simply sleep in the street. If these events occur, intoxicated assault victims will be more likely to use an emergency department than sober victims, even if their injuries are the same. The result will be that intoxicated persons will be over-represented among emergency department assault victims, making it appear that alcohol use increases the risk of assault-related injury. This form of bias was pointed out by Berkson (1946); he noted that two diseases can falsely appear to be associated in a hospital-based study because each independently affects the likelihood of admission. This bias will arise with only some exposures; if the exposure of interest is bicycle safety helmets, then aside from the presence or absence of a head injury, it seems doubtful that helmet-use status would influence the decision to come to a hospital. The crucial point is that one should try to select cases in a way that is not influenced by the exposure, aside from the exposure's influence on the likelihood of injury.

Selection of Controls

In principle, controls should be a sample of persons from the same population from which the cases were derived. They are persons who would have been ascertained as cases had they suffered the injury under study (Rothman, 1986, pp. 64–8; Wacholder et al., 1992a, b). Collecting a suitable group of controls is often a vexing problem. Population-based community studies, which may obtain controls by random digit dialing (Potthoff, 1994) or by canvassing neighborhoods on foot (Kellermann et al., 1993; Rivara et al., 1997), can be very expensive. In some populations, a roster of members can simplify control selection; for example, a list of persons in a health plan (Cummings et al., 1997) or employees of a large company.

Locating controls at the site where the injury occurred has been a method used in some studies (Haddon et al., 1961; Smith and Houser, 1994). For example, McCarroll and Haddon (1962) had information regarding the blood alcohol level of 43 drivers who died in crashes in New York City. In 1960 they returned to the site of each crash on the same day of the week and at about the same time of day as the crash. Using a random method, they had police officers stop six passenger vehicles for each case and requested that drivers submit to a breath alcohol test. Remarkably, only one of 259 drivers refused to cooperate with the study.

The first case–control study of bicycle helmets chose as cases people who came to a group of emergency departments in Seattle, Washington, with a head injury sustained in a bicycle crash (Thompson et al., 1989). The authors felt their ideal control group would be selected from bicyclists who crashed and who would have attended a study emergency department had they suffered a head injury. But most cyclists who crash never seek medical attention, because they have no or only minor injuries. The investigators therefore turned to a group that they felt would approximate the prevalence of helmet wearing and other characteristics of the ideal controls: they sought information from persons who came to the same emergency departments with cycling injuries that did not involve the head.

Some cyclists who crash will avoid a serious injury because they were wearing a helmet, and therefore they will not be ascertained in an emergency department based study (Cummings et al., 1998). Will this bias the results? We have created hypothetical data for a population of bicycle crash victims (Table 11.3). Cyclists in column A have serious head injuries and they should be identified as cases in the emergency departments (or by the medical examiner). The goal is to compare the prevalence of helmet use in head injury victims (0.2, say) with that of cyclists who crash without head injury (columns B + C). Cyclists in group B have some other injury, so they will be seen in emergency departments, where their helmet use can be determined. Persons in group C avoided a serious injury, so they will not be available. However, it is reasonable to expect that a comparison of helmet-wearing behavior between groups B and C would show little difference, because we would not expect helmet use to increase or decrease the risk of injury

Table 11.3 Hypothetical data from a case–control study of bicyclists who crashed. Each cell shows the number of cyclists and the proportion in each column who were helmeted or not. The column headings A through C designate each cyclist's injury classification

	Head injury	*No head injury*	
		(B)	(C)
	(A)	*Other injury*	*No other injury*
Helmeted	200 (0.2)	1000 (0.5)	100,000 (0.5)
Not helmeted	800 (0.8)	1000 (0.5)	100,000 (0.5)

to body sites other than the head. The total experience of the ideal controls, groups B + C, should be reasonably approximated by the experience of group B alone.

Our discussion of emergency department controls has been limited to an exposure which is thought to protect one body region, allowing control selection from persons engaged in the same activity who have an injury to another anatomical site. More commonly, we would like to assess the association between an exposure, such as seat belts, and injury to any part of a person's anatomy. As seatbelts might prevent injuries to any body part, the cases would be all persons brought to an emergency department after a car crash, plus persons who died at the scene. The ideal controls would be a random sample of persons in the community who are in a car crash, who would have come to the study emergency departments if they needed treatment; but only a few of these will come to any emergency department (Cummings et al., 1995). An investigator committed to using emergency department controls might try to eliminate from that group any conditions for which it is plausible to assume a possible association with the use of seat belts in a crash; for example, there is evidence that intoxicated drivers are less likely to use seat belts than other drivers, so the study might exclude intoxicated patients. Other people attending emergency departments for chest pain, fever, work injuries, and other problems may use seat belts as often as persons in the community who were occupants of a vehicle that crashed. If prevalence of seat belt use were similar in these groups, this would suggest that none of these conditions is associated with belt use. If the investigator discovered, after collecting the data, an unexpected association with any condition in the controls, consideration could be given to eliminating that group. However, we still could not entirely rule out the possibility that restraint use was atypical in people with all of the selected conditions, compared with the ideal control group.

If we wanted to study the association between drinking alcohol and assault, control selection in an emergency department would be unwise. So many health conditions may be related to the use of or abstinence from alcohol, that we are concerned that no group of emergency patients is likely to accurately represent the use of alcohol among the population that produced the cases.

In selecting cases or controls from one or more hospitals or emergency departments, one may want to remove referral bias introduced by a regional system of trauma care (Payne and Waller, 1989; Waller, 1989). One option would be to use a group of hospitals that provides care to essentially all persons in a given geographic region and exclude from selection any patients transferred from outside that defined area. Alternatively, one could limit the study to the members of a large health maintenance organization. The cases and controls would then be health plan members who used any study hospital.

Special Case–Control Designs
Proportional Mortality Studies

Some studies of traffic crashes have utilized information only from vehicle occupants who were dead (Zador and Ciccone, 1993; Braver et al., 1997). Imagine, for example, that we want to estimate the effect of air bags on the risk of death in a crash. Air bags are designed to operate and protect an occupant in a frontal crash, but not when the impact affects a vehicle from the side or rear. We now estimate two proportions: (1) among dead front-seat occupants who were exposed to air bags, what proportion of the deaths were in frontal crashes (as opposed to nonfrontal crashes)?; and (2) among dead front-seat occupants who were not exposed to air bags, what proportion died in frontal crashes? If air bags really work, we would expect that some deaths would be prevented, and therefore not appear as counts in our data, in frontal crashes; as a result, the first proportion should be smaller than the second.

In the epidemiology literature, this design is sometimes referred to as a proportional mortality study. As others have pointed out (Kelsey et al., 1996, pp. 179–83; Rothman and Greenland, 1998, pp. 76–7), these studies can be thought of as a type of case–control study. The cases are persons who died from an injury for which we believe the risk of death may be influenced by the presence or absence of the exposure of interest. In our example, the cases would be vehicle occupants who died in a frontal crash only. The ideal controls would be a random sample of other persons in similar crashes who did not die. These people are not available in fatal crash data, but if dashboard air bags do not protect or injure the passenger when a vehicle is struck from the side or the rear, air bags may not be associated with death in a nonfrontal crash. Therefore, the air bag exposure history of persons killed in nonfrontal crashes may serve as a reasonable estimate of the exposure of the ideal controls. Braver et al. (1997) studied front-seat passengers in 1992 through 1995 model-year cars (Table 11.4). The relative risk of death in a frontal crash was 0.82 (95% confidence interval, 0.67–1.00) for passengers exposed to an air bag compared with other passengers. By thinking of a proportional mortality study as a case–control study, authors can consider and possibly control for potential confounders in their data.

Case-crossover Studies

Maclure (1991) described the case-crossover study design. For short-term exposures that may acutely change the risk of an outcome, each case can serve as their

Table 11.4 Data from a study of car passenger deaths, classified according to presence of a passenger air bag and whether the crash was frontal or not. Column proportions shown in parentheses

Passenger air bag	Angle of impact	
	Frontal (case)	Not frontal (control)
Yes	336 (0.33)	288 (0.38)
No	668 (0.67)	470 (0.62)

own control. The exposure status of the case in some time interval before the injury outcome is compared with the same person's exposure status during some other suitable time period. The major advantages of this design are once the cases have been identified, no extra effort is needed to find the controls, and the study design can easily control for characteristics of individuals that do not change over a short time period. Case-crossover studies have examined transient factors that may be associated with myocardial infarction, such as physical exertion (Mittleman et al., 1993) and sexual activity (Muller et al., 1996). The case-crossover design seems suitable for many studies of injury, because many injury-related exposures are intermittent and brief, but to date only a few injury studies have used this method (Roberts et al., 1995a; Vinson et al., 1995; Barbone et al., 1998). Redelmeier and Tibshirani (1997) studied 699 drivers with cellular telephones who were in collisions; they compared the use of these telephones during the 10 minutes before the crash, as judged from computerized billing records, with use while driving during the same interval on the previous day. The proportion of drivers who had used their cellular telephone was 0.24 before the crash and only 0.05 on the previous day. The adjusted relative risk of a crash, given cellular telephone use, was 4.3 (95% confidence interval 3.0–6.5).

Confounding

Our goal is to estimate the association between an exposure and an outcome; specifically, we want an accurate relative risk estimate. When that estimate is erroneous because of failure to account for the effects of a third factor, we say that confounding is present. A confounding factor may obscure a true association when one exists, or create an apparent association when none is truly present. For a factor to confound an association, it must be associated with the outcome; that is, the risk of the outcome must differ for different levels of the confounding factor. Furthermore, a confounding factor must be associated with the exposure of interest. In conducting a case–control study, much effort usually goes into collecting information about potential confounding factors, and then examining these factors in the analysis, controlling for any that are found to be confounders in the collected data.

Imagine that in our hypothetical study of life vests and drowning (Table 11.2), we also had data regarding weather (Table 11.5). Predictably, boaters in stormy

Table 11.5 Results of a hypothetical case–control study of boaters and life vest use, stratified by weather

| | Outcome during 1 year | | | |
| | Stormy weather | | Calm Weather | |
Life vest use	Drowned	Controls	Drowned	Controls
Always	15	20	10	111
Never	15	10	135	384
Relative risk within stratum	RR = 0.50 (95% CI 0.18–1.40)		RR = 0.26 (95% CI 0.13–0.50)	
Adjusted relative risk	RR = 0.30 (95% CI 0.17–0.52)			

weather were more likely to drown compared with those in calm weather; 30 drowned in stormy weather and 30 control boaters were observed in similar rough weather, compared with 145 cases who died in calm weather and their 495 controls: relative risk 3.4. And the relative prevalence of vest use was sixfold greater among boaters in bad weather compared with boaters in calm weather. The crude relative risk of drowning among boaters with vests, compared with those without, was 0.50; we obtained this from the data in Table 11.2. But when we computed relative risks within each strata and summarized them using Mantel–Haenszel methods, the adjusted relative risk estimate was 0.30 (Table 11.5); the association of vest use with drowning was, therefore, confounded by weather.

The Use of Matching

Matching has been used in several case–control studies of injuries. For example, some studies have selected controls from other persons at road sites where a driver crashed (McCarroll and Haddon, 1962) or at the beach or harbor where a person drowned (Smith and Houser, 1994). Other studies matched closely on neighborhood of residence and other individual characteristics (Kellermann et al., 1992, 1993).

Matching can be done on an individual basis in which each case is matched to one or more controls. Alternatively, frequency matching may be done in which groups of controls are selected to be similar groups of cases, according to designated strata of a matching variable.

The justification for matching is related to both confounding and study efficiency. If a potential confounder is distributed in such a way that most cases are in one or several categories of the confounder and most controls are in other categories, study power may be compromised if the analysis must control for this factor. Study power may be enhanced if we use matching to force the cases and controls to overlap more in regard to the potential confounder.

Imagine, for example, that we wished to study the association between swimming lessons and drowning among children aged 1 through 4 years. Mortality due to drowning is higher among 1 year olds compared with 4 year olds. On the other hand,

4 year old children probably receive more swimming instruction than 1 year old children. As age is related to both the outcome and the exposure, it may confound the association that we hope to measure, and we may need to control for age in our analysis. Study power may be enhanced if the controls were distributed in age in a manner similar to the cases. The degree to which matching on age or any other factor may enhance, or impair, study efficiency is a function of the cost of finding controls, the cost of collecting the information, the distribution of the exposure and outcome with respect to the matching factor, and the degree to which the matching factor really is a confounder in the data. It is rare that the investigator will know all of this information with accuracy, but estimates may help in deciding whether matching is worthwhile or not.

There is no guarantee that matching will enhance efficiency; as one-to-one or one-to-many matching will usually require additional money and effort, we prefer to avoiding matching unless there is evidence that the extra effort will be rewarded. If matching is done, we suggest that it be limited to no more than one or two factors. If matching criteria are too numerous or stringent, the pool of potential controls may not even have a match; this will result in a loss of study power, as cases without controls will not contribute to the results.

In a randomized clinical trial, or a cohort study, matching the exposed and unexposed populations on one or more characteristics can decrease bias in the planned comparison. In a case–control study, however, we match those with and without the outcome; by selecting as controls only those who are like the cases in some respects, we may actually introduce bias in our measurement of exposure among noncases (MacMahon and Trichopoulos, 1996; Rothman and Greenland, 1998). Fortunately, as long as the analysis of the data accounts for any matching that occurred, relative risk estimates from case–control studies will not be biased by any matching that was done.

Exposure Measurement

Once we have selected our cases and controls, we must measure their exposure history (Armstrong et al., 1992). Any case–control study may find difficulty in eliciting accurate information about exposure; studies of injury are not special in this regard. Injury studies may differ, however, in that they sometimes need to examine very short periods of exposure. In a study of child pedestrian injury, Roberts and Lee-Joe (1993) classified traffic flow as large or small depending on whether or not 600 or more vehicles per hour passed the collision site in a given time interval. When the time interval was 24 hours, the relative risk of being struck was 5.6, but when the time interval was only the 3 hours that centered on the time the collision occurred, the relative risk estimate was much larger, 14.5. This suggests that traffic flow near the actual time of the collision is more relevant to the risk of being hit than traffic flows at all hours of the day.

Sometimes a case–control study is fortunate in that the information about exposure was recorded before the outcome; differential recall of information about the cases and controls is not of concern. If the exposure information is already entered into a computer, the investigator may have the luxury of analyzing the data either as a case–control or cohort study (Cummings et al., 1994; Scholer et al., 1997). More commonly, however, information about cases and controls must be obtained from self-report. Self-report may be inaccurate because events may be forgotten, admirable behaviors may be exaggerated, and behaviors that are socially unacceptable may be denied. Thus, for example, drivers might forget about their recent use of a medication, exaggerate their use of seat belts, and deny their use of alcohol while driving. When errors in recall are not systematically different between cases and controls, a study will erroneously classify some exposed persons as unexposed and visa versa. Except in certain circumstances (Dosemeci et al., 1990; Wacholder, 1995), nondifferential misclassification of exposure will tend to bias the relative risk estimate toward the null value of 1.

Differential misclassification of exposure may arise if the case subjects, by virtue of their injury, devote considerable thought to their exposure history, while the controls, who have no special stimulus to promote recall, devote less energy to recalling past details of their lives. This type of information bias, sometimes called recall bias, can cause the estimate of association to deviate in either direction from the correct value.

In the interest of obtaining accurate exposure information, investigators resort to several strategies. Interview forms and technique should be standardized as much as possible for cases and controls. Questions about the key exposures may be placed among other questions so that the study subject does not focus unduly on the most critical exposures. Indeed, the exposure of greatest interest may not be explicitly stated to the study subjects and the interviewers. If asking about behaviors that are illegal or not socially acceptable, questions may be introduced with a permissive statement (Kellermann et al., 1993): for example, Many people have quarrels or fights. Has anyone in this household ever been hit or hurt in a fight in the home?

Unlike some studies of cancer, the interval between disease onset and death is usually very short for studies of injury. For studies with fatal cases, therefore, information must be obtained from relatives or other proxies for the case. Proxies might report different information than the cases themselves would report if they were available. For example, if a man died, his wife might be more forthcoming about his heavy drinking habit than he would have been himself; or she might not be aware of his use of illicit drugs. Depending on the exposure, the proxies might systematically report more or less exposure than the case would have reported. For this reason, some investigators have used proxy respondents both for the dead cases and the living controls (Walker et al., 1988; Nelson et al., 1990).

Analysis

Case-control studies are designed to generate odds ratios that approximate the desired relative risk estimates. Generating an odds ratio from a 2×2 table is easy and formulas for the appropriate confidence intervals are described in many texts

(Breslow and Day, 1980; Kleinbaum et al., 1982; Schlesselman, 1982; Rothman and Greenland, 1998). When matching has been used and exposure is classified into only two categories, this can still be accounted for in a 2×2 table; the table now shows the counts of agreement and disagreement in exposure for the four categories of case–control status and exposure status. Only the counts of the discordant pairs contribute to the odds ratio estimate.

When confounders must be controlled in an analysis, Mantel-Haenszel stratified methods provide an excellent method for doing this (Emerson, 1994). In Table 11.5, data regarding drowning and life vest status were presented in two tables, one for each stratum of weather. A separate odds ratio was generated within each stratum, and these odds ratios were then summarized using a Mantel-Haenszel weighted average. A stratified analysis of this type is an excellent choice for many studies. Even if logistic regression methods are to be used, examining stratified tables of the data can help guide the analysis and presenting these tables may help the reader understand the results. Software for carrying out the computations is available for free in Epi Info, a DOS-based software package developed by the Centers for Disease Control and Prevention in Atlanta, Georgia; the software can be downloaded from http://www.cdc.gov

Logistic regression is often used for the analysis of case–control data (Breslow and Day, 1980; Kleinbaum, 1992). When specific case patients are matched to specific control patients, conditional logistic regression can account for this matching. These regression methods provide the analyst with considerable flexibility in expressing exposure and controlling for confounding (Greenland, 1995).

In studies of nonfatal injuries, a study subject might appear as a case more than once. In order to account for the fact that observations may be clustered within an individual, and not independent in a statistical sense, the analyst can use robust variance estimators in logistic regression; this is sometimes referred to as the sandwich or Huber–White estimator (Greene, 1997, pp. 503–6), or the linearization method (Levy and Lemeshow, 1999, pp. 365–70). The estimate of association will be the same, but the estimated variance will usually be greater. This variance estimator is widely used in the survey literature.

Conclusions

Because of their relative efficiency compared with other study designs, case–control studies will continue to provide useful information about factors that cause or prevent injuries. Variations on this design, such as the case-crossover study, will likely become more common. In planning these studies, investigators should try to define the population, even if hypothetical, from which the cases arise. The step in the causal chain that is being studied should be defined. Cases should be selected in a manner that is not influenced by exposure history, independent of the exposure's effect on the outcome. Controls should be selected to represent the exposure of the study population members that are not cases. Matching controls to cases may be justified if it promises to enhance study efficiency or to control for factors that cannot otherwise be measured.

References

Armenian HK (ed.) (1994) Applications of the case–control method. Epidemiol Rev 16(1).

Armstrong BK, White E, Saracci R (1992) Principles of Exposure Measurement in Epidemiology. New York: Oxford University Press.

Ballard JE, Koepsell TD, Rivara F (1992) Association of smoking and alcohol drinking with residential fire injuries. Am J Epidemiol 135(1):26–34.

Barbone F, McMahon AD, Davey PG, Morris AD, Reid IC, McDevitt DG, MacDonald TM (1998) Association of road-traffic accidents with benzodiazepine use. Lancet 352:1331–6.

Berkson J (1946) Limitations of the application of fourfold table analysis to hospital data. Biometrics 2:47–53.

Braver ER, Ferguson SA, Greene MA, Lund AK (1997) Reductions in deaths in frontal crashes among right front passengers in vehicles equipped with passenger air bags. JAMA 278:1437–9.

Brent DA, Perper JA, Allman CJ, Moritz GM, Wartella ME, Zelenak JP (1991) The presence and accessibility of firearms in the homes of adolescent suicides: a case–control study. JAMA 266(21):2989–95.

Brent DA, Perper JA, Moritz G, Baugher M, Schweers J, Roth C (1993) Firearms and adolescent suicide: a community based case–control study. Am J Dis Child 147:1066–71.

Breslow NE, Day NE (1980) Statistical Methods in Cancer Research. Volume 1 – The Analysis of Case–Control Studies. Lyon, France: International Agency for Research on Cancer.

Cornfield J (1951) A method of estimating comparative rates from clinical data. Applications to cancer of the lung, breast, and cervix. J Natl Canc Inst 11:1269–75.

Cummings P, Koepsell TD (1998) Does owning a firearm increase or decrease the risk of death? JAMA 280(5):471–3.

Cummings P, Theis MK, Mueller BA, Rivara FP (1994) Infant injury death in Washington State, 1981 through 1990. Arch Pediatr Adolesc Med 148:1021–6.

Cummings P, Koepsell TD, Mueller BA (1995) Methodological challenges in injury epidemiology and injury prevention research. Annu Rev Public Health 16:381–400.

Cummings P, Rivara FP, Boase J, MacDonald JK (1996) Injuries and their relation to potential hazards in child day care. Injury Prev 2:105–8.

Cummings P, Koepsell TD, Grossman DG, Savarino J, Thompson RS (1997) The association between purchase of a handgun and homicide or suicide. Am J Public Health 87:974–8.

Cummings P, Koepsell TD, Weiss NS (1998) Studying injuries with case–control methods in the emergency department. Ann Emerg Med 31(1):99–105.

Dosemeci M, Wacholder S, Lubin JH (1990) Does nondifferential misclassification of exposure always bias a true effect toward the null value? Am J Epidemiol 132(4):746–8.

Emerson JD (1994) Combining estimates of the odds ratio: the state of the art. Stat Methods Med Res 3:157–78.

Greenberg ER (1990) Random digit dialing for control selection: a review and a caution on its use in studies of childhood cancer. Am J Epidemiol 131(1):1–5.

Greene WH (1997) Econometric Analysis, 3rd edn. Upper Saddle River, NJ: Prentice Hall.

Greenland S (1995) Dose-response and trend analysis in epidemiology: alternatives to categorical analysis. Epidemiology 6:356–65.

Haddon W Jr, Valien P, McCarroll JR, Umberger CJ (1961) A controlled investigation of the characteristics of adult pedestrians fatally injured by motor vehicles in Manhattan. J Chronic Dis 14:655–78.

Hartge P, Brinton LA, Rosenthal JF, Cahill JI, Hoover RN, Waksberg J (1984) Random digit dialing in selecting a population-based control group. Am J Epidemiol 120(6): 825–33.

Holcomb RL (1938) Alcohol in relation to traffic accidents. J Am Med Assoc 111(12):1076–85.

Inter-Governmental Working Party on Swimming Pool Safety. (1988) Preschool Drowning in Private Swimming Pools. East Perth, Australia: Health Department of Western Australia.

Kellermann AL, Rivara FP, Somes G, Reay DT, Francisco J, Banton JG, Prodzinski J, Fligner C, Hackman BB (1992) Suicide in the home in relation to gun ownership. N Engl J Med 327(7):467–72.

Kellermann AL, Rivara FP, Rushforth NB, Banton JG, Reay DT, Francisco JT, Locci AB, Prodzinski J, Hackman BB, Somes G (1993) Gun ownership as a risk factor for homicide in the home. N Engl J Med 329(15):1084–91.

Kellermann AL, Rivara FP, Lee RK, Banton JG, Cummings P, Hackman BB, Somes G (1996) Injuries due to firearms in three cities. N Engl J Med 335:1438–44.

Kelsey JL, Whittemore AS, Evans AS, Thompson WD (1996) Methods in Observational Epidemiology, 2nd edn. New York: Oxford University Press.

Kleinbaum DG (1992) Logistic Regression: a Self-Learning Text. New York: Springer-Verlag.

Kleinbaum DG, Kupper LL, Morgenstern H (1982) Epidemiologic Research: Principles and Quantitative Methods. New York: Van Nostrand Reinhold.

Levy PS, Lemeshow S (1999) Sampling of Populations: Methods and Applications, 3rd edn. New York: John Wiley.

Maclure M. (1991) The case-crossover design: a method for studying transient effects on the risk of acute events. Am J Epidemiol 133:144–53.

MacMahon B, Trichopoulos D (1996) Epidemiology: Principles and Methods, 2nd edn. Boston: Little, Brown.

Mantel N, Haenszel W (1959) Statistical aspects of the analysis of data from retrospective studies. J Natl Cancer Inst 22:719–48.

McCarroll JR, Haddon W Jr (1962) A controlled study of fatal automobile accidents in New York City. J Chronic Dis 15:811–26.

Mittleman MA, Maclure M, Tofler GH, Sherwood JB, Goldberg RJ, Muller JE (1993) Triggering of acute myocardial infarction by heavy physical exertion: protection against triggering by regular exertion. N Engl J Med 329(23):1677–83.

Muller JE, Mittleman MA, Maclure M, Sherwood JB, Tofler GH (1996) Triggering myocardial infarction by sexual activity: low absolute risk and prevention by regular physical exertion. JAMA 275:1405–9.

Nelson LM, Longstreth WT Jr, Koepsell TD, van Belle G (1990) Proxy respondents in epidemiologic research. Epidemiol Rev 12:71–86.

Payne SR, Waller JA (1989) Trauma registry and trauma center biases in injury research. J Trauma 29:424–9.

Potthoff RF (1994) Telephone sampling in epidemiologic research: to reap the benefits, avoid the pitfalls. Am J Epidemiol 139(10):967–78.

Redelmeier DA, Tibshirani RJ (1997) Association between cellular-telephone calls and motor vehicle collisions. N Engl J Med 336(7):453–8.

Rivara FP, Mueller BA, Somes G, Mendoza C, Rushforth NB, Kellermann AL (1997) Alcohol and drug abuse and the risk of violent death in the home. JAMA 278(7):569–75.

Roberts I (1995) Methodologic issues in injury case–control studies. Epidemiology 1(1):45–8.

Roberts I, Lee-Joe T (1993) Effect of exposure measurement error in a case–control study of child pedestrian injuries. Epidemiology 4(5):477–9.

Roberts I, Marshall R, Lee-Joe T (1995a) The urban traffic environment and the risk of child pedestrian injury: a case-crossover approach. Epidemiology 6(2):169–71.

Roberts I, Norton R, Jackson R (1995b) Driveway-related child pedestrian injuries: a case–control study. Pediatrics 95(3):405–8.

Rothman KJ (1986) Modern Epidemiology, 1st edn. Boston: Little, Brown and Company.

Rothman KJ, Greenland S (1998) Modern Epidemiology, 2nd edn. Philadelphia: Lippincott-Raven.

Runyan CW, Bankdiwala SI, Linzer MA, Sacks JJ, Butts J (1992) Risk factors for fatal residential fires. N Engl J Med 327:859–63.

Schieber RA, Branche-Dorsey CM, Ryan GW, Rutherford GW Jr, Stevens JA, O'Neil J (1996) Risk factors for injuries from in-line skating and the effectiveness of safety gear. N Engl J Med 335:1630–5.

Schlesselman JA (1982) Case–control Studies: Design, Conduct, Analysis. New York: Oxford University Press.

Scholer SJ, Mitchel EF Jr, Ray WA (1997) Predictors of injury mortality in early childhood. Pediatrics 100(3):342–7.

Smith GS, Houser J (1994) Risk factors for drowning: a case–control study [abstract], p. 323. Abstracts of the 122nd Annual Meeting of the American Public Health Association. Washington, DC: American Public Health Association.

Thompson DC, Rivara FP, Thompson RS (1996) Effectiveness of bicycle helmets in preventing head injuries: a case–control study. JAMA 276(24):1968–73.

Thompson RS, Rivara FP, Thompson DC (1989) A case–control study of the effectiveness of bicycle safety helmets. N Engl J Med 320:1361–7.

Vinson DC, Mabe N, Leonard LL, Alexander J, Becker J, Boyer J, Moll J (1995) Alcohol and injury: a case-crossover study. Arch Fam Med 4:505–11.

Wacholder S (1995) When measurement errors correlate with truth: surprising effects of non-differential misclassification. Epidemiology 1995(6):157–61.

Wacholder S, McLaughlin JK, Silverman DT, Mandel JS (1992a) Selection of controls in case–control studies. I. Principles. Am J Epidemiol 135:1019–28.

Wacholder S, Silverman DT, McLaughlin JK, Mandel JS (1992b) Selection of controls in case–control studies. II. Types of controls. Am J Epidemiol 135:1029–41.

(1992c) Selection of controls in case–control studies. III. Design options. Am J Epidemiol 135:1042–50.

Walker AM, Velema JP, Robins JM (1988) Analysis of case–control data derived in part from proxy respondents. Am J Epidemiol 127:905–14.

Waller JA (1989) Methodologic issues in hospital-based injury research. J Trauma 28:1632–6.

Zador PL, Ciccone M (1993) Automobile driver fatalities in frontal impacts: air bags compared with manual belts. Am J Public Health 83:661–6.

12

Ecologic Studies

Ralph Hingson, Jonathan Howland, Thomas D. Koepsell, and Peter Cummings

Introduction

Ecologic studies are investigations in which groups, rather than individuals, are the units of analysis (Morgenstern, 1995). Typically, the groups under study are the resident populations of geopolitical areas such as states, counties, or census tracts; but in principle, studies of other kinds of groups, such as students in certain schools or employees in certain workplaces, would also qualify as ecologic. Studies that involve random assignment of social groups en bloc to alternative conditions also fit our definition of ecologic studies, but for convenience we consider them to be a special kind of randomized trial, as discussed in Chapter 9; here, we consider only observational ecologic studies. Morgenstern (1982, 1995, 1998) has written useful reviews of the ecologic study design.

As an introductory example, Anderson et al. (1998) studied neighborhood environmental factors in relation to the incidence of injuries resulting in hospitalization or death among Hispanic and non-Hispanic white children in Orange County, California. During 1991–92, injury surveillance was conducted at eight local hospitals and in the county coroner's office. Child injuries by age and ethnicity were counted for each of 594 census block groups, which ranged from three to 20 city blocks in size. The estimated number of children at risk and certain sociodemographic characteristics of each block group, including household crowding and the proportion of families with income below the federal poverty level, were obtained from the U.S. census data. Poisson regression was then used to examine the relationship of injury incidence in each block group to its sociodemographic characteristics. Among non-Hispanic white children, high levels of household crowding and of poverty proved to be the strongest correlates of injury incidence across block groups, while rates among Hispanic children were essentially unrelated to neighborhood crowding and were actually lower in poorer neighborhoods. The researchers concluded that neighborhood environmental risk factors for injury may vary importantly by ethnicity. Other examples of ecologic studies of injury include studies by Jacobsen et al. (1992, 1993) of the association between water fluoridation and hip fracture rates and by Killias (1993) of the relation between firearm ownership and rates of homicide and suicide.

Uses of the Ecologic Study Design
Study of Group-level Associations as a Surrogate for Individual-level Associations

Often the primary goal of injury research involves determining whether persons with a certain exposure differ from other persons in their risk of experiencing a certain injury-related outcome. Although scientific interest may focus on the association between exposure and outcome at the individual-person level, data on exposure and outcome for a sufficient number of individuals may be unavailable and obtainable only at high cost. Group-level data on the exposure and outcome, however, may be much less costly to obtain. Injury mortality data, for example, are routinely collected and readily available. Aggregate data regarding many exposures, such as ownership of smoke detectors, may be available from routinely conducted population surveys. It may then be relatively inexpensive to study whether geographic areas with a high prevalence of smoke detectors also have low mortality due to household fires. Prentice and Sheppard (1995) also noted that within-area variation in exposure may sometimes be inadequate to permit adequate estimation of individual-level associations within populations, particularly in the presence of measurement error, while between-area variation in exposure may be much greater, favoring an ecologic study design. Exploratory ecologic studies may also be a useful source of hypotheses about individual-level associations that can be followed up in studies that use individuals as the units of measurement and analysis.

Study of Individual Exposures that Affect Risk to Others

Many people are injured because of the behavior of others. For example, half of the 13,000 people who died in crashes involving speeding drivers in 1997 were persons other than the speeding drivers (NHTSA, 1998a), and 40% of people who died in crashes involving drinking drivers were persons other than the drinking driver (Hingson, 1996). In a similar vein, the full population impact of smoke detectors may not be revealed by a study that examines only individual- or household-level associations between presence of a smoke detector and fire injury, because a smoke detector in one dwelling unit may prevent injuries in other nearby units. Under these circumstances, a narrow focus on individual-level associations may miss important spillover effects. Ecologic studies, in contrast, may detect them.

Study of Group-level Exposures

Communities or states often enact legislation or promulgate regulations designed to influence behavioral risk factors for injury. Examples include changes in speed limits, safety belt and child restraint laws, drunk driving legislation, boating laws, requiring fencing around swimming pools, fire codes, gun regulations, alcohol control laws, drug laws, and penalties for intentional assaults and murder. Likewise, community-based intervention programs often target all residents of a certain area or members of some predefined social group. Studies of the effectiveness of these interventions may thus involve determining whether presence of the law, policy, or program in a population is associated with a lower rate of adverse outcomes in that population. Because primary scientific interest focuses on group-level associations, ecologic studies are well matched to this purpose.

Use of ecologic study designs for evaluation of laws and policies is a particularly important application of this methodology in injury research because of the attractiveness of legal intervention as a strategy for injury control. There are many instances of the use of laws to prevent injuries where educational programs alone had proven ineffective. For example, prior to the passage of seat belt laws, years of educational programs in the United States had produced belt use rates of only about 20% among motor-vehicle occupants. Forty-nine states have since adopted mandatory safety belt legislation, and safety belt use is currently over 60% nationwide and averages 70% in states that permit police to stop vehicles whenever they observe unbelted occupants (NHTSA, 1998b). Such findings are consistent with deterrence theory, which posits that people will be less likely to engage in a particular behavior if they believe they are likely to be apprehended and that penalties for engaging in the behavior are certain, swift, and severe (Ross, 1982). The deterrent effect of laws may reduce both the likelihood of initiating a dangerous behavior and the likelihood of resuming that behavior after having been punished for an initial infraction (Hingson, 1996a). Public debate that precedes passage of a law can also increase public awareness and salience of the injury issue in question, educate the public about behaviors that contribute to an injury, and disseminate the rationale for making those behaviors illegal. Sometimes legal interventions are aimed at institutional rather than individual behavior, as when safety standards are directed at manufacturers of automobiles, guns, recreational equipment, and other products.

Design Considerations in Ecologic Studies
Types of Ecologic Studies

Morgenstern (1995) has classified ecologic studies into three broad categories.

Multiple Groups Studied Cross-sectionally in Time

As applied to injury, the first category includes multiple-group studies that compare injury rates among several areas at the same point or period of time. The study described above by Anderson et al. (1998) of injuries in Hispanic and non-Hispanic children in California exemplifies this kind of ecologic study. In the context of evaluating laws, another example could involve comparing traffic crash mortality rates in a given year among several states, each classified according to the relative stiffness of penalties for driving while intoxicated.

As in other kinds of observational studies, there is a risk of being unable to control for potential confounding factors that may influence the frequency of the injury under study beyond the laws of interest, such as demographic characteristics, cultural norms regarding alcohol, or effects of other laws. Morgenstern (1982) points out that studying a larger number of smaller areas can offer advantages over studying a few large areas in terms of statistical power and ability to control for confounding factors.

Single Group Studied Over Time

The second category includes studies that compare injury rates over time in a single defined population. For example, Jacobsen et al. (1993) found that the incidence of hip fracture in Rochester, Minnesota was about 37% lower during the 10 years after fluoridation of the city's water supply, compared with the preceding 10 years. Chiu et al. (1997), found that the frequency of clinic visits in Barrow, Alaska, was strongly related to changes in local laws about whether alcohol could be legally sold in the village. By using the study population as its own control over time, this kind of ecologic study helps avoid confounding by factors that may vary across communities. However, it may be difficult to exclude the possibility that other historical factors besides changes in the law or other exposure of main interest account for part or all of the observed change in injury rates.

Multiple Groups Studied Over Time

The third category includes studies that combine features of the first two categories. Hingson et al. (1994) used such a design to study whether lowering the legal blood alcohol limit for young drivers reduced the proportion of fatal crashes that involved only a single vehicle and occurred at night, these being much more likely than other crash types to be alcohol-related. Twelve states that had enacted lower limits were matched to 12 other nearby states without such laws. Pre-law and post-law changes in crash types were then calculated in states that had enacted a law and compared with concurrent changes in the matched states that had not. The findings suggested sharp reductions in nighttime single-vehicle crashes among young drivers in states that had enacted 0.00% or 0.02% limits, with little change in the matched comparison states. Little change was observed in crash types for adults above the ages targeted by the new laws.

When suitable data are available, this design can be further strengthened by statistical modeling of secular trends in injury rates or other outcomes in exposed and nonexposed areas. For example, Cummings et al. (1997) studied the effect of state laws that make gun owners criminally liable for injuries inflicted by children who gain unsupervised access to a gun. Annual child deaths due to firearms and population-size data by age, gender, and race were obtained for all 50 states and the District of Columbia for the years 1979–94. After statistical adjustment for temporal trends, unintentional firearm-related deaths in children were 23% lower than expected in states with safe-storage laws during the years when the laws were in effect.

Measurement of Exposure, Outcome, and Covariates

When measurements on all study variables are available only at the group level, their joint distribution at the individual level is unknown. However, just because the exposure may be measured ecologically does not mean all other variables must also be measured in that way. Morgenstern (1995) has argued that it is advantageous to have individual-level data on as many relevant measures as possible. For example, in the study of gun safe storage laws just described, the age, gender, and race of each victim were known, as was the demographic composition of each state. Thus, it was possible to gain better control over these potentially confounding factors than would have been possible had only aggregate data been available.

Analysis

Although several statistical approaches have been used for analysis of ecologic data, some potential pitfalls of relatively simple methods have not always been appreciated. Fortunately, newer methods of analysis make it easy to avoid these pitfalls. Imagine a study of seat belt use in relation to crash fatality for drivers. Group-level data are available for 25 regions on the number of drivers killed, the number of crashes, and the number of drivers in crashes who were restrained by a seat belt. A simple form of ecologic analysis would use a linear regression model in which the dependent (or outcome) variable is the region-specific proportion of drivers who died, and the independent (or exposure) variable is the region-specific proportion of drivers who were belted. One problem with this analysis is that the numbers of eligible drivers are likely to differ among regions, resulting in variable levels of precision in the group-level proportions being used in the regression, which violates the homoscedasticity assumption. In principle, this problem can be circumvented by weighted regression. Yet a subtler problem is that the analysis is based on two ratios for each region, one representing the proportion of drivers who die, the other the proportion of drivers who are restrained. Each ratio has the same denominator: the number of drivers involved in a crash. The use of ratios with common (or even related) denominators can create spurious correlations (Kronmal, 1993). Fortunately, regression models for count data, such as Poisson or negative binomial regression, avoid this source of artifact. This preferred statistical approach, as described in the chapter by Cummings and Norton (this volume), would use the count of deaths as the outcome, the count of belted drivers as the exposure of interest, and the number of crashes as an offset variable.

When at least some individual-level data are available, the statistical analysis can become more complex but also potentially more informative. Multi-level modeling (Bryk and Raudenbush, 1992; Von Korff et al., 1992; Morgenstern, 1998) provides flexible statistical tools for analysis of data in which measurements are made at the individual, group, and perhaps additional levels.

Threats to Validity in Ecologic Studies

Campbell and Stanley (1966), in their classic book on experimental and quasi-experimental designs, identified several kinds of potential bias that need to be considered when choosing among alternative study designs. We focus here on concerns of special relevance to ecologic studies, particularly when they are used for evaluating legal interventions, drawing freely on the Campbell and Stanley formulation.

Ecologic Bias

Associations observed at one level of aggregation do not necessarily imply corresponding associations at other levels. Ecologic bias (also sometimes called the ecologic fallacy or cross-level bias) occurs when an investigator incorrectly interprets group-level associations as reflecting individual-level relationships. This problem was first identified nearly 50 years ago by Robinson (1950).

A classic injury-related example of ecologic bias is based on the work of Emile Durkheim (1951), a nineteenth century sociologist who investigated the relationship between religion and suicide in Prussian provinces. The example is discussed in detail by Morgenstern (1995). Briefly, Durkheim found that suicide rates in these provinces had a strong positive association with the proportion of Protestants in each province. The ecologic data suggest about an eightfold increase in suicide risk associated with Protestantism. However, each province consisted of a known mixture of Protestants and non-Protestants, and data were available on the religion of each suicide victim. When Durkheim recalculated suicide rates by religion, the suicide rate among Protestants was only about twice that of members of other religious groups – still in the same direction, but a substantially weaker association. These apparently discrepant findings can be reconciled by noting that many suicides in predominantly Protestant provinces were in fact committed by non-Protestants (mainly Catholics) and accounted in large part for the higher rates.

Firebaugh (1978) showed that, under certain assumptions, a necessary and sufficient condition for absence of ecologic bias is that the group mean level of exposure (which, for a dichotomous exposure, would be its population prevalence) has no effect on outcome after controlling for exposure status at the individual level. Greenland and Morgenstern (1989) considered the more complex case in which the effect of exposure at the individual level varies by group (effect modification) and showed that ecologic bias can appear, even if the group-level exposure variable is unrelated to outcome. Unfortunately, individual-level data are often unavailable in ecologic studies, so that the degree to which ecologic bias is present in a grouped analysis cannot be determined from the available data alone. Our confidence that a grouped analysis may yield valid information at the individual level must therefore often rest on information from outside sources. One way to minimize ecologic bias is to keep the studied groups as small as possible; for example, one would expect less ecologic bias in a study conducted at the county, rather than state, level.

Because laws are population-based interventions, ecologic bias may be a less serious concern because the group-level associations themselves are of main interest. However, one must be cautious not to overinterpret such associations as indicating mechanisms of effect at the individual level. For example, tougher penalties for persons repeatedly arrested for drunk driving may not necessarily act by getting habitual offenders who are directly affected by the penalties off the road; instead, such laws may deter others from a first offense.

Measurement Error

As in other study designs, invalid and/or unreliable measures of exposure, outcome, or key covariates can bias the results of an ecologic study. In non-ecologic studies of individuals, nondifferential misclassification of exposure or disease classically tends to bias results toward the null. By contrast, in ecologic studies, Brenner et al. (1992), showed that nondifferential misclassification of a dichotomous exposure within groups can lead to bias away from the null, and sometimes markedly so. Greenland and Brenner (1993) described a method to correct for such misclassification if sensitivity and specificity characteristics of the measure in question are known.

A special problem can arise when the social climate in which information is collected changes, even if the actual measuring technique remains constant. This can occur, for example, when evaluating a new law or regulation that is intended to change behaviors about which there are strong social norms. If a population is surveyed about a risky behavior both before and after implementation of a legal intervention, the behavior in question may be legal before the law is passed but illegal afterwards. The survey questions may be the same, but the social desirability of the response has changed. Direct observation of behavior can help address this issue. Thus, observing seat belt use before and after a new belt law goes into effect may be preferable to interviewing subjects about their belt use.

Confounding

As discussed in the chapter on selecting a study design for injury research, confounding is present to the extent that the estimate of association between an exposure and an outcome is biased by failure to account for the effects of a third factor. Confounding may distort a measure of association in either direction: it can obscure a true association when one exists or create an apparent association when none is truly present.

Confounding can more than live up to its name in ecologic studies: confounders can be individual-level factors, group-level factors, or both. For example, in a multigroup cross-sectional ecologic study of mandatory motorcycle helmet laws, part of the difference in head injury death rates between jurisdictions with such a law versus those without it could stem from demographic differences in their populations. Age and gender, which are individual-level characteristics, might thus be confounding factors unless properly accounted for in the analysis. In addition, states with helmet laws could differ from those without them with regard to other laws that could affect head injury deaths in motorcyclists, such as speed limit laws or daytime headlight laws. Presence or absence of these other laws would be group-level confounding factors. Demographic characteristics or other laws could also be confounding factors in an ecologic study of the same question involving one or more jurisdictions over time if the demographic mix in jurisdictions changes or if other relevant laws are enacted or repealed during the study period. Campbell and Stanley (1966) referred to the influence of other concurrent events as bias due to "history," but it can also be considered a special case of confounding.

In an ordinary individual-level analysis, confounding can often be controlled fairly easily by stratification or regression. If a substantial change is found in the estimate of association after such adjustment, confounding is present and the adjustment leads to an estimate of association that is closer to the truth. Unfortunately, controlling for confounding is not always so simple in ecologic studies (Morgenstern, 1995, 1998). A variable may have no association with the exposure within groups (and therefore cannot be a confounder at the individual level), but it may be associated with exposure across groups. In this situation, adjusting for the variable will actually introduce bias into any estimate of association that we wish to apply at an individual level. Alternatively, a variable may be a true confounder at the individual level within each group, but if it is not associated with the exposure level across groups, adjusting for it in a grouped analysis will not control confounding. Unfortunately, without individual-level data or some external source of information, the investigator cannot determine whether confounding has been increased or reduced by adjustment for a group-level variable.

Some recently developed statistical techniques can simultaneously evaluate both group effects and individual effects and can accommodate covariates measured at both levels. These analyses generally treat the individual as the unit of analysis while accounting for the correlation structure imposed by individuals being clustered in defined geographic population units (Diggle et al., 1994). These techniques can be applied when information is available both at the geopolitical area and individual level.

Multicollinearity

Sociodemographic characteristics that are correlated at the individual level tend to be more strongly correlated at the group level (Connor and Gillings, 1984). This phenomenon can create complications when attempting to control for two or more such covariates at the group level in an ecologic study. In effect, the multivariate modeling method is being expected to separate the effects of factors that are strongly associated with each other. The result can be relatively unstable estimates of the effect of exposure, with wide confidence limits.

Regression to the Mean

Rates of most outcomes fluctuate over time due to factors which we cannot measure. We may think of short-term rate estimates as reflecting an underlying true rate, coupled with some chance variation in the expression of that underlying rate. Regression to the mean refers to the tendency of rates to shift back toward the underlying true value after unusual peaks and dips. If more stringent criminal penalties were adopted because of a chance increase in homicide rates, then it could be difficult to ascertain whether post-law declines were the result of the stiffer penalties or simply due to regression to the mean. Potential bias due to regression to the mean can be reduced by examining rates over long periods of time before and after the new laws are passed. In addition, one can examine the data to see whether there is any evidence of a peak in injury rates just before the intervention, as was done by Cummings et al. (1997) in the study of state safe gun storage laws mentioned earlier.

Inadequate Statistical Power

Ecologic studies implicitly involve two kinds of sample sizes: the number of groups and the number of individuals in each group. In multiple-group ecologic studies of legal interventions, statistical power may be low if only a few jurisdictions have enacted the law of interest, or if nearly all have done so, leaving few controls. The precision of an observed injury rate in any given group also depends on both the size of the population at risk within the group and on the frequency of the injury events of interest. Small populations can have relatively extreme rates, reflecting high random variability. Some types of injury, such as fatal head injuries among bicyclists, may also occur too rarely in communities of modest size to be feasible for use as an outcome measure. In such situations, investigators may instead need to rely on a more proximal behavioral outcome, such as helmet-wearing, that are already known to be strongly linked to injury risk.

Multiple Comparisons

As in other kinds of studies, statistical testing applied to many possible exposure–outcome relationships increases the risk of finding spurious associations. A specific risk in ecologic studies of laws can occur when the expected time lag between enactment of a law and its effects on injury outcomes is not specified a priori. If enough possible lag times are tried, apparent effects of laws on injuries can emerge by chance alone. This risk can be kept low by hypothesizing a lag time in advance for the primary analyses.

Migration

Finally, migration into and out of study groups can affect the findings of an ecologic study. In- and out-migrants may differ from long-term residents with regard to injury rates, and they may have much less exposure to aspects of the community environment being examined as potential determinants of injury risk.

Conclusions

Ecologic studies can offer a rapid and inexpensive approach to studying potential determinants of injury occurrence and outcomes when group-level data are available. Because they are susceptible to several special threats to validity, especially when used to infer individual-level biologic or behavioral mechanisms, they must often be interpreted with special caution. Nonetheless, ecologic studies are the most suitable study design for interventions designed to affect entire populations, such as legal changes intended to change environmental factors or behaviors that contribute to injury.

References

Anderson CL, Agran PF, Winn DG, Tran C (1998) Demographic risk factors for injury among Hispanic and non-Hispanic white children: an ecologic analysis. Injury Prev 4:33–8.

Brenner H, Savitz DA, Jockel K-H, Greenland S (1992) Effects of non-differential exposure misclassification in ecologic studies. Am J Epidemiol 135:85–95.

Bryk AS, Raudenbush SW (1992) Hierarchical Linear Models: Applications and Data Analysis Methods. Newbury Park, CA: Sage Publications.

Campbell DT, Stanley JC (1966) Experimental and Quasi-experimental Designs for Research. Chicago: Rand McNally.

Chiu AY, Perez PE, Parker RN (1997) Impact of banning alcohol on outpatient visits in Barrow, Alaska. JAMA 278:1775–7.

Connor MJ, Gillings D (1984) An empiric study of ecological inference. Am J Public Health 74:555–9.

Cummings P, Grossman D, Rivara F, Koepsell T (1997) State gun safe storage laws and child mortality due to firearms. JAMA 278:1084–6.

Diggle P, Liang K, Zeger S (1994) Analysis of Longitudinal Data. New York: Oxford University Press.

Durkheim E (1951) Suicide: A Study in Sociology. New York: Free Press.

Firebaugh G (1978) A rule for inferring individual-level relationships from aggregate data. Am Sociol Rev 43:557–72.

Greenland S, Brenner H (1993) Correcting for non-differential misclassification in ecologic analyses. Appl Stat 42:117–26.

Greenland S, Morgenstern H (1989) Ecological bias, confounding, and effect modification. Int J Epidemiol 18:269–74.

Hingson R (1996a) Prevention of drinking and driving. Alcohol Health and Research World 20:219–26.

Hingson R, Heeren T, Winter M (1994) Lower legal blood alcohol limits for young drivers. Public Health Rep 109:738–44.

Hingson R, Mc Govern T, Heeren T, Winter M, Zaleaco R (1996) Reducing alcohol impaired driving in Massachusetts: The Saving Lives program. Am J Public Health 86:791–7.

Jacobsen S, Goldberg J, Cooper C, Lockwood S (1992) The association between water fluoridation and hip fracture among white women and men aged 65 years and older: A national ecologic study. Ann Epidemiol 2:617–26.

Jacobsen S, OFallon WM, Melton LJ III (1993) Hip fracture incidence before and after the fluoridation of the public water supply, Rochester, Minnesota. Am J Public Health 83:743–5.

Killias M (1993) International correlations between gun ownership and rates of homicide and suicide. CMAJ 148:1721–5.

Kronmal RA (1993) Spurious correlation and the fallacy of the ratio standard revisited. J R Stat Soc A 156:379–92.

Morgenstern H (1982) Uses of ecologic analysis in epidemiologic research. Am J Public Health 72:1336–44.

Morgenstern H (1995) Ecologic studies in epidemiology: concepts, principles, and methods. Annu Rev Public Health 16:61–81.

Morgenstern H (1998) Ecologic studies. In: Rothman KJ, Greenland S. Modern Epidemiology. Philadelphia: Lippincott-Raven.

National Highway Traffic Safety Administration (1998a) Traffic Safety Facts 1997: Speeding. Publication DOT HS 808 775. Washington, DC: NHTSA.

(1998b) Traffic Safety Facts 1997: Occupant protection. Publication DOT HS 808 768. Washington, DC: NHTSA.

Prentice RL, Sheppard L (1995) Aggregate data studies of disease risk factors. Biometrika 82:113–25.

Robinson WS (1950) Ecologic correlations and the behavior of individuals. Am Sociol Rev 15:351–7.

Ross HL (1982) Deterring the Drinking Driver: Legal Policy and Social Control. Lexington, MA: Lexington Books.

Von Korff M, Koepsell T, Curry S, Diehr P (1992) Multi-level analysis in epidemiologic research on health behaviors and outcomes. Am J Epidemiol 135:1077–82.

13

Case Series and Trauma Registries

Charles Mock

Introduction

Case series are one of the original and most basic forms of medical research, dating back to our earliest attempts to understand illness and its origins. Until recently, much of our knowledge of the clinical manifestations of disease was based on descriptions of persons with similar sets of symptoms, often seen or cared for by one individual.

Case series are usually considered a less rigorous means of investigation than more analytic strategies, such as case–control or cohort studies. However, it is important to point out the importance of case series to the advancement of knowledge through the years. As a brief example, Sir Percival Pott described the occurrence of an unusual disease, scrotal cancer, in chimney sweeps in eighteenth century England and inferred an etiologic relationship with their occupation. This was a case series and represented the first description of carcinogenesis (Pott, 1778; Cummings and Weiss, 1998). In modern times, the global epidemic of acquired immune deficiency syndrome was heralded by a case series of homosexual men with the unusual combination of Kaposi's sarcoma and *Pneumocystis carinii* pneumonia (Centers for Disease Control, 1981). Likewise, in the study of injury, the first indications of the risks associated with air bags came from individual case reports and small case series (Ingram, 1991; Rimmer and Shuler, 1991; Huelke et al., 1992; Blacksin, 1993; Lancaster et al., 1993).

This chapter will explore the uses of case series data for the assessment of clinical care, as well as understanding the etiology of injuries. It will consider the spectrum from individual case reports to case series to trauma registries. The chapter will examine the advantages and disadvantages of these data sources and will consider methods to improve their usefulness.

Uses in Clinical Care

The case series is the most common type of publication that addresses clinical care of trauma patients. As discussed in both chapters by Koepsell (this volume), the ideal source of information about clinical care is the prospective randomized controlled trial. The second best is a study in which there is a prospective, but nonrandomized, control group. The third most desirable source of data is a study in which

168

comparisons are made retrospectively, as in a typical case series (Guyatt et al., 1995; Chestnut, 1997; Kirkpatrick, 1997).

The preponderance of such observational or case series data for the evaluation of clinical trauma care is most likely due to the difficulty in standardizing operative treatment, especially for large groups of patients, many of whom have very different and unique constellations of injuries. The randomized controlled trials that have been performed in trauma care usually address administration of medications, more so than operative interventions (Cochrane Collaboration Websites, 1999). Examples include trials of steroids for spinal cord injury (Bracken et al., 1992) and trials of various types of intravenous fluid resuscitation (Vassar et al., 1993; Bickell et al., 1994).

Hence, in evaluating the effectiveness of different treatments in trauma care, the preponderance of studies involve observational case series, in which patients are treated in different ways for varying reasons, such as the clinician's choice. The outcomes of the different groups are then compared in retrospect or against generally accepted values derived from the literature.

For example, Barone et al. (1999) reviewed 33 patients aged 55 or greater who had sustained a splenic injury. In this 3-year review, the authors addressed the question of whether nonoperative treatment of splenic injuries was safe in these older patients. They compared the mortality rates of two groups: patients who had undergone immediate operation versus those who had undergone initial observation. They also compared the proportion of observed patients who eventually required operation to the same proportion reported in the literature for other age groups (Barone et al., 1999). As another example, Wall et al. (1998) reported a series of 30 patients who underwent pulmonary tractotomy for penetrating pulmonary injuries. There was no control group in this case series. The authors compared the mortality and complication rate in their series with the values obtained from other reported case series in which tractotomy or other operative techniques were used (Wall et al., 1998).

In addition, case series data can be useful for evaluating diagnostic tests. For example, cases presenting with certain mechanisms of injury or symptoms are reviewed for the diagnostic tests they received. By knowing the diagnoses that were eventually uncovered, one may be able to calculate the sensitivity, specificity, as well as positive and negative predictive values. Such estimates are most valuable if the workup is standardized, so that test results are available on all patients. However, one must also beware that test results themselves may influence assignment of a final diagnosis.

In trauma care, the accuracies of many of the commonly used diagnostic tests are known through case series data. For example, Yoshii et al. (1998) reviewed 1239 patients with blunt abdominal trauma who had received abdominal ultrasound as a diagnostic test over a 14-year period. Likewise, Jhirad and Boone (1998) reviewed 55 patients with blunt abdominal trauma who received abdominal computer tomography over a 1-year period. Both of these studies were case series. Both calculated sensitivity and specificity rates, in which repeat tests, other diagnostic studies, the results of surgery, and the ultimate outcome of patients with negative studies were used as gold standards for evaluation of the accuracy of the initial tests (Jhirad and Boone, 1998; Yoshii et al., 1998).

Finally, many case series present descriptive data on patients with certain types of injuries. From these, ideas on the clinical presentation, clinical course, and prognostic indicators can be gleaned. For example, Ghali et al. (1999) reviewed 40 ureteric injuries over a 5-year period. They presented data on the clinical presentation, methods of diagnosis, technique of repair, and outcome in terms of renal salvage. Although not undertaking analytic comparisons of diagnostic modalities or treatment options, this case series provided data that allow clinicians caring for patients with ureteric injuries to understand better the nature and outcome of this injury (Ghali et al., 1999).

Uses in Understanding Injury Etiology

Case series provide only numerator data, without having access to the denominator of uninjured persons who do not come to attention. Nonetheless, case series data can provide some important insights into injury etiology that are useful for injury prevention work. This is principally because injuries, unlike many other diseases, are traditionally subclassified by mechanisms, by use of E-codes, in addition to classification by anatomic type of injury (Jones et al., 1996).

When getting an idea of the relative importance of different mechanisms of injury in a geographic area, the cases treated at local hospitals can serve as an important foundation. Even when injury researchers know more exact injury incidence rates from other sources, use of data from local hospitals can be helpful to bring public and political attention to injury prevention priorities (The National Committee for Injury Prevention and Control, 1989; Robertson, 1998).

Case series data can also provide insights into the etiology of injuries and into the effectiveness of injury prevention efforts. Although the data are not as valid as those derived from population-based studies, the case series can help to corroborate such studies. For example, several studies from trauma centers have shown decreased frequency and severity of head injuries in motorcyclists wearing helmets compared with unhelmeted motorcyclists (Offner et al., 1992; Orsay et al., 1995). Likewise, hospital-based studies have shown decreases in the number of motorcyclists admitted for head injuries after the institution of mandatory helmet laws (Mock et al., 1995b).

Although the case series is usually a descriptive study, it can evolve toward a more analytic study when internal comparisons are made. For example, Mock et al. (1995a) looked at the injuries in persons hospitalized at a rural African hospital. In addition to the numbers of persons admitted for different mechanisms, the injury prevention priorities in the area could be identified by comparing the case fatalities rates and disability rates resulting from different mechanisms. Further details on internal comparisons within case series are to be found in the chapter on selecting a study design for injury research.

Case series are also excellent sources of data for the generation of hypotheses about injury causation, which then form the basis for later, more analytic studies (Cummings and Weiss, 1998).

Trauma Registries

An extension of the case series is the trauma registry. Such registries generally consist of all trauma patients admitted to a given hospital over a specified period. Such data are similar to those from case series, except that data are gathered in a more standardized fashion and on an ongoing basis. Registries are the prime sources of information for continuous quality improvement activities (see Maier and Rhodes, this volume). Registry data also offer many advantages for injury research, usually providing the best source of data about severe, nonfatal injuries (Pollock and McClain, 1989). Summary data on all admitted trauma patients in a given area are one of the main components for assessing the "burden" of injury, along with mortality rates, emergency department records, and long-term followup of disabilities (Rice et al., 1989).

Registries are the best source of in-depth data on the anatomic nature and physiologic consequences of injuries for large numbers of people. Hence, registries are also the best existing source of data to allow comparisons of outcome on large groups of patients, adjusted for injury severity. When making comparisons between groups of patients with any disease, a major issue to be addressed is to what extent differences in initial severity of illness influence any observed differences in outcome. Most trauma registry studies currently utilize a similar method of analysis: the Major Trauma Outcome Study (MTOS) as a source of national norms about expected outcomes; and TRISS methodology for injury severity adjustment (Flora, 1978; Boyd et al., 1987; Champion et al., 1990).

The MTOS was coordinated by the American College of Surgeons (Champion et al., 1990). It was primarily designed for use in quality assurance, but has been used for many other research purposes as well. Data were collected on hospitalized patients and included demographics, etiologies, specific injuries, Abbreviated Injury Scores (AIS), Injury Severity Score (ISS) (Copes et al., 1988; Association for the Advancement of Automotive Medicine, 1990), and outcomes in the form of in-hospital mortality. The study ran from 1982 to 1989 and collected data on approximately 160,000 trauma patients admitted to 140 U.S. and Canadian hospitals (Champion et al., 1990), by far the largest and most comprehensive trauma case series to date.

The statistical basis for most outcome comparisons using trauma registry data involves a comparison of proportions, most commonly the proportion of admitted trauma patients who die in hospital (Flora, 1978). Simplistically, one could compare such a proportion to the national proportion of mortality in MTOS without accounting for severity. However, a further refinement is to estimate the proportion of patients who would have survived in the national norm or population, had they had the same injury severity as the patients in the observed group (Flora, 1978).

For patients in the MTOS, the outcome predictors include: ISS, as the indicator of the anatomic extent of injury (Copes et al., 1988; Association for the Advancement of Automotive Medicine, 1990); Revised Trauma Score, as the indictor of physiologic derangement (Champion et al., 1989); and age (see also Jurkovich and O'Keefe, this volume; Maier and Rhodes, this volume). These variables are used to derive the probability of survival for a given individual based on national norms. This is equivalent to estimating the percent survival among all patients with the same ISS, same Revised Trauma Score, and same age group, in the MTOS data. The TRISS methodology then uses the aggregate of all individual survival probabilities for a group of patients, as in an individual hospital trauma registry, to estimate the expected number of in-hospital deaths (Boyd et al., 1987; Champion et al., 1990). A so-called z statistic is then calculated and used to obtain a p-value that gives the probability that the observed number of deaths would occur by random chance, if that hospital's mortality rate was indeed the same as the national norm. In essence, it indicates whether that hospital's mortality rate is significantly lower or higher than the national norm.

Although the comparisons with MTOS using the TRISS methodology have been the mainstay of severity adjusted outcomes analysis, other methods have been used. For example, the frequent lack of physiologic data for calculation of the revised trauma score has led some to use ISS and age alone in deriving standardized mortality ratios for comparisons among different patient populations (Sampalis et al., 1992). Similarly, some have used ICD-9-CM (International Classification of Diseases, Ninth Revision, Clinical Modification) codes as the basis for severity adjustment (Jones et al., 1996; Rutledge et al., 1998). More detail on severity adjustment can be found in Jurkovich and O'Keefe (this volume).

Hence, some of the main advantages of trauma registries for such outcomes analysis, as well as for other injury research related purposes include:

- most registries have a similar format for the data, which facilitates comparisons;
- statistical comparisons using TRISS methodology and the MTOS norms remove some of the subjectivity of analyses of individual cases;
- in comparison with administrative databases, there may be more detail on injuries, which makes severity adjustment possible;
- case series in general are relatively inexpensive, compared with other forms of research. Even though the cost of maintaining a trauma registry may be fairly high (Pollock and McClain, 1989; Shapiro et al., 1994), the large databases that are created allow analysis for many purposes in addition to the quality assurance role for which they were originally created.

Limitations of Case Series and Trauma Registries

The main difficulties with analysis of case series data, in general, and with trauma registry data in particular, are in attempting to make generalizations about all injury victims and about injury risk factors from patients admitted to one hospital.

Both problems arise from considering patients in trauma registries as a representative sample of all patients with qualifying injuries. Trauma registry data are hospital-based and almost always limited to inpatients. Hence, registries contain no data about persons who sustain minor injuries that do not require treatment, persons who are treated in emergency departments as outpatients, nor persons who die at the scene of the injury (Payne and Waller, 1989; Pollock and McClain, 1989; Waller et al., 1995). These biases are more extreme in the registries of trauma centers which receive a higher proportion of referred patients, as they are more likely to receive a higher proportion of multiply injured patients and patients with severe head, cardiovascular, spine, and extremity injuries requiring specialized attention. Furthermore, there are many other factors that influence the likelihood of a patient being transferred from a smaller hospital to a trauma center. These include the patient's insurance status, geographic distances, the clinical expertise and facilities available at the referring hospital, and probably a variety of factors that are not fully understood (Payne and Waller, 1989; Waller et al., 1995).

Patients who are referred differ considerably from those who are taken to a hospital directly from the scene of an injury, who may be more representative of the characteristics of the population of all injured persons in a geographic area. The purpose of many studies that use hospital-based data is to describe the characteristics of a typical injured person. This is usually taken to mean typical of the community or population, not typical of the hospital. To the extent that a significant proportion of hospitalized patients are referred and to the extent that referred patients are different from non-referred patients, such descriptive analyses will be biased.

As an example, in a comparison of local and referred injured patients at a trauma center in Vermont, Waller et al. (1995), found that only 5% of local patients were hospitalized, with the remainder treated in the emergency department. The percentage of referred patients who were hospitalized was much higher (22%). Referred patients accounted for 15% of the total patient population studied, but accounted for nearly half (44%) of admitted patients. There were also considerable differences between local and referred patients in their injury severity and pattern. Only 4% of local patients had an AIS of 3 or higher, compared with 14% of referred patients. Only 0.5% of local patients had an ISS of 16 or greater, compared with 5% of referred patients. Local patients were more likely to have extremity injuries and referred patients more likely to have head, spine, and chest injuries. Referred patients were older and had more underlying medical problems than local patients. There were also differences in mechanism of injury, with local patients having more household-related injuries and referred patients having more transport-related injuries (Waller et al., 1995).

Because of such differences, it has been suggested that, when attempting to discern injury patterns in the population, trauma registry data should be disaggregated into direct admissions and referred patients, something that is not usually done (Payne and Waller, 1989; Waller et al., 1995). Differing proportions of referred patients in different trauma registries can likewise influence interpretation of analyses on outcomes and quality of medical care (Jurkovich and Mock, 1999).

Problems in the interpretation of trauma registry data especially arise when there are several trauma centers in a given area, with overlapping catchment areas. The triage patterns of the regional emergency medical system and patient preference may change over time. Hence trends in injuries recorded in the registries of individual hospitals might be misleading (Payne and Waller, 1989; Pollock and McClain, 1989; Waller et al., 1995).

Hospital-based data can occasionally be used to derive population-based injury incidence rates, if the catchment area is well defined and not served by other hospitals, as in more isolated areas. However, hospital trauma registries are not usually able to define the populations from which the injured persons came, thus limiting their ability to provide population-based incidence rates. This problem is compounded in circumstances in which there are several trauma centers in the same area (Payne and Waller, 1989; Waller et al., 1995; Robertson, 1998).

Difficulties with using trauma registry data to make generalizations about the population as a whole especially apply to mortality. Even in a well developed trauma system, the majority of trauma deaths still occur in the prehospital setting (Mock et al., 1998). Hence, the deaths recorded in a hospital setting reflect only a minority of all trauma deaths. Moreover, a sizeable minority of trauma deaths occurs after hospital discharge, particularly among elderly patients (Gubler et al., 1997; Mullins et al., 1998). Mullins et al. (1998) studied this issue using statewide hospital discharge data linked with death certificates. They found that of a total of 1269 trauma deaths in the study, 182 (14%) occurred within 30 days after discharge. The people who died after discharge were primarily older individuals (mean age 77 years) with extremity injuries (75%). These deaths would not be included in traditional trauma registries (Mullins et al., 1998).

Trauma registry data are also problematic in attempts to look at exposure to injury risk factors. For example, Orsay et al. (1995) examined the protective effect of motorcycle helmets. They used trauma center based data to show that the proportion of admitted motorcyclists who sustained head injury was higher among unhelmeted (51%) than among helmeted (30%) patients (Orsay et al., 1995). It was subsequently argued that, although this study does add corroborating evidence of the efficacy of motorcycle helmets, such data cannot be used to elucidate fully the protective effect of helmets (Mock et al., 1995b). To do so would require knowing about the denominator of all persons, helmeted and unhelmeted, involved in motorcycle crashes. Knowledge of the numbers of uninjured would allow calculation of rates, such as head injuries per crash for helmeted and unhelmeted riders. Case series data cannot provide this, as uninjured persons are not included (Lowenstein, 1996).

As discussed previously, registry data are useful for evaluating outcomes of trauma care and provide the best mechanism for adjusting for injury severity in such outcome assessment. Even here, however, there are a number of difficulties that must be addressed.

1. Most registries have considerable proportions of missing data. For example, among patients in the MTOS database, 11% had insufficient

information to calculate a TRISS score, primarily because of missing respiratory rates (Centers for Disease Control, 1988; Gilliott et al., 1989; Champion et al., 1992).

2. Any large database may have problems with miscoded data. It is often difficult to discern the extent of such miscoding. An example of how likely this is to be a problem in trauma registry work is to be found in the use of registry data for quality assurance purposes. Many involved in trauma quality assurance work have had the experience of reviewing trauma deaths that have been detected by audit filters such as deaths with ISS < 15. It is not infrequent that many, or even most, of these are due to miscodings. Usually, the injuries were more severe than initially coded. There is no easy way for such problems to be detected when large datasets are used (Jurkovich and Mock, 1999).

3. There are often differences in the manner in which injury severity coding is done at different hospitals. This may greatly influence the interpretation of outcome comparisons, by skewing the assessment of the underlying severity of injury of the patients. This is especially an issue when different hospitals perform autopsies on different proportions of deaths, as autopsy data usually increase the calculated ISS. For example, Shackford et al. (1987) and Sampalis et al. (1992) reported similar trauma registry studies in which they compared their outcomes with MTOS, with adjustment for ISS. In Shackford's study, all trauma deaths received an autopsy, with the findings then used to derive an ISS. In Sampalis's study, an unspecified number of autopsies were performed, with none of the findings used to derive ISSs. This represents a potential, significant information bias. It could be expected that the ISSs in Shackford's study would be skewed higher and those from Sampalis's study would be skewed lower than those in the MTOS, in which hospitals performing varying numbers of autopsies pooled their data (Shackford et al., 1987; Sampalis et al., 1992).

Statewide Trauma Registries

Many of the problems of generalizability and representativeness of hospital-based trauma registries might be solved by combining data from all hospitals caring for trauma patients in a given geographic area. This would create a type of trauma surveillance system and would have the potential for providing population-based data. This would thus overcome some of the selection biases of individual hospital registries.

It might be thought that the MTOS database could serve this function. However, this database was created by voluntary submission of data from selected hospitals throughout North America. Although hospitals from many geographic areas were included, they were not randomly selected and, hence, this database is not truly population based (Boyd et al., 1987; Champion et al., 1990). Moreover, the data were collected over a limited time period, making the database not suitable for use for surveillance.

However, many states have instituted statewide trauma registries. The first of these originated in Illinois in the 1970s (Goldberg et al., 1980; Shapiro et al., 1994). Currently, 24 states have some form of statewide trauma registry. The potential for use of these registries to further injury prevention and to improve trauma care is immense. In a survey of state EMS directors in 1992, 58% of states with registries indicated that the registry data had influenced legislation (Shapiro et al., 1994).

There are several limitations to statewide trauma registries as currently instituted, however. In the review of statewide registries, it was found that case criteria for entry into the registry varied considerably among states (Shapiro et al., 1994). Participation in submission of data was mandatory in most (63%) of states with registries, but voluntary in 37%. Moreover, states varied as to the types of hospitals from which data were requested or required. The majority of states with registries required only designated trauma centers (71%) to submit data, with the remainder (29%) requiring all acute care hospitals to do so. Only one state included data on out-of-hospital deaths. Data on the completeness of reporting were available only for 17 states. For these states, compliance with reporting was estimated at 80%, defined as the number of patients reported divided by the number of patients meeting case criteria (Shapiro et al., 1994).

In order for a statewide trauma registry to be useful for surveillance and for calculation of population-based rates, the registry would need to receive data from all acute care hospitals, not just trauma centers. Compliance with reporting would need to be near complete. Moreover, all out of hospital deaths would need to be included. Hence, despite the realized and potential usefulness of statewide trauma registries, they do not, in general, have sufficient data to calculate true population-based rates of injury incidence (Shapiro et al., 1994; Robertson, 1998).

Ways to Improve the Usefulness of Case Series and Trauma Registry Data

As they currently exist, both individual hospital trauma registries and statewide registries represent a considerable input of manpower and contain large amounts of very useful information. However, their usefulness is constrained by the above noted limitations. Moreover, comparisons involving data from different registries are often limited by differences in inclusion criteria and in the data elements gathered. Comparability of data from different registries might be improved by several means, in terms of both data collection and data analysis.

The CDC has recommended case criteria for hospital trauma registries (Centers for Disease Control, 1988; Pollock and McClain, 1989). These include a trauma-related diagnosis based on ICD-9 codes, and either admission as an inpatient or transfer to or from another acute-care facility or death in a hospital. As of yet, however, there is still considerable variability in the inclusion criteria used by different hospital and statewide trauma registries (Pollock and McClain, 1989; Shapiro et al., 1994). In addition, trauma registries use a variety of different software programs and may or may not include a wide variety of data elements.

Greater standardization of core data content, data definitions, and coding has been advocated in an effort to overcome these technical problems (Centers for Disease Control, 1988; Pollock and McClain, 1989). The American College of Surgeons has recently organized the National Trauma Data Bank (NTDB). This is similar to the MTOS database of the 1980s, but is intended to continue as an ongoing, nationwide trauma registry. An emphasis has been placed on the standardization of the data elements and their coding (American College of Surgeons, 1996).

The utility of trauma registries for estimating population-based rates and for undertaking analytic study of risk factors for injury can be improved by linking to other databases. This is especially true for statewide trauma registries, as they encompass defined populations. Some of these other databases include death certificates, police crash reports, hospital discharge data from hospitals not participating in the registry, and emergency medical service reports (Pollock and McClain, 1989; Shapiro et al., 1994). Linking with death certificate data would allow a more complete assessment of overall trauma mortality. As indicated above, the majority of trauma deaths occur in the prehospital setting and hence are not recorded by traditional hospital-based trauma registries. Likewise, a small but significant proportion of post-discharge trauma deaths are also missed by such hospital-based registries, particularly among the elderly.

Linking with police crash reports may allow greater validity of efforts to use registry data to estimate the magnitude of the effects of injury risk factors. For example, such linking would allow data on head injuries among helmeted and unhelmeted motorcyclists (e.g., registry data) to be compared with data on the number of collisions occurring to helmeted and unhelmeted motorcyclists (e.g., police crash reports). This would allow a more accurate measurement of the increased risk of head injury to unhelmeted motorcyclists who are involved in a collision (Shankar et al., 1992; Lowenstein, 1996). Use of hospital discharge data allows a more complete understanding of all injuries leading to hospitalization, especially in states which do not have statewide trauma registries or where these registries only receive data from designated trauma centers and not all acute care hospitals (Pollock and McClain, 1989; Shapiro et al., 1994).

Linking can be technically difficult (see chapter on data sets and data linkage). Unless the linking is set up prospectively as the databases are designed, matching of subjects between databases may be incomplete and unreliable. Arrangements for concurrent linking with other databases is done in a minority of state trauma registries. In their review of state trauma registries, Shapiro et al. found that of the 24 states with statewide registries, only eight (33%) linked with death certificates; only seven (29%) with crash reports; and only seven (29%) with hospital discharge data (Shapiro et al., 1994).

Use of registry data for analyses seeking to infer characteristics about the population of all injured persons might be improved by taking into account potential sampling biases in these registries. For example, analyzing referred patients and directly admitted patients separately would help to eliminate one of the major sampling biases. As indicated previously, these two patient populations can be very different (Payne and Waller, 1989; Waller et al., 1995). When attempting to obtain

Table 13.1 Summary of benefits and limitations of case series and trauma registries

Case reports/case series		Trauma registries	
Benefits	Limitations	Benefits	Limitations
Often represent the first report of a clinical problem or entity.	Represents only numerator data.	Maintained already for quality assurance work.	Large proportions of referred patients may bias analysis of the "typical" trauma patient.
Low cost	Cannot be used to calculate incidence rates.	Detailed information on injuries and similar data format allow comparisons between registries.	Lack of data on prehospital and postdischarge deaths.
Most common type of study addressing diagnostic workup and treatment of trauma patients.	Comparisons of outcomes between different groups do not involve randomization and are usually retrospective.	Registry-based analysis using TRISS and MTOS norms is the most common method of severity adjusted, outcome comparison for large groups of injured persons.	Frequent lack of physiologic data precludes use of TRISS methodology for many patients.
Can identify injury prevention priorities in a specific locality.	Not able to look at risk factors unless they are very strong.	If catchment area well known, population-based incidence rates can be calculated.	Usually, ill defined catchment areas preclude calculation of true population-based rates.
Can be used to get a preliminary idea of injury risk factors.		Usefulness of data can be expanded by linking to other databases.	Differences in injury coding at different institutions may influence interpretation of outcome comparisons.

TRISS, Trauma and injury severity score; MTOS, Major Trauma Outcome Study.

data on the full spectrum of injuries occurring in a given community or area, supplemental data on minor injuries will be needed. Such data are not usually included in registries of admitted patients. Some form of sampling of cases treated only in the emergency department or in other ambulatory settings is needed (Payne and Waller, 1989; Waller et al., 1995).

Finally, the use of case series data could be improved by regarding this study methodology on a more fundamental level. It has been argued that case series are, in essence, a type of case–control study, in which the controls are implied to be the population at large. This viewpoint is especially useful when trying to make inferences about the etiology of injury from case series data. Such inferences about the injury–exposure relationship can be made by assuming that the exposure is fairly well known in the population at large. Hence, if the exposure among injured subjects is very different from the population, it can be recognized as aberrant. Approaching a case series in this light allows one to better recognize its strengths and weaknesses. Case series can suspect a strong association but cannot provide an estimate of the actual relative risk of injury (Cummings and Weiss, 1998) (see also chapter on case–control studies).

Moreover, looking at case series in this light allows one to address the same methodologic issues that can weaken case–control studies, such as selection bias, information bias, and confounding. Selection bias may occur when the exposure being studied increases the chance that a case would be included, independent of the exposure's effect on disease or injury causation. For example, facial injuries suffered after a crash in which an air bag deployed are more likely to be noticed by injury researchers and denoted as potentially due to the air bag. Information bias can arise when greater attention is directed towards ascertaining the exposure history of cases than into controls. In case series, such exposure would be assumed to be low among the general public and assumed to be common knowledge (Cummings and Weiss, 1998).

In conclusion (Table 13.1), data from case series has a long history of contributing to medical research. This form of study has been used extensively in the study of trauma care. It has also been used to discern mechanisms of injury that are common in a given geographic area. Trauma registries are an extension of case series and offer many advantages to both clinical care and the study of injury mechanisms. However, for both case series and trauma registry studies, considerable caution must be exercised in attempting to make inferences about injury risk factors and about injury characteristics of the population. There is a tendency to draw conclusions that cannot be supported by such numerator data. As Pollock indicated in his 1989 review of trauma registries, "The tendency to view registries as research gold mines should be tempered with a realistic assessment of the nature of the data." (Pollock and McClain, 1989).

References

American College of Surgeons (1996) National Trauma Data Bank Data Dictionary. Chicago: American College of Surgeons.

Association for the Advancement of Automotive Medicine (1990) The Abbreviated Injury Scale: 1990 Revision. DesPlaines, Illinois: Association for the Advancement of Automotive Medicine.

Barone JE, Burns G, Svehlak SA et al. (1999) Management of blunt splenic trauma in patients older than 55 years. J Trauma 46:87–90.

Bickell WH, Wall MJ, Pepe PE (1994) Immediate vs. delayed fluid resuscitation for hypotensive patients with penetrating torso injuries. N Engl J Med 331:1105–09.

Blacksin MF (1993) Patterns of fracture after air bag deployment. J Trauma 35:840–3.

Boyd CR, Tolson MA, Copes WS (1987) Evaluating trauma care: The TRISS method. J Trauma 27:370–8.

Bracken MB, Shepard MJ, Holford TR et al. (1992) Administration of methylprednisolone for 24 or 48 hours or tirilazad mesylate for 48 hours in the treatment of acute spinal cord injury: results of the third national acute spinal cord injury randomized controlled trial. JAMA 277:1597–604.

Centers for Disease Control (1981) Kaposi's sarcoma and Pneumocystis pneumonia among homosexual men in New York City and California. MMWR 30(25):305–8.

   (1988) Report from the 1988 Trauma Registry Workshop, including recommendations for hospital-based trauma registries. J Trauma 29:827–34.

Champion HR, Sacco WJ, Copes WS, Gann DS, Gennarelli TA, Flanagan ME (1989) A revision of the Trauma Score. J Trauma 29:623–9.

Champion HR, Copes WS, Sacco WJ et al. (1990) The Major Trauma Outcome Study: Establishing national norms for trauma care. J Trauma 30:1356–65.

Champion HR, Sacco WJ, Copes WS (1992) Improvement in outcome from trauma center care. Arch Surg 127:333–8.

Chestnut RM (1997) Guidelines for the management of severe head injury: what we know and what we think we know. J Trauma 42:S19–22.

Cochrane Collaboration Websites: (1999) http://www.updateusa.com/clibip/clib.htm and http://hiru.mcmaster.ca/cochrane/

Copes WS, Champion HR, Sacco WJ, Lawnick MM, Keast SL, Bain LW (1988) The Injury Severity Score revisited. J Trauma 28:69–77.

Cummings P, Weiss NS (1998) Case series and exposure series: the role of studies without controls in providing information about the etiology of injury or disease. Injury Prev 4:54–7.

Flora JD (1978) A method for comparing survival of burn patients to a standard survival curve. J Trauma 18:701–5.

Ghali AMA, El-Malik EMA, Ibrahim AIA, Ismail G, Rashie M (1999) Ureteric injuries: diagnosis, management, and outcome. J Trauma 46:150–8.

Gilliott AR, Thomas JM and Forrester C (1989) Development of a statewide trauma registry. J Trauma 29:1667–72.

Goldberg J, Gelfand HM, Levy PS et al. (1980) An evaluation of the Illinois Trauma Registry. Med Care 18:520–31.

Gubler KD, Davis R, Koepsell T, Soderberg R, Maier RV, Rivara FP (1997) Long-term survival of elderly trauma patients. Arch Surg 132:1010–14.

Guyatt GH, Sackett DL, Sinclair JC, Hayward R, Cook DJ, Cook RJ (1995) Users' guides to the medical literature IX: A method for grading health care recommendations. JAMA 274:1800–4.

Huelke DF, Moore JL, Ostrom M. (1992) Air bag injuries and occupant protection. J Trauma 33:894–8.

Ingram HJ (1991) Airbag keratitis. N Engl J Med 324:1599–600.

Jhirad R, Boone D (1998) Computed tomography for evaluating blunt abdominal trauma in the low-volume nondesignated trauma center: the procedure of choice? J Trauma 45:64–8.

Jones MK, Schmidt KM, Aaron WS (1996) ICD-9-CM Code Book. Reston, VA: St Anthony's Publishing Co.

Jurkovich GJ, Mock CN (1999) A systematic review of trauma system effectiveness based on registry comparisons. J Trauma 47(Suppl):S46–55.

Kirkpatrick PJ (1997) On guidelines for the management of the severe head injury. J Neurol Neurosurg Psychiatry 62:109–11.

Lancaster GI, DeFrance JH, Borruso JJ (1993) Air-bag-associated rupture of the right atrium. N Engl J Med 328:358.

Lowenstein S (1996) Trauma registries: tarnished gold. Ann Emerg Med 27:389–91.

Mock CN, Adzotor E, Denno D, Conklin E, Rivara F (1995a) Admissions for injury at a rural hospital in Ghana: Implications for prevention in the developing world. Am J Public Health 85:927–31.

Mock CN, Maier R, Pilcher S, Boyle E, Rivara F (1995b) Injury prevention strategies to promote helmet use decrease severe head injury at a level I trauma center. J Trauma 39:29–35.

Mock CN, Jurkovich GJ, nii-Amon-Kotei D, Arreola-Risa C, Maier RV (1998) Trauma mortality patterns in three nations at different economic levels: implications for global trauma system development. J Trauma 44:804–14.

Mullins RJ, Mann NC, Hedges JR et al. (1998) Adequacy of hospital discharge status as a measure of outcome among injured patients. JAMA 279:1727–31.

Offner PJ, Rivara FP, Maier RV (1992) The impact of motorcycle helmet use. J Trauma 32:636–42.

Orsay E, Holden JA, Williams J, Lumpkin JR (1995) Motorcycle trauma in the state of Illinois: analysis of the Illinois Department of Public Health Trauma Registry. Ann Emerg Med 26:455–60.

Payne SR, Waller JA (1989) Trauma registry and trauma center bias in injury research. J Trauma 29:424–9.

Pollock DA, McClain PW (1989) Trauma Registries: Current status and future prospects. JAMA 262:2280–3.

Pott P (1778) The Chirurgical Works of Percival Pott, FRS. Dublin: James Williams.

Rice DP, MacKenzie EJ et al. (1989) Cost of Injury in the United States: A Report to Congress. San Francisco: Institute for Health & Aging, University of California and Injury Prevention Center, The Johns Hopkins University.

Rimmer S, Shuler JD (1991) Severe ocular trauma from a driver's side airbag. Arch Ophthalmol 109:774.

Robertson LS (1998) Injury Epidemiology. New York: Oxford University Press.

Rutledge R, Osler T, Emergy S, Kromhout-Schiro S (1998) The end of the Injury Severity Score (ISS) and the Trauma and Injury Severity Score (TRISS): ICISS, an International Classification of Diseases, ninth revision-based prediction tool, outperforms both ISS and TRISS as predictors of trauma patient survival, hospital charges, and hospital length of stay. J Trauma 44:41–9.

Sampalis JS, Lavoie A, Williams JI, Mulder DS, Kalina M (1992) Standardized mortality ratio analysis on a sample of severely injured patients from a large Canadian city without regionalized trauma care. J Trauma 33:205–12.

Shackford SR, Mackersie RC, Hoyt DB et al. (1987) Impact of a trauma system on outcome of severely injured patients. Arch Surg 122:523–7.

Shankar BS, Ramzy AI, Soderstrom CA, Dischinger PC, Clark CC (1992) Helmet use, patterns of injury, medical outcome, and costs among motorcycle drivers in Maryland. Accid Anal Prev 24:385–96.

Shapiro MJ, Cole KE, Keegan M, Prasad CN, Thompson RJ (1994) National survey of state trauma registries – 1992. J Trauma 37:835–42.

The National Committee for Injury Prevention and Control (1989) Injury Prevention: Meeting the Challenge. New York: Oxford University Press.

Vassar MJ, Fischer RP, O'Brien PE et al. (1993) A multicenter trial for resuscitation of injured patients with 7.5% sodium chloride. The effect of added dextran 70. Arch Surg 128:1003–11.

Wall MJ, Villavicencio RT, Miller CC et al. (1998) Pulmonary tractotomy as an abbreviated thoracotomy technique. J Trauma 45:1015–23.

Waller JA, Skelly JM, Davis JH (1995) Trauma center-related biases in injury research. J Trauma 38:325–9.

Yoshii H, Sato M, Yamamoto S et al. (1998) Usefulness and limitations of ultrasonography in the initial evaluation of blunt abdominal trauma. J Trauma 45:45–51.

14

Systematic Reviews of Injury Studies

Frances Bunn, Carolyn G. DiGuiseppi, and Ian Roberts

Introduction

The identification of effective strategies for the prevention, treatment, and rehabilitation of injury is essential, and the importance of taking evidence into account is increasingly recognized. However, sifting through the available research is a vast undertaking. Systematic reviews, through an evaluative process, identify and synthesize research, and present it in a manageable, accessible format for health care professionals, researchers, service planners, and consumers.

What is a Systematic Review?

A systematic review is a summary of the best available evidence that addresses a sharply defined question (Sackett and Haynes, 1992). Conducting a review is a structured process involving several steps:

- a careful formulation of the question
- a comprehensive data search
- an unbiased selection and abstraction process
- a critical appraisal of data
- synthesis of data.

It is now recognized that the same scientific principles that apply to conducting original research should apply to reviewing research (Chalmers, 1995). A systematic review seeks to draw together the totality of evidence using rigorously applied scientific criteria.

Systematic reviews should not be mistaken for meta-analyses. Meta-analysis is a quantitative method for combining and summarizing the results of different studies, which may or may not be employed in a systematic review.

Why do a Systematic Review?
Reducing Selection Bias

A systematic review of the literature aims to reduce the likelihood of biased conclusions. Such bias may come from several sources. A language bias can be

Table 14.1 Examples of electronic databases and other electronic resources for preparation of systematic reviews

Acronym or abbreviated name	Full name or source	Web address or access	Comment
Medical and health-related databases			
CCTR	Cochrane Controlled Trials Register	By subscription from The Cochrane Library at hiru.mcmaster.ca/cochrane/	Published and unpublished controlled trials. Systematic reviews also accessible
mRCT	meta Register of Controlled Trials	www.controlled-trials.com/search/cct.htm	Ongoing and published trials
MEDLINE	MEDLARS On-Line	www.ncbi.nlm.nih.gov/PubMed and by subscription[a]	Biomedicine, pharmacology, dentistry (National Library of Medicine)
EMBASE	Excerpta Medica	By subscription[a]	Biomedicine, pharmacology
CINAHL	Cumulative Index to Nursing and Allied Health Literature	By subscription[a]	Nursing, allied health
PsycLIT	Subset of PsycINFO ® Database	By subscription[a]	Psychology
ISTP	Index of Scientific and Technical Proceedings	By subscription[a]	Science, technology proceedings from ≥ 4000 conferences/year
SCISEARCH	Science Citations Indices and Current Contents Series	By subscription[a]	Indices to biomedicine, science, technology, social sciences, humanities literature
WHOLIS	World Health Organization Library Information System	unicorn.who.ch	Public health
–	Systematic Reviews of Childhood Injury Prevention Interventions	weber.u.washington.edu/~hiprc/childinjury	Reviews organized by injury topic
DARE	Database of Abstracts of Reviews of Effectiveness	nhscrd.york.ac.uk	Systematic reviews of health-care topics
CHID	Combined Health Information Database	chid.nih.gov	U.S. government health information and health education resources
Other Databases			
ERIC	Education Resource Information Center	www.ericse.org/ericsys.html and by subscription[a]	Education literature from U.S. Department of Education-sponsored clearinghouse

–	Dissertation Abstracts	By subscription[a]	≥ 1000 academic institutions worldwide
IBSS	International Bibliography of the Social Sciences	By subscription[a]	Social sciences
EI Compendex	Engineering Index	By subscription[a]	Engineering articles, proceedings, technical reports
–	Child Abuse and Neglect	Free to qualifying institutions from www.nics.com	> 26,000 records on child maltreatment
–	Electronic Highway Safety Library	www.albany.edu/sph/injr_012.html	Organized by injury topic
TRIS	Transport Research Information Services	www.nas.edu/trb/about/tris.html	Published, unpublished transportation research
TRANSPORT	–	By subscription[a]	> 650,000 transport-related records from TRIS, other databases
TRL	Transport Research Laboratory	www.trl.co.uk	Transport-related records, reports
FIREDOC	Fire Research Information Services	www.bfrl.nist.gov/fris	> 50,000 fire research documents
LRC	U.S. Fire Administration Learning Resources Center	www.usfa.fema.gov/lrc	Fire and emergency management
FEDRIP	Federal Research in Progress	By subscription[a]	U.S. government-sponsored research in progress
NRR	UK National Research Register	www.doh.gov.uk/research/nrr.htm	U.K. government-sponsored ongoing, completed research
Other electronic resources			
–	Traffic Safety/Injury Prevention Web Sites	apocalypse.berkshire.net/traffic.safety/Safelink.htm	Guide to traffic safety, injury prevention web sites
OMNI	Organizing Medical Networked Information	www.omni.ac.uk	Internet resources in medical, biomedical, allied health, and related topics
NTIS	National Technical Information Service	www.ntis.gov/index.html	Source for ordering U.S. government health and safety-related publications

[a] e.g., SilverPlatter (www.silverplatter.com/catalog.htm); OVID (www.ovid.com/db/all-page.htm); NISC (www.nisc.com); Dialog Corporation (library.dialog.com). Provide on-line catalogs describing available databases.

introduced if only studies published in English are included. For example, authors of studies conducted in German speaking Europe are more likely (odds ratio = 3.75; 95% confidence interval 1.25–11.3) to publish statistically significant findings in English language journals than in German language journals (Egger et al., 1997a). If only English language studies are used, treatment differences may be systematically exaggerated. Systematic reviews that review the literature without any language restrictions are less susceptible to language bias.

Another possible source of bias is publication bias, where research with statistically significant findings is more likely to be published than is work with null or nonsignificant findings. For example, National Institutes of Health-funded trials with "significant" results were more than twice as likely to be published as were those showing "nonsignificant" results (Dickersin and Min, 1993). Among ethics committee-approved studies at Oxford in the United Kingdom, those with statistically significant results were more than twice as likely to be published as studies with null results (Easterbrook et al., 1991). In subgroup analyses, publication bias was greater for non-randomized trials (odds ratio = 10.3; confidence interval 1.8–59.8) and observational studies (odds ratio = 3.8; confidence interval 1.5–9.8) (Easterbrook et al., 1991). Easterbrook et al. (1991) found no apparent publication bias among randomized trials, but effect estimates were imprecise due to small numbers.

Importantly, the quality of study design has not been shown to be associated with publication (Easterbrook et al., 1991; Dickersin and Min, 1993; Elvik, 1998). Instead, the most common reason why trials went unreported was that the investigators thought the results "uninteresting," or else they "did not have enough time."

Searching for unpublished studies is one way that systematic reviews seek to minimize publication bias. The Medical Editors Trial Amnesty was initiated to encourage registration of unpublished research (Smith and Roberts, 1997). Two bibliographic databases, the CCTR and mRCT (see Table 14.1), include unpublished or ongoing trials. Because there have not been extensive efforts to identify and build similar registers of unpublished observational studies, additional effort may be required to identify such studies, and the risk of publication bias is increased.

Publication bias may also operate within individual studies when investigators selectively report outcomes with significant results. For example, in a systematic review of randomized trials of the effectiveness of home-based social support in the prevention of childhood injury, the pooled odds ratio for the eight identified trials was 0.74 (95% confidence interval 0.54–1.03) (Hodnett and Roberts, 1999). All eight were published trials. In two trials, however, the data on injury outcomes were not published and were obtained only after contacting the authors. These two trials had the least promising intervention effects. The pooled odds ratio from the other six trials that did report injury outcomes was 0.59 (95% confidence interval 0.40 – 0.88), suggesting that failure to include the data on unpublished outcomes would have substantially overstated the effectiveness of home visiting. Contacting investigators to request information on unpublished outcomes can reduce bias and is therefore an important aspect of systematic reviews.

Increasing Precision

When a systematic review pools quantitative data in a meta-analysis, this creates a larger sample of study subjects, which can increase the precision of the effect estimate. Moderate effects can be difficult to assess reliably because large numbers are required for them to be apparent. Meta-analysis, by bringing together all available evidence, can provide more precise estimates of effect.

Exploring Heterogeneity and Generalizability

Systematic reviews allow the reviewer to assess heterogeneity among the study results and investigate the influences of specific differences between studies (Thompson, 1995). Unless heterogeneity is explored, diverse studies may be inappropriately combined and yield misleading results. Investigations of heterogeneity may also guide the development of new research hypotheses.

Systematic reviews, by including all available relevant evidence, usually comprise varied types of participants, exposures, and outcomes. Variations between studies provide an opportunity to examine the consistency of the results across types of studies and exposures, and their applicability in a range of subjects and settings (Mulrow et al., 1997).

Giving an Overview of the Evidence

Systematic reviews provide an overview of the evidence. For example, many randomized controlled trials have compared the administration of albumin with no administration, or with administration of crystalloid solution, in critically ill or injured patients. A systematic review was conducted to quantify the effects of albumin administration on mortality (Cochrane Injuries Group Albumin Reviewers, 1998). The results suggested that albumin use may actually increase the risk of death. This disturbing finding might have been detected as early as 1983, had there been a periodically updated systematic review of the available clinical trials (Figure 14.1).

How to do a Systematic View
Formulating the Question and Specifying Inclusion Criteria

A well focused question allows clear decisions to be made about what research to include in the systematic review and how to summarize it (Mulrow and Oxman, 1997). As with any research, preparing a protocol is essential. The protocol should specify the types of participants, exposures or interventions, outcomes, and study designs to be included in the review. Eligible participants may be defined by age, sex, setting, or other factors. Restrictions in types of participants should be based on biological or sociological justification – for example, restricting a review of

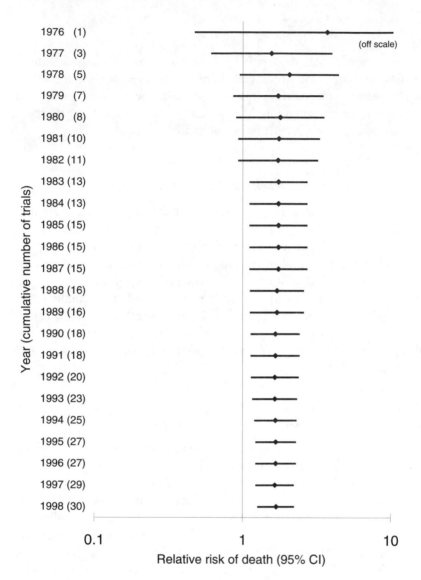

Figure 14.1 Cumulative meta-analysis of the effect on mortality of albumin administration in critically ill and injured patients.

driver education interventions to studies in adolescents (Vernick et al., 1999). Inclusion criteria for exposures might specify type, dosage, duration, setting, etc. In specifying outcomes, the reviewer should include all outcomes likely to be meaningful to decision makers (i.e., clinicians, patients, policy makers).

Another key protocol decision is what study designs to include. Randomized controlled trials are generally considered the optimal study design for unbiased estimates of intervention or treatment effects (see the chapter on selecting a study design for injury research). For certain interventions, however, no controlled trials have been conducted, and a systematic review of the best available literature will necessarily involve other study designs. In particular, studies of the effects of community programs, engineering changes, product modification, and legislation are rarely evaluated using randomized trials because the decisions about which product or area receives the intervention are determined by factors, such as politics or economics, that are beyond the investigator's control. For example, a systematic review of the best available evidence on the effects of pool fencing on drowning consisted solely of case–control studies (Thompson and Rivara, 1998). Study designs other than trials may also be appropriate, or even preferable, for answering certain types of research questions, including the assessment of etiology or risk factors (e.g., pedestrian exposure to high traffic volume), accuracy of diagnostic tests (e.g., screening for problem drinking), or natural history (e.g., functional outcomes of minor head injury). Inclusion criteria may also define other methodologic aspects, such as type of control group (e.g., placebo-controlled), method of outcome assessment or duration of follow-up. Reviewers should consider in advance which study designs are likely to provide valid, reliable data for answering the research question and define their inclusion criteria accordingly.

Conducting the Data Search

There are many sources for identifying published literature. Among the most commonly used are electronic bibliographic databases. Consultation with an experienced librarian will help identify electronic databases likely to contain citations relevant to the specific research questions. Examples of potentially useful databases are shown in Table 14.1. These databases have different foci, hence many studies may appear in only one. For example, although EMBASE and MEDLINE both index biomedical literature, the overlap in journals covered is only 34% (Smith et al., 1992).

Because the injury field is so broad, incorporating, for example, education, criminology, sociology, and engineering, it is important to cast a wide net when searching for injury studies. General databases useful for identifying relevant studies include ERIC, Dissertation Abstracts, IBSS, and EI Compendex (Table 14.1). Specialized databases may be identified by discussions with expert librarians, contacts with organizations, and internet searches. Lists of available databases have been published (Armstrong and Fenton, 1996) and are available online from OMNI, commercial suppliers (e.g., SilverPlatter, OVID, NISC, Dialog), and other web sites (Table 14.1). Many government and other national organizations sponsor specialized databases that can be located by searching their web sites (e.g., FIREDOC, LRC).

Search strategies should be developed in consultation with librarians experienced in electronic searching. It is important to be as comprehensive as possible, without retrieving an overwhelming number of irrelevant articles. Combining content terms with methodologic terms can help narrow the search. A variety of methodologic filters (e.g., for prognostic studies, diagnostic studies, randomized controlled trials) can be downloaded from www.ihs.ox.ac.uk/library/filters.html#list. All search strategies should be documented in enough detail to allow others to replicate the search.

Reference lists of trials and other reviews, contacts with investigators, experts, and organizations, and manually (as opposed to electronically) searching conference proceedings and abstract books, will help identify technical, internal, unpublished, and ongoing studies. Electronic databases of reviews, such as the Cochrane Library and DARE, as well as MEDLINE and similar databases, can identify previously published reviews. Older published studies may be identified from these sources and by manually searching Index Medicus, which includes citations from 1879, and Excerpta Medica, with citations from 1948.

To illustrate, we reviewed controlled trials of interventions to promote smoke alarms (C. DiGuiseppi, 1999, personal communication). Among 25 eligible trials, nine appeared in at least two health-care databases. One trial appeared only in PsycLIT, four were found only in Dissertation Abstracts, and one appeared only in ERIC. We identified seven ongoing trials and three completed trials (including one trial in press and one manuscript in preparation) through contact with experts ($n = 1$) and government organizations ($n = 5$), and examination of conference abstracts ($n = 3$) and bibliographies of published reviews ($n = 1$). Thus, 10 of 25 relevant trials were not found in any of 11 electronic databases searched, and six were found in one electronic database each.

Selecting Studies and Abstracting Data

Once identified, studies must be assessed to determine whether they meet inclusion criteria. Titles, abstracts, and keywords may be sufficient to exclude many studies. The full text of questionable studies should be reviewed, and in some cases authors should be contacted, to determine eligibility. At each stage of the selection process one should err toward overinclusiveness because once excluded, studies are rarely reconsidered.

The protocol should establish who will review (more than one reviewer, experts vs. non-experts), whether the reviewers will be blinded to author, journal, etc., and how disagreements will be handled. It is useful to pilot test the inclusion criteria on a sample of articles. A database system helps track the retrieval status of studies identified through searches and identifies duplicates. Either reference management databases or general database programs or spreadsheets may be used.

For data extraction, a paper or electronic data collection form must be developed. The data collection form: (1) visually represents the review question and planned appraisal of included studies; (2) records decisions taken during the review process; and (3) records outcomes data to be analyzed (Mulrow and Oxman, 1997). Key items include the review name, reviewer, study author, year, and journal, a check list to verify eligibility, study characteristics (e.g., participants, exposures, outcomes, methods), and results. The form should be pilot tested on a sample of trials. A library of data collection forms is available (Mulrow and Oxman, 1997).

Critically Appraising Studies

There is increasing evidence that the quality of studies included in systematic reviews can influence effect estimates. Hence, it is appropriate to assess study quality. Randomization methods and double-blinding have been analyzed for their influence on effect estimates in meta-analyses. Randomization should involve both the generation of an unpredictable assignment sequence and the concealment of that sequence until allocation to study group occurs (Schulz et al., 1995). Of these, the concealment of allocation appears most important. Analyzing 250 trials from 33 meta-analyses, Schulz et al. (1995) found that, compared with trials with adequate allocation concealment, odds ratios were exaggerated by 41% for inadequately concealed trials and by 30% when the adequacy of concealment was unclear. In a similar study, inadequate allocation concealment exaggerated the effect estimate by 37% (Moher et al., 1998). Neither study found an overall effect of the method of randomization generation. However, among adequately concealed trials and trials that did not clearly report about concealment, inadequate methods of sequence generation exaggerated effects by 25% and failure to double-blind, by 17% (Schulz et al., 1995). There is debate about how to take account of quality assessment in a systematic review. Many scales and checklists designed to assess the validity and quality of randomized controlled trials have been identified (Moher et al., 1995). However, serious doubts remain about the usefulness of many of these scales and it may be more appropriate to assess the impact on the effect estimates of the specific methodologic factors known to be associated with bias.

Non-randomized studies tend to overestimate treatment effects compared to randomized studies (Chalmers et al., 1977), probably due to inadequately controlled biases. Observational studies are also at increased risk for bias, because such studies can control only for known and measured confounding variables. Nevertheless, as described in the section on formulating the question and specifying inclusion criteria, there may be good reasons for including nonrandomized trials and observational studies. A number of attempts have been made to develop criteria for assessing the quality of such studies (Feinstein and Horwitz, 1982; Freemantle et al., 1999).

To date studies have shown conflicting results on the impact blinding of reviewers has on quality assessment. Two studies (Jadad et al., 1996; Berlin et al., 1997) found that summary quality scores were lower when the reviewers were blinded, while a third study (Moher et al., 1998) reported that quality scores where higher when reviewers were blinded. The importance of blinded assessment of trials for inclusion is therefore not established and the effort involved may not be justified.

Data Synthesis

To decide whether it is appropriate to combine data quantitatively in a meta-analysis, researchers must judge the relevance to the results of heterogeneity in participants, interventions, design, and outcomes. This judgement may take into account, for example, known effect modifiers, biologic plausibility, methodologic

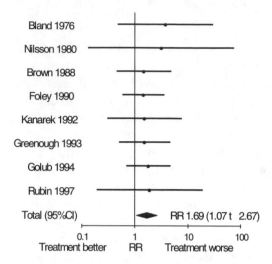

Figure 14.2 Meta-analysis of the effect on mortality of albumin supplementation in critically ill and injured patients.

quality, relevance of outcomes, clinical experience, or other factors. Ideally, all these issues were considered when formulating the research question and choosing inclusion criteria.

When judged to be appropriate, performance of a meta-analysis can contribute importantly to a systematic review. Combining the results from similar randomized trials will increase the precision of the effect estimates, and may allow the reliable estimation of even modest effects. There are several methods for pooling study results, all of which take a weighted average of the study-specific effect estimates, with the weights being inversely proportional to the variance of the effect estimates. Methods to combine observational studies are similar to those used for trials (Greenland, 1998). Clearly, in order to combine data, information on the effect estimate and its variance must be available and poor reporting of study results can therefore be an important obstacle to meta-analysis (Wagenaar, 1999).

Figure 14.2 shows a meta-analysis of randomized controlled trials of the effect of albumin supplementation on mortality in critically ill and injured patients. Each of the eight trials showed a nonsignificant increase in mortality in the albumin-treated group. In other words, in each trial the excess of deaths in the albumin-treated group was easily compatible with the play of chance. However, the fact that all eight trials showed an effect in the same direction is less compatible with the play of chance, and this information is embodied in the pooled relative risk with its much narrower confidence intervals (Cochrane Injuries Group Albumin Reviewers, 1998).

Assessing the Potential for Selection Bias

Various methods have been developed to assess the presence of publication and other selection biases in identifying studies (Begg and Mazumdar, 1994; Egger et al.,

1997b). For example, in a funnel plot, the treatment effect from each trial, the log odds ratio, is plotted against the precision of the treatment effect (the inverse of the standard error), which is largely a function of sample size. A regression test of funnel plot asymmetry has been developed to test for the statistical likelihood of selection bias (Egger et al., 1997b).

The Cochrane Injuries Group

The Cochrane Injuries Group is part of a wider organization known as the Cochrane Collaboration (Bero and Rennie, 1995). This is an international network that prepares, maintains, and promotes the accessibility of high-quality peer-reviewed systematic reviews of the effects of health-care interventions. Protocols for systematic reviews and completed reviews are peer reviewed and published in the Cochrane Library, where they are open to public and professional scrutiny. The Cochrane Library is published quarterly on CD-ROM and the internet (see Table 14.1), and is distributed by subscription. With electronic publication, reviews can be updated or amended in response to post-publication criticism or new information.

The Injuries Group produces reviews on the prevention, treatment, and rehabilitation of traumatic injury. Researchers interested in preparing reviews as part of the Injuries Group can obtain assistance with protocol development, literature searches, software, peer reviews, and other aspects of conducting systematic reviews by contacting the Cochrane Injuries Review Group Co-ordinator (Frances Bunn), Department of Epidemiology and Public Health, Institute of Child Health, 30 Guilford Street, London WC1N 1EH, UK; +44 020 7242 9789 ext 2655 or f.bunn@ich.ucl.ac.uk

Conclusions

Systematic reviews identify and summarize the best available research evidence in order to answer specific questions about prevention, treatment, or rehabilitation. Systematically reviewing the literature decreases the likelihood of bias in evaluating existing research. When results can be combined, systematic reviews also allow greater precision in estimating the effects of intervention. The methodology for systematic reviews can be applied to injury research as to other areas of health-care. However, the wider context of injury research dictates the casting of a wide net to identify all relevant evidence on a given research question. Whether embarking on a new area of injury research, or an injury intervention program, the first step to take should be a systematic review of the relevant evidence.

Acknowledgements

We gratefully acknowledge the assistance of Phil Alderson with the cumulative meta-analysis of albumin studies and of Reinhard Wentz in identifying data sources.

References

Armstrong CJ, Fenton RR (1996) World Databases in Biosciences and Pharmacology. (World databases Series ISBN 1-85739-068-7.) London: Bowker Saur.

Begg CB, Mazumdar M (1994) Operating characteristics of a rank correlation test for publication bias. Biometrics 50:1088–101.

Berlin JA, Miles CG, Crigliano MD (1997) Does blinding of readers affect the results of meta-analyses? Results of a randomized trial. Online J Curr Clin Trials Document no. 205.

Bero L, Rennie D (1995) The Cochrane Collaboration. Preparing, maintaining, and disseminating systematic reviews of the effects of health care. JAMA 274:1935–8.

Chalmers I In: Chalmers I, Altman DG (eds) (1995) *Systematic Reviews.* London: BMJ Publishing Group.

Chalmers TC, Matta RJ, Smith H, Kunzler AM (1977) Evidence favoring the use of anticoagulants in the hospital phase of acute myocardial infarction. N Engl J Med 297:1091–6.

Cochrane Injuries Group Albumin Reviewers (1998) Human albumin administration in critically ill patients: systematic review of randomized controlled trials. Br Med J 317:235–40. Also available in: The Cochrane Library, Issue 3 1998 Oxford: Update Software.

Dickersin K, Min YI (1993) NIH clinical trials and publication bias. Online J Curr Clin Trials Apr 28: Doc No. 50.

Easterbrook PJ, Berlin JA, Gopalan R, Matthews DR (1991) Publication bias in clinical research. Lancet 337:868–72.

Egger M, Zellweger-Zahner T, Schneider M, Junker C, Lengeler C, Antes G (1997a) Language bias in randomized controlled trials published in English and German. The Lancet 350:326–9.

Egger M, Davey Smith G, Schneider M, Minder C (1997b) Bias in meta-analysis detected by a simple graphical test. Br Med J 315:629–34.

Elvik R (1998) Are road safety evaluation studies published in peer reviewed journals more valid than similar studies not published in peer reviewed journals? Accid Anal Prev 30:101–18.

Feinstein AR, Horwitz RI (1982) Double standards, scientific methods, and epidemiologic research. New Engl J Med 307(26):1611–17.

Freemantle N, Bero L, Grilli R et al. (eds) (1999) *Effective Professional Practice Module, Cochrane Database of Systematic Reviews.* The Cochrane Library. Issue 2. Oxford: Update Software.

Greenland S (1998) Meta-analysis. In: Rothman KJ, Greenland S (eds), Modern Epidemiology, Chapter 32. Philadelphia: Lippincott-Raven.

Hodnett ED, Roberts I (1999) Home-based social support for socially disadvantaged mothers. The Cochrane Library. Issue 1. Oxford: Update Software.

Jadad AR, Moore RA, Carroll D et al. (1996) Assessing the quality of reports of randomized clinical trials: Is blinding necessary? Control Clin Trials 17:1–12.

Moher D, Jadad AR, Nichol G, Penman M, Tugwell T, Walsh S (1995) Assessing the quality of randomized controlled trials: an annotated bibliography of scales and checklists. Controlled Clin Trials 16(1):62–73.

Moher D, Pham B, Jones AL et al. (1998) Does quality of reports of randomized trials affect estimates of intervention efficacy reported in meta-analyses? Lancet 352:609–13.

Mulrow C, Langhorne P, Grimshaw J (1997) Integrating heterogeneous pieces of evidence in systematic reviews. Ann Intern Med 127:989–95.

Mulrow CD, Oxman AD (eds) (1997) Formulating the Problem. Cochrane Collaboration Handbook [updated September 1997]. Section 4. In: The Cochrane Library [database of disk and CDROM]. The Cochrane Collaboration. Oxford: Update Software; (1999), Issue.

Sackett DL, Haynes RB (1992) On the need for evidence-based medicine. A new approach to teaching the practice of medicine. JAMA 268:2420–5.

Schulz KF, Chalmers I, Hayes RJ, Altman DG (1995) Empirical evidence of bias: dimensions of methodological quality associated with estimates of treatment effects in controlled trials. JAMA 273:408–12.

Smith BJ, Darzins PJ, Quinn M, Heller RF. (1992) Modern methods of searching the medical literature. Med J Aust 157:603–11.

Smith R, Roberts I (1997) An amnesty for unpublished trials. Br Med J 315:62.

Thompson SG (1995) Why sources of heterogeneity in meta-analysis should be investigated. In: Chalmers I, Altman DG (eds), *Systematic Reviews* pp. 48–63. London: BMJ Publishing Group.

Thompson D, Rivara F (1998) Pool fencing for drowning prevention. (Cochrane Review). In: The Cochrane Library, Issue 3. Oxford: Update Software.

Vernick JS, Li G, Ogaitis S, MacKenzie E, Baker SP, Gielen AC (1999) Effects of high school driver education on motor vehicle crashes, violations, and licensure. Am J Prev Med 16:40–6.

Wagenaar AC (1999) Importance of systematic reviews and meta-analyses for research and practice. Am J Prev Med 16(S):9–11.

15

Evaluating an Injury Intervention or Program

Robert S. Thompson and Jeffrey J. Sacks

Introduction

Evaluation is defined by Last's Dictionary of Epidemiology as a "process that attempts to determine as systematically and objectively as possible, the relevance, effectiveness, and impact of activities in light of their objectives. Several varieties of evaluation can be distinguished; e.g., evaluation of structure, process, and outcome." (Last et al., 1995).

No single definition captures all the aspects of program evaluation. Evaluation research shares some themes with outcomes research and with efforts to measure the quality of healthcare (Petitti, 1998; Petitti and Amster, 1998). With outcomes research, it shares a focus on effectiveness (intervention under everyday circumstances) more often than on efficacy (the effect of the intervention under ideal and tightly controlled conditions). With quality of care research, it shares the use of structural, process, and outcome (health effects) measures to examine program/intervention effects.

We emphasize the importance of linking an intervention with an evaluation plan at the outset. Without this linkage, it is often impossible to design an evaluation post hoc that will provide valid process and outcome information.

Performing Program Evaluation
Purpose of Evaluation

Evaluation is often described as having one or more of three purposes: (1) to establish or clarify program effectiveness; (2) to improve program implementation; and (3) to address administrative needs. This chapter addresses the first two purposes. Generally evaluation indicates how effectively the program was implemented (process), what it has accomplished (outcomes), and how effective it was for health (outcome) (Dannenberg and Fowler, 1998; Thompson and McClintock, 1998).

By working with the program's stakeholders, one should generate a list of the specific questions to be answered by the evaluation. The overall purpose of the evaluation will embody the goals of the program, while the specific questions should target specific measurable outcomes to be evaluated.

Intervention Model Specification as a Basis for Program Evaluation

A logic model is a diagrammatic representation of the universe of determinates, intermediate outcomes, potential interventions, and health outcomes (i.e., automobile crash) known and hypothesized for the outcome of interest (Clinical Practice Guideline Development: Methodology Perspectives, 1994). Similarly, but usually narrower in scope, a causal model is a diagram of the main linkages in the central causal pathway (Koepsell, 1998). Generally, logic or causal models, or specifically for injury, the Haddon Matrix (Runyan, 1998), all of which lay out the individual, family, population, including intervention subpopulations, cultural, environmental, health-care system, and legal system determinates of major injury outcomes, can be quite helpful in suggesting which linkage points in a causal chain offer the most promise for specific intervention. In brief, these models suggest where to intervene. Subsequently, it is helpful to have the specific implementation intervention strategies developed on the basis of conceptual planning models (Green and Kreuter, 1991; Walsh and McPhee, 1992; Thompson, 1996; Goodman, 1998; Curry and Kim, 1999). These models provide the framework for spelling out the how of a specific intervention. The planning model chosen must then be populated with the evidence-based intervention tools available and best suited to the situation (Thompson, 1996; Thomson, 1998a, b, c, d).

One useful intervention implementation model is the Precede/Proceed model (Green and Kreuter, 1991), which specifies three categories of factor (predisposing, enabling, and reinforcing) supporting behavior change. Predisposing factors influence a person's willingness to change, the possession of, and the confidence (sense of self-efficacy) in, his or her skills to perform a task, and the provider's or patient's (depending on the issue) knowledge, attitudes, beliefs (KAB), and personal health behaviors or experiences. Prochaska's Stages of Change model may be incorporated into the Precede/Proceed model, depending on the issue to be addressed and the magnitude of the behavioral component (Prochaska et al., 1998). Enabling factors, such as supportive policies or computer systems, are environmental factors at the practice, organizational, or community-level, which make change possible. Reinforcing factors, such as measurement and feedback, amplify the intervention.

Public health and community-based models for program delivery and continuous evaluation have been described by Walsh and McPhee (1992), Dever (1997), Durch et al. (1997), and Goldstein et al. (1998). All of the models described, when successfully applied, involve the application of behavior change techniques at the individual level for patients, or clinical practitioners or public health practitioners, and application of the same general principles at the organizational or community change level (Skinner and Botelho, 1999; Curry and Kim, 1999). Figure 15.1 illustrates a systems approach model incorporating many of these concepts (e.g., Green and Kreuter, 1991; and Dever, 1997).

Initially, a conceptual framework for intervention implementation (step 1a) and the intervention components from the "tool kit" (step 1b) are chosen. The "tools" (e.g., the use of opinion leaders) listed in the figure are based on systematic reviews and empirical practices. The intervention (step 2) is concurrently directed

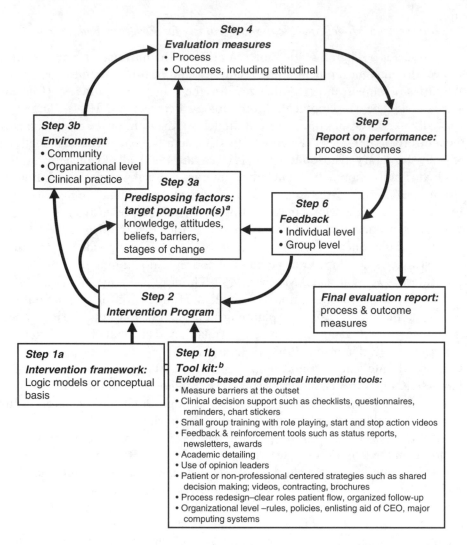

Figure 15.1 A systems model for: continuous program implementation, outcome measurement, feedback, and improvement. a. Practitioners.

to the predisposing factors of the target population (step 3a) and environmental enabling factors (step 3b). The enabling factors may be addressed at the practice level, the organizational level, or the broader community. Interventions may then lead to changes in processes, KAB, or other health outcomes that can be measured (step 4), summarized (step 5), and fed back into the intervention process (step 6).

The take home message is that interventions and implementation strategies based on conceptual models can lead to more coherent programs and to the development of prespecified evaluation measures tied directly to the planning model.

Planning Issues

Involve the stakeholders in the evaluation planning process early. Stakeholders include decision-makers, insiders from the intervention delivery groups, and representatives from the target population (Centers for Disease Control and Prevention, 1998). This is important in a small group setting, but becomes virtually mandatory for large-scale community-based interventions (Goodman, 1998). It is then helpful to refine the objectives of the evaluation and the use of the results (Carey and Lloyd, 1995; Dever, 1997; Goodman, 1998; Thompson and McClintock, 1998).

Methods for Evaluation
Intervention Level to be Evaluated

The level (practice, organization, and/or community) at which the intervention is applied plays a major part in dictating the design of the evaluation.

The Practice Level

Because this level addresses the interface of the 1 : 1 provider patient interaction, randomized clinical trials, case–control, case-cohort, and cohort designs are all possible.

The Organizational Level

In integrated health-care systems, combination strategies come into play. The level of randomization may be the clinic, while the level of analysis may be the clinic, provider, and/or individual patient levels. The effects of group randomization on variance must be taken into account in estimating study power and in the analysis. While randomized controlled trials with individuals as the unit of randomization are possible, group randomization may be preferable for effectiveness trials (Thompson et al., 2000).

The Community-level

There are two broad types of community intervention models – the social experiment, which is mainly externally driven, where the community participates because of the anticipated gains for community health or general knowledge; and the grass roots program, which arises mainly from the community and its members working together to address perceived community needs. Evaluation needs and strategies are likely to be quite different based on the model used.

"In community trials, there are at least two kinds of sample sizes to consider (number of communities and number of individuals per community) and two kinds of variability to be estimated in study planning and accommodated during data analysis (within community variance, and across community variance)" (Koepsell, 1998). If community-level variance is not taken into account, effect estimation is driven in the nonconservative direction, leading to the suggestion of intervention effects when there are no effects.

Several recent reviews are helpful for further information about community-level trials: designing community intervention trials (Koepsell, 1998); general principles of evaluation for community intervention trials (Goodman, 1998); proposed indicator sets for community health profiles (Durch et al., 1997); and analytic issues for group randomized trials including the issue of community-level variance (Murray, 1997, 1998; Feldman, 1997; Koepsell, 1998).

Evaluation Design

The "gold standard" for experimental designs in clinical medicine is the randomized controlled trial (RCT). Quasi-experimental designs, time series designs, exposure series, or designs using an external comparison group, while weaker, can also provide useful information (Cummings and Weiss, 1998).

Without a comparison group to evaluate injury interventions, it can be difficult to determine how much of any intervention effect is due to the intervention and how much is due to secular trend (Hancock et al., 1997; Green, 1997). A one-intervention, one-control community design confounds community-level variation with treatment group status. Use of several control communities mitigates this problem.

Cohort study designs lend themselves well to assessment of injury programs when the outcome is relatively common as, in this design, the specification is on the exposure (Breslow and Day, 1987).

Well-designed case–control studies can yield highly meaningful evaluative information (Rothman and Greenland, 1998). The case crossover methodology has promise for injury evaluation research. Redelmeier and Tibshirani (1997) used this technique to demonstrate a fourfold increased risk for motor vehicle collisions associated with the use of cell phones in cars (see chapter on selecting a study design for injury research).

Types of Evaluation

There are several types of program evaluation. Some classification schemes separate program evaluation into the following sequential phases: pilot testing, formative evaluation, summative evaluation, process evaluation, impact evaluation, outcome evaluation, and structural evaluation (Thompson and McClintock, 1998; Petitti and Amster, 1998, p. 301). While useful for some investigators, for others it will seem needlessly complex.

We use just two broad categories to describe evaluation: (1) process evaluation, where the measures reflect what was done to implement the intervention, and what was done to, for, or by the target population (Feldman, 1997); and (2) outcome evaluation, which indicates changes in KABs, and health states associated with the intervention. Under our definition, impact measures, which assess whether a broad community message reached the target subjects, are a form of process measure. KABs are viewed as a form of outcome measure.

Process Evaluation

An example of process evaluation measures at the practice level would be enumerating discount coupons distributed for bicycle safety helmets; or, at the community-level, the presence and application of regulations to require lower hot water heater temperatures. Process evaluation measures can be defined for individuals, organizations, and communities or broader areas.

Process measurement may be especially applicable for the ongoing assessment of programs. This evaluation may incorporate concepts of continuous quality improvement as the focus is on decreasing variation (Carey and Lloyd, 1995). In this situation, quality control sampling methods that utilize small numbers are often used, and the process will undoubtedly include feedback of newly measured information into the modification of the overall process (Reinke, 1991; Carey and Lloyd, 1995; Shahian et al., 1996; Dever, 1997). Evaluative information of this type then becomes part of the intervention itself.

W. Edwards Deming and other quality managers have for many years maintained that approximately 85% of the opportunities for improvement in processes are in system changes such as role assignments, and policy changes (often what we would now call guidelines) and 15% rests with individual people (Carey and Lloyd, 1995; Skinner and Botelho, 1999).

In our view, process evaluation should begin as soon as the program begins operation. This helps to identify any early problems, shows how well procedures and materials are working, and allows for modification of materials and adjustments in resources. Ultimately process evaluation indicates how well the program is achieving its intermediate goals such as increased bicycle safety helmet use or increased use of seat belts by motor vehicle occupants.

Outcome Evaluation

Outcome evaluation measures the KAB and the health and/or well being of patients or populations (Table 15.1). It may include relevant healthcare outcomes such as death, disease, disability, discomfort, and dissatisfaction (Elinson, 1987).

Most injuries can be thought of as short "incubation period" illnesses (e.g., a motorcycle crash). As such they lend themselves well to outcome evaluations early in the program history. However, this may not apply to more chronic and recurrent problems such as domestic violence.

The decision to use process or outcome measures is part of an ongoing debate (National Committee for Injury Prevention and Control, 1989; Hancock et al., 1997; Green, 1997). For example, process measurements for quality are espoused by Robert Brook and others from the Rand Corporation while the Foundation for Accountability (FACCT) recommends the use of outcome measures for measuring quality (Petitti and Amster, 1998, p. 307). Process measures are more under the control of the interventionist (i.e., doctor) and are more sensitive to change. However, they are not necessarily strong predictors of outcome (Petitti and Amster, 1998, p. 302). Outcomes are much less under the control of the interventionist (e.g.,

Table 15.1 Potential health outcomes

- Death
- Length of life
- Complications of disease
- Complications of medical care (harms of any intervention)
- Physical function
- Psychosocial function
- Role Function (e.g., returning to work)
- Quality of life
- Cost of care
- Service utilization (e.g., length of stay, physician visits)
- Patient preferences

Adapted from Iezzoni (1994) and Petitti (1998).

consider death from handguns), are more difficult to assign to a particular intervention because of time effects, and because these are rare events, the power of a study to show important differences is often lacking (Petitti and Amster, 1998, p. 303).

We feel that both process measures and other outcomes should be measured on a regular basis for ideal program implementation. If the measurements are well planned, these same data can provide the basis for periodic overall program evaluation reports.

Choice of Evaluation Measures: Case Studies from Injury Interventions

To demonstrate some of the choices entailed in selecting process and outcome measures, we summarize the Seattle, Washington area bicycle safety helmet campaign and the statewide injury prevention program (SCIPP) in Massachusetts.

Bicycle Safety Helmets

The Seattle campaign begun in 1986 was designed to increase the use of bicycle safety helmets in children 5–15 years of age. The campaign was spearheaded by the Harborview Injury Prevention and Research Center (HIPRC) of the University of Washington and included 18 different community groups. The community campaign included repeated radio and TV spots, newspaper stories, provision of lapel buttons ("Wear a Bicycle Helmet") for primary care physicians, discount helmet coupons given out in doctors' offices, schools, and grocery stores, and distribution of quality helmets at discount through health maintenance organizations. The broad community efforts focused on increasing parental awareness of the significance of bicycle-related head injuries, on convincing children that helmet wearing was "cool" and "non-nerdy," and advocating for decreased helmet costs with manufacturers (DiGuiseppi et al., 1990; Bergman et al., 1990).

When this was a new community campaign, a broad menu of potential evaluation measures was considered at various levels from the practice setting to the whole community. The actual evaluation measures chosen included: a 1986 parental and child KAB survey, which was instrumental in indicating initial barriers to be addressed (DiGuiseppi et al., 1990), and part of the formative process for the campaign; repeated assessments of observed helmet wearing by riders [with Portland, Oregon as a comparison community (DiGuiseppi et al., 1989)]; safety helmet sales in the area and redemption rates for discount coupons for helmets (Bergman et al., 1990); bicycle-related head injury (BRHI) incidence rates measured at GHC, as a minipopulation laboratory, to reflect the broader community effect (Rivara et al., 1994); and a cost-effectiveness analysis of helmet subsidies (Thompson et al., 1993).

The evaluation measures chosen were relatively objective and directly observable. This approach, combined with parsimony of choice, is preferable when feasible. All the measures listed fall within the broad framework of process and outcome measures.

Example 2: The Statewide Childhood Injury Prevention Program (SCIPP)

The SCIPP intervention project was a social experiment conducted in nine intervention and five comparison communities in Massachusetts with a total population of 286,676 in the late 1970s and early 1980s (Gallagher et al., 1982, 1984; Guyer et al., 1989). The focus was on parents with children 18 years of age or younger. The overall intervention, delivered over a period of 22 months, consisted of five components: (1) injury counseling for parents of young children by pediatricians; (2) school and community burn prevention education; (3) household injury hazard identification and control through regular home safety inspections; (4) community-wide promotion of the poison control system's telephone information service and public education about poison prevention; and (5) promotion of child automobile restraint use, especially for children less than 5 years of age. The study targeted five injuries: motor vehicle occupant injuries, poisonings, burns, falls, and suffocation.

The unit of allocation and intervention for the study was the community, as was the level of intervention. "Because it was impractical to randomize communities," communities were matched on socioeconomic and demographic variables. Measurements were performed pre- and postintervention using telephone surveys and a hospital-based injury surveillance system. The analysis was performed at the level of the community with adjustment for an index of socioeconomic status (SES). Evaluation measures consisted of process measures – determination of exposure to the intervention components, and outcome measures including changes in safety knowledge and practices, and changes in target injury rates.

The main health outcome result, after adjusting for SES, was that the incidence of motor vehicle occupant injuries decreased by 54% in the intervention communities while it rose in the control communities. This intervention employed parsimoniously selected process (participation) and outcome (KAB and injury rates) measures for evaluation. Analysis was performed at the community-level as a means of avoiding violation of statistical independence.

Specific Measures for Use in Evaluation

Potential process and outcome measures for evaluating interventions or programs for injury control are listed in Table 15.2.

Measurement categories and some individual measures are further described below.

Table 15.2 Partial list of evaluation measures for consideration

Measures	References
Process measures	
HEDIS (Health Plan Employer Data and Information Set)	HEDIS, 1999
When a process measure may substitute for a health outcome	Schulman et al. (PICARD), 1998
	MacKenzie (this volume)
Outcomes	
Knowledge, attitudes, beliefs (KAB)	
Self-efficacy (confidence)	Bandura, 1995
	Curry & Kim, 1999
Stages of change	Willey et al., 1996
	Prochaska et al., 1998
	Skinner and Botelho, 1999
Cognitive, behavioral, environmental factors	Curry and Kim, 1999
Harms from the intervention	Fisher and Welch (generic), 1999
	Graham et al. (air bags), 1997
Health status	
Injury severity: AIS, ISS, and other injury severity scores	Fingerhut and McLoughlin (this volume)
	Jurkovich and O'Keefe (this volume)
Health Status – Short Form (SF)	McDowell and Newell, 1996
36 Questionnaire	Stewart et al., 1988
	Ware, 1994, 1995
Sickness Impact Profile (SIP)	DeBruin et al., 1992
	McDowell and Newell, 1996
	Jurkovich et al. (injury application), 1995
Functional outcome assessment	MacKenzie (this volume)
Quality of well-being	Clancy and Eisenberg, 1998
	Chenn et al., 1975
	Kaplan and Anderson, 1988
	Petitti, 1998
Years of potential life lost	Committee on Trauma Research, 1985
	Rice et al., 1989
Cost-benefit (CBA); cost-effectiveness (CEA) and cost-utility analysis (CUA)	Haddix et al., 1996
	Gold et al., 1996
	Petitti, 1994
	Graham and Segui-Gomez (this volume)
Concept of value in health care	Lawrence, 1992
	Halvorson, 1993

Process Measures

Process measures reflect the quantity of inputs into or products produced by the intervention. Included are those things done to people (e.g., given a smoke alarm), done by people (e.g., wore a seat belt), or done to the environment (e.g., seat belt laws, air bags, posters in practice locations). Process measures are those features of the care process believed to be integrally linked to the outcome(s) of interest. Examples would be supplying smoke alarms to all those who do not have them (Mallonee et al., 1996). The strong relationship between bicycle helmet use and BRHIs is another example of linkage (Rivara et al., 1994). Taking this linkage one step further, the Centers for Disease Control and Prevention has developed methods to estimate the numbers of avoided fatal and nonfatal cases of BRHI and associated economic costs (Schulman et al., 1998) given helmet usage rates pre- and postprogram as the only directly measured data. This method is potentially generalizable to other injury problems.

Outcome Measures
Knowledge, Attitudes and Beliefs (KAB):

- Increased knowledge by itself does not seem to predict individual behavior change. In most areas of health, knowledge is thought to be necessary but not sufficient for change (Davis et al., 1992, 1995; Freemantle et al., 1998). For injuries, changes in knowledge seem to correlate especially poorly with changes in behavior. [See Grossman and Garcia (1999) on educational approaches for increasing automobile restraint use by young children; Vernick et al. (1999) on drivers' education courses for high school aged people; or Hardy et al. (1996) on gun safety education for preschoolers.]
- Self-efficacy is a measure of the belief (confidence) that one has the skills and the ability to carry out the targeted behavior successfully. Self-efficacy is influenced by performance accomplishment, i.e., realizing that you can accomplish the action often through role-playing or rehearsal. To a lesser degree, self-efficacy is positively influenced by vicarious experiences and verbal persuasion but is negatively influenced by tasks that are emotionally draining. Self-efficacy is an important predictor of behavior change (Bandura, 1995; Clark and Becker, 1998, pp. 16–17). Self-efficacy is generally measured by questionnaire using a set of questions (commonly with a five-point scale for choices) that are associated with a domain designated for the concept. Often, these questions can be distilled to a few that are highly predictive.
- Stages of Change. The Transtheoretical model of behavior change, also called the Stages of Change model, is generalizable to a broad range of behaviors. These include, substance abuse, alcohol use patterns, adolescent delinquent behaviors, and other risk behaviors (Prochaska et al., 1995, 1998; Willey et al., 1996). The model delineates five stages that generally follow one upon another. Not every person goes through all stages and people also relapse and repeat stages passed through previously. Situational self-efficacy occurs when people believe they can

cope with high-risk situations without relapsing. In general, the further along in the Stages of Change a person is, the higher their situational self-efficacy.

The stages of change are:

- Precontemplation. These individuals have not thought of change and are not intending to take action within the next 6 months.
- Contemplation. These individuals are seriously considering making a change in the next 6 months. They are aware of the pros of changing, but also acutely aware of the cons. This is a time of behavioral cost–benefit assessment by the individual.
- Preparation. Individuals are planning to change in the next 30 days and usually have a plan for action.
- Action. This is measured as having changed in the last 6 months. People must have made a significant enough change that experts would agree that the risk of injury is diminished by the change.
- Maintenance. Person has made the change and maintained it for over 6 months. People in this phase are working to prevent relapse and are increasingly more confident (self-efficacy) in their ability to continue the changes. Maintenance is estimated by Prochaska and colleagues (1998) to last from 6 months up till 5 years. For example, smoking relapse after 1 year of abstinence is 43%, but by 5 years the rate is only 7%.
- Termination. In this phase, individuals have little temptation to engage in the behavior, have essentially complete self-efficacy and little chance of relapse.

The Stages of Change model is increasingly being used to focus stage-specific interventions (Prochaska et al., 1995, 1998; Willey et al., 1996; Curry and Kim, 1999; Skinner and Botelho, 1999). Stages of Change predicts who will quit smoking cigarettes or will reduce problem drinking, so linkage between stages and the probability of action is being increasingly established (Prochaska et al., 1998; Skinner and Botelho, 1999). To our knowledge, no studies have demonstrated a graduated, or dose–response linkage between various stages of change in target populations or individuals and injury outcomes. Understanding the characteristics of the population with respect to the stages-of-change provides a basis for more appropriate planning and delivery of targeted health interventions (Willey et al., 1996). Furthermore, these findings force us to rethink the manner in which we evaluate injury and public health interventions. Based predominately on the tobacco cessation literature, the data indicate that assisting individuals in progressing from one stage to the next doubles the probability that they will take action in the ensuing 6 months (Prochaska et al., 1998). These findings seem promising for application to the evaluation of injury control programs, for example, assessing gun owners' shift from pre-contemplation to contemplation/preparation for the safe storage of firearms. Examining the intervention effect on the population with respect to the stages of change at baseline and at follow-up may prove to be a useful outcome measure.

Health Outcomes:

Information on mortality and hospitalization is generally available as outcome measures (see chapter on data sets and data linkage). Hospitalization data are generally available in automated format and can be categorized by International Classification of Disease diagnosis codes, and E-codes for cause of injury (DHHS, 1998; Fingerhut and McLoughlin, this volume). Though less generally available in automated format, primary care utilization is very important for describing the total burden of disease, for example, 50% of head injuries in children are cared for in primary care (Rivara et al., 1989). Other important health outcomes to consider include shifts in severity of injury (see Jurkovich and O'Keefe, this volume) and changes in mid- and long-term disability from injury (see MacKenzie, this volume).

• Harms. As we consider program effects on health, both positive outcomes and negative outcomes (harms) must be take into account. The issue of harm from the side-effects of various interventions has been insufficiently considered and quantified in injury evaluation work. While harms have been considered for the side-effects of automobile air bags on children (Graham et al., 1997), several thousand publications on automobile passenger safety revealed very little information on harms resulting from other interventions, such as mandatory seat belt laws.

At a more general level, Fisher and Welch (1999) demonstrate harms from medical care entailing: more use of home monitoring in pregnancy; more anti-arrhythmic medications; more coronary angioplasty instead of medical management; more capacity for general care in both the inpatient and outpatient arenas, invasive management of coronary artery disease, structured discharge procedures of patients with diabetes, heart disease, or chronic obstructive pulmonary disease. Harms as well as benefits should be routinely ascertained for medical, general public health, and injury interventions. This is a concept that is long overdue.

Other ways of describing the impact of diseases or injuries include the use of:

• Health status measures. The reviews by Patrick and Erickson (1993) and McDowell and Newell (1996) are highly recommended. The Short Form (SF) 36 developed by Rand is a classic for this purpose (Stewart et al., 1988; Ware, 1994, 1995). Another generic health status measure is the well-validated Sickness Impact Profile (SIP), which has been applied to a wide range of disease entities (DeBruin et al., 1992; McDowell and Newell, 1996). It has been applied to burn injuries, spinal cord injuries and lower extremity fractures (Jurkovich et al., 1995). The reader should consult MacKenzie (this volume) for a more detailed discussion of health status measures and functional outcome assessment.

• Quality of well-being. The SF 36 and the SIP offer little insight into the meaning of a particular health state. For example, scores on the SIP can range from 0 to 100, which is valuable for categorization, but not explanatory in terms of what the score means to the individual (Clancy and Eisenberg, 1998).

Well-being scales are being developed to permit assessments of the perceived value of health states (Chenn et al., 1975; Kaplan and Anderson, 1988; Clancy and Eisenberg, 1998).

• Costs and cost-effectiveness. The concept of using years of potential life lost as an outcome measure gained prominence in 1985 through its use in the book, Injury in America (Committee on Trauma Research, 1985). As injuries have a disproportionate impact on younger people, this method of analysis serves to emphasize one of the important impacts of injuries. For example, injuries in the United States account for 4.1 million years of life lost, while cancer accounts for 1.7 million and heart disease 2.1 million years of life lost annually in the U.S. population (Committee on Trauma Research, 1985; Rice et al., 1989). Interventions can be evaluated by examining the number of years of life saved through implementation of a program. Further elaboration of this general theme extends to cost–benefit analysis (CBA), cost-effectiveness analysis (CEA) and cost utility analysis (CUA) (Petitti, 1994; Gold et al., 1996; Haddix et al., 1996; Graham and Segui-Gomez, this volume).

• Concept of value. In economic circles, value is defined as the health benefit divided by cost. However, as used by health-care delivery organizations (Lawrence, 1992; Halvorson, 1993), value is the best balance between: (1) health outcomes; (2) member or patient satisfaction; (3) practitioner or practice team satisfaction; and (4) costs. This approach requires thinking of outcomes for health, satisfaction (members, providers), and costs simultaneously. Interventions positively affecting health outcomes and satisfaction while decreasing costs, have the greatest prospect for future widespread application.

Data Definitions and Sources

The next step is to define the target population operationally in terms of the data sources available. This includes definitions of the denominators, for example, in-line skaters 15–24 years of age, and numerators such as the age group, number of skaters wearing wrist-guards (process measure), or number with wrist fractures (outcome).

Data sources need to be defined. Will it be medical records, telephone interviews, state death tapes, hospitalization, and emergency room utilization tapes for the Medicaid population, or linkages to state patrol records for single occupant motor vehicle crashes? (See Mueller and Grossman, and Runyan and Bowling, this volume, for details.)

Data collection instruments should be designed and pilot tested (McDowell and Newell, 1996). If these are newly developed instruments to be used for chart abstraction or for telephone interviews, we recommend a pilot assessment of a minimum of 30 individuals. This is a great help for finalization of the format and content of the instrument. Other evaluation procedures should also be described and piloted.

Data quality should be assessed initially and over time. This may require a comparison of medical record information and automated data. (For methodologic considerations, see Mullooly, 1996; Mullooly et al., 1999.)

If KABs are to be measured in the evaluation process, it is useful to pilot the questionnaire on a group similar to but separate from the intervention group. Where possible, use previously developed and utilized instruments or questions as a part of the evaluation process. This will provide information that can be compared with external groups. In addition, work on validity (does the instrument measure the phenomenon it is said to measure) and reliability (the extent to which the instrument achieves the same results on repeated administration to the same person) may have already been performed. For more detailed examination of the issues entailed in assessing validity and in designing questionnaires, see Kim and Mueller (1978a, b), Carmines and Zeller (1979), and Runyan and Bowling (this volume).

A key part of data collection is collecting information on potential confounders (Petitti, 1998). A confounding variable is one that is (1) causally associated with the outcome under study independent of the exposure (or the intervention) of interest, and (2) is associated with the exposure of interest, but is (3) not a consequence of the exposure. Confounding may occur because of differences in age, gender, ethnicity, or other risk status variables (e.g., alcohol use patterns), and income, for example. In outcome studies, severity of illness and co-morbidity are major additional sources of confounding to consider. Potential confounders should be measured to the extent possible in all injury intervention studies. This is especially critical when nonexperimental study designs are used.

Finally, once data sources have been delineated, data collection schedules, responsibilities, and role specification are necessary steps (Carey and Lloyd, 1995).

Data Analysis

Data analysis will frequently have two purposes: (1) to provide immediate and ongoing process information as feedback for amplifying or modifying the implementation of the intervention (Carey and Lloyd, 1995; Thompson, 1996; Dever, 1997; Thomson et al., 1998b, c), and (2) to provide periodic process and outcome analyses. We recommend that the analytic plan for the data be pre-specified, shell tables be constructed and the actual analyses be piloted early to provide the opportunity to modify the plan should significant problems be found.

For intervention analysis, we usually specify three time periods for data collection: (1) baseline or pre-intervention; (2) intervention implementation; and (3) short and long-term periods post-implementation. If automated data are used for evaluation, measurement may be performed across all three of these time periods. If primary data collection is involved, measurement may be feasible only in the baseline and post-implementation periods.

Analyses should control for possible confounding, especially for nonrandomized studies. For dichotomous outcomes, logistic regression analysis is appropriate (Breslow and Day, 1980; Clayton and Hills, 1993). For cohort analyses where time to outcome is examined, Cox proportional hazards models are commonly employed (Breslow and Day, 1987; Clayton and Hills, 1993). For more complex study designs involving randomization or matching of communities or groups (e.g., medical clinics), a variety of analytic approaches have been developed in recent years (Murray 1997, 1998; Koepsell, 1998). To avoid violations of statistical independence assumptions, one approach is to analyze data at the level of the community by aggregating individual-level observations to the level of the community. This approach was used in the analysis of the SCIPP studies (Guyer et al., 1989). Another approach is to adjust an individual-level analysis for clustering (Donner and Klar, 1994). A two-stage analysis can be performed where the first stage ignores clustering effects, and the second stage takes community-level covariates into account through the use of ANOVA or ANCOVA (Zucker et al., 1995). Finally, an individual level analysis for correlated data can be performed. These models use mixed models of variance or covariance, or may employ general estimating equations (GEE) to take clustering effects into account (Zeger and Liang, 1986; Grossman et al., 1997).

Reporting the Results of the Program Evaluation

The effects of the intervention should be presented as both an absolute or actual change, and a relative or percentage change (Eddy, 1996). For example, consider bicycle-related head injuries (BRHI) rates in 10–14 year olds, before (188/100,000) and after (61/100,000) a major community helmet campaign. The absolute effect is an actual decrease of 127/100,000. The relative or percentage change is 67.6% (188–127)/188) (Rivara et al., 1994).

Relative outcome differences between intervention and comparison groups are often expressed as relative risks or odds ratios. For example, the risk for BRHIs in helmet wearers is only 15% of that for non-wearers (odds ratio of BRHI is 0.15, 95%CI 0.07 to 0.29). Alternatively stated, non-wearers are at 6.6-fold increased risk for BRHIs compared to helmet wearers (Thompson et al., 1989).

Public health interventions are likely to reach more people than clinical interventions: clinical interventions are often more effective, but reach a much smaller portion of the overall population. This can be quantified as program impact, the product of absolute effectiveness × the percentage of the population affected by the program (Velicer et al., 1999). While this concept of impact is intuitively appealing, it is more familiar to epidemiologists as the population attributable risk (PAR) (Morgenstern and Bursic, 1982; Haddix et al., 1996). See Kraus (this volume) for a further discussion of these concepts.

Once the data have been analyzed, it is important to reflect upon the findings. What are the central findings? For internal organizational purposes, what recommendations for program changes should be made? What will your organization do differently now to improve the program? What are the implications of these findings? What will these findings mean to others? Are the findings generalizable? Should the findings be published? Is a formal or informal dissemination plan called for? What should be included in the plan?

Conclusions

Evaluation should be part of any injury intervention program. Before a program is launched, there should be a clear conceptualization of what the program will do, how it works, and what the specific objectives are. The purpose of program evaluation and the anticipated use of the results should be defined at the outset. As a part of this, we strongly recommend early involvement of key stakeholders in the process. Table shells of process and outcome measures to answer the questions posed should be prepared before evaluation is initiated. While evaluation to determine program effectiveness is familiar to many, a more continuous evaluation to improve program implementation is less familiar. Because of the broad scope of many injury interventions, the unit of randomization for research is likely to be the cluster (community or clinic). Harms, as well as benefits, should be assessed. With the development of experimental designs and statistical methods to quantitate and adjust for variance across communities in the analysis, it should be possible increasingly to employ experimental or quasi-experimental designs in measuring effectiveness of injury interventions.

Acknowledgements

Eve Adams for manuscript preparation. Fred Rivara, David Grossman, Steven Woolf, Edward Wagner, and three anonymous National Center for Injury Prevention and Control employees for their constructive reviews.

References

Bandura A (1995) Self-efficacy in Changing Societies, pp. 1–45. New York: Cambridge University Press.

Bergman AB, Rivara FP, Richards DD, Rogers LW (1990) The Seattle Children's Bicycle Helmet Campaign. Am J Dis Child 144:727–31.

Breslow NE, Day NE (1980) Statistical Methods in Cancer Research, Volume I – The Analysis of Case–Control Studies. Lyon, France: International Agency for Cancer Research.

(1987) Statistical Methods in Cancer Research, Volume II – The Design Analysis of Cohort Studies. Lyon, France: International Agency for Cancer Research.

Carey RG, Lloyd RC (1995) Measuring Quality Improvement in Healthcare: A Guide to Statistical Process Control Applications. New York: The Kraus Organization Limited.

Carmines EG, Zeller RA (1979) Reliability and Validity Assessment. Sage University Paper series on Quantitative Applications in the Social Sciences, 07-017 Newbury Park, CA: Sage Publications.

Centers for Disease Control and Prevention (1998) Practical Evaluation of Public Health Programs Workbook. Available at http://www.cdc.qov.phtn/pract_eval/workbook.htm

Chenn MM, Bush JW, Patrick DL (1975) Social indicators for health planning and policy analysis. Policy Sci 6:71–89.

Clancy CM, Eisenberg JM (1998) Outcomes research: measuring the end results of health care. Science 282:245–6.

Clark NM, Becker MH (1998) Theoretical models and strategies for improving adherence and disease management. In: Shumaker SA, Schron EB, Ockene JK, McBee WL (eds), The

Handbook of Health Behavior Change, 2nd edn, pp. 5–33. New York: Springer Publishing.

Clayton D, Hills M (1993) Statistical Models in Epidemiology. New York: Oxford Science Publications.

Clinical Practice Guideline Development: Methodology Perspectives (1994) AHCPR Pub No. 95-0009, pp. 105–13. Rockville, MD: US Department of Health and Human Services, Agency for Health Care Policy Research.

Committee on Trauma Research, Foege WH (chair) Commission on Life Sciences, National Research Council, Institute of Medicine. (1985) Injury in America: A Continuing Public Health Problem. Washington (DC): National Academy Press.

Cummings P, Weiss NS (1998) Case series and exposure series: the role of studies without controls in providing information about the etiology of injury or disease. Injury Prev 4:54–7.

Curry SJ, Kim EL (1999) A public health perspective on addictive behavior change interventions: conceptual frameworks and guiding principles. In: Tucker JA, Donovan DM, Donovan GA (eds), Changing Addictive Behavior: Moving Beyond Therapy Assisted Change. New York: Guilford Publications.

Dannenberg AL, Fowler CJ (1998) Evaluation of interventions to prevent injuries: an overview. Injury Prev 4:141–7.

Davis DA, Thomson MA, Oxman AD, Haynes RB (1992) Evidence for the effectiveness of CME: a review of 50 randomized controlled trials. J Am Med Assoc 268:1111–7.

(1995) Changing physician performance: a systematic review of the effect of continuing medical education strategies. J Am Med Assoc 274:700–5.

DeBruin AF, DeWitte LP, Stevens F, Diedricks JP (1992) Sickness impact profile: The state of the art of a generic functional status measure. Soc Sci Med 35:1003–14.

Dever GEA (1997) Improving Outcomes in Public Health Practice: Strategy and Methods. Gaithersburg, MD: Aspen Publishers.

DHHS (1998) International Classification of Diseases, 9th Revision, Clinical Modification 6th edn. DHHS Publication No. (PHS), pp. 98–1260. Washington DC: US Department of Health and Human Services, CDC and Health Care Financing Administration.

DiGuiseppi CG, Rivara FP, Koepsell TD, Polissar L (1989) Bicycle helmet use by children: evaluation of a community-wide helmet campaign. J Am Med Assoc 262:2256–61.

DiGuiseppi CG, Rivara FP, Koepsell TD (1990) Attitudes toward bicycle helmet ownership and use by school-age children. Am J Disab Child 144:83–6.

Donner A, Klar N (1994) Methods for comparing event rates in intervention studies when the unit of allocation is a cluster. Am J Epidemiol 140:279–89.

Durch JS, Bailey LA, Stoto MA (eds) (1997) Improving Health in the Community: A Role for Performance Monitoring. Washington DC: National Academy Press.

Eddy DM (1996) Clinical Decision Making: From Theory to Practice, p. 53. Boston, MA: Jones and Bartlett Publishers.

Elinson J (1987) Advances in health assessment discussion panel. J Chronic Dis 40(Suppl. 1): 835–915.

Feldman HA (1997) Selecting end point variables for a community intervention trial. Annals of Epidemiology S7:S78–88.

Fisher ES, Welch HG (1999) Avoiding the unintended consequences of growth in medical care: how might more be worse? JAMA 281:446–53.

Freemantle N, Harvey EL, Wolf F, Grinshaw JM, Grilli R, Bero LA (1998) Printed educational materials to improve the behaviour of health care professionals and patient outcomes (Cochrane Review). In: The Cochrane Library, Issue 2. Oxford: Update Software.

Gallagher SS, Guyer B, Kotelchuck M, Bass J, Lovejoy FH, McLoughin E, Mehta K (1982) A strategy for the reduction of childhood injuries in Massachusetts: SCIPP. N Engl J Medicine 307:1015–8.

Gallagher SS, Finison K, Guyer B, Goodenough S (1984) The incidence of injuries among 87,000 Massachusetts children and adolescents: results of the 1980–81 Statewide Childhood Injury Prevention Program Surveillance System. Am J Public Health 74:1340–7.

Gold MR, Siegel JE, Russell LB, Weinstein MC (eds) (1996) Cost-effectiveness in Health and Medicine. New York: Oxford University Press.

Goldstein MG, DePue J, Kazura A, Niaura R (1998) Models for provider–patient interaction: applications to health behavior change. In: Shumaker SA, Schron EB, Ockene JK, McBee WL (eds), The Handbook of Health Behavior Change, 2nd edn, pp. 85–113. New York: Springer Publishing.

Goodman RM (1998) Principles and tools for evaluating community-based prevention and health promotion programs. In: Brownson RC, Baker EA, Novick LF (eds), Community-based Prevention: Programs that Work, pp. 211–27. Gaithersburg, MD: Aspen Publishers.

Graham J, Thompson KM, Goldie SJ, Segui-Gomez M, Weinstein MC (1997) The cost effectiveness of airbags by seating position. J Am Med Assoc 278:1418–25.

Green LW (1997) Community health promotion: applying the science of evaluation to the initial sprint of a marathon. Am J Prev Med 13:225–8.

Green L, Kreuter M (1991) Application of PRECEDE/PROCEED in Community Settings: Health Promotion Planning: An Educational and Environmental Approach. Mountain View, CA: Mayfield.

Grossman DC, Neckerman HJ, Koepsell TD, Liu PY, Asher KN, Beland K, Frey K, Rivara FP (1997) Effectiveness of a violence prevention curriculum among children in elementary school. A randomized controlled trail. J Am Med Assoc 277:1605–11.

Grossman DC, Garcia CC (1999) Effectiveness of health promotion programs to increase motor vehicle occupant restraint use among young children. Am J Prev Med 16(1S):12–22.

Guyer B, Gallagher SS, Chang BH, Azzara CV, Cupples LA, Colton T (1989) Prevention of childhood injuries: evaluation of the Statewide Childhood Injury Prevention Program (SCIPP). Am J Public Health 79:1521–7.

Haddix AC, Teutsch SM, Shaffer PA, Dunet DO (eds) (1996) Prevention Effectiveness: A Guide to Decision Analysis and Economic Evaluation. New York: Oxford University Press.

Halvorson GC (1993) Strong Medicine. New York: Random House Publishers.

Hancock L, Sanson-Fisher RW, Redman S, Burton R, Burton L, Butler J, Girgis A, Gibberd R, Hensley M, McClintock A, Reid A, Schofield M, Tripodi T, Walsh R (1997) Community action for health promotion: a review of methods and outcomes 1990–1995. Am J Prev Med 13:229–39.

Hardy MS, Armstrong FD, Martin BL, Strawn KN (1996) A firearm safety program for children: they just can't say no. J Dev Behav Pediatr 17:216–21.

HEDIS 1999, Vol. 2, Technical Specifications (1999) Washington, DC: National Committee for Quality Assurance (NCQA).

Iezzoni LI (1994) Risk Adjustment for Measuring Health Care Outcomes. Ann Arbor, MI: Health Administration Press.

Jurkovich G, Mock C, MacKenzie E, Burgess A, Cushing B, deLateur B, McAndrew M, Morris J, Swiontkowski M (1995) The Sickness Impact Profile as a tool to evaluate functional outcome in trauma patients. J Trauma Injury Infect Crit Care 39:625–31.

Kaplan RM, Anderson JP (1988) A general health policy model: update and applications. Health Services Research 23:203–35.

Kim JO, Mueller CW (1978a) Introduction to Factor Analysis. Sage University Paper series on Quantitative Applications in the Social Sciences, 07-013. Newbury Park, CA: Sage Publications

(1978b) Factor Analysis – Statistical Methods and Practical Issues. Sage University Paper series on Quantitative Applications in the Social Sciences, 07-014. Newbury Park, CA: Sage Publications.

Koepsell TD (1998) Epidemiologic issues in the design of community intervention trials. In: Brownson RC, Petitti DB (eds), Applied Epidemilogy: Theory to Practice, pp. 177–212. New York: Oxford University Press.

Last JM, Abramson JH, Friedman GD, Porta M, Spasoff RA, Thuriauz M (eds) (1995) A Dictionary of Epidemiology, 3rd edn. New York: Oxford University Press.

Lawrence D (1992) Kaiser Quality Journey (E_2) Presented at Institute for Health Improvement Annual Meeting, December 8–9, 1992.

Lohr KN, Yordy KD, Thier SO (1988) Current issues in quality of care. Health Affairs 7:5–18.

Mallonee S, Istre GR, Rosenberg M, Redddish-Douglas M, Jordan F, Silverstein P, Tunnell W (1996) Surveillance and prevention of residential-fire injuries. N Engl J Med 335:27–31.

McDowell I, Newell C (1996) Measuring Health: A Guide to Rating Scales and Questionnaires, 2nd edn, pp. 446–56. New York: Oxford University Press.

Morgenstern H, Bursic ES (1982) A method for using epidemiologic data to estimate the potential impact of an intervention on the health status of a target population. J Community Health 7:292–309.

Mullooly JP (1996) Misclassification model for person-time analysis of automated medical care databases. Am J Epidemiol 144:782–92.

Mullooly J, Drew L, DeStefano F, Chen R, Okoro K, Swint E, Immanuel V, Ray P, Lewis N, Vadheim C, Lugg M (1999) Quality of HMO vaccination databases used to monitor childhood vaccine safety Vaccine Safety DataLink Team. Am J Epidemiol 149:186–94.

Murray CJL, Lopez AD (eds) (1996a) The Global Burden of Disease. 1st edn. Boston, MA: Harvard University Press.

Murray CJL, Lopez AD (eds) (1996b) Summary: The Global Burden of Disease. Boston, MA: Harvard University Press.

Murray DM (1997) Design and analysis of group-randomized trials: a review of recent developments. Ann Epidemiol 7(Suppl):S69–77.

(1998) Design and Analysis of Group-Randomized Trials. New York: Oxford University Press.

National Committee for Injury Prevention and Control (1989) Injury prevention: meeting the challenge. Program design and evaluation. Am J Prev Med 5(Suppl):63–88.

Patrick DL, Erickson P (1993) Types of health related quality of life assessments. In: Health Status and Health Policy, pp. 113–42. New York: Oxford University Press.

Petitti DB (1994) Meta-analysis, Decision Analysis, and Cost-effectiveness Analysis. New York: Oxford University Press.

(1998) Epidemiologic issues in outcomes research. In: Brownson RC, Petitti DB (eds), Applied Epidemiology: Theory to Practice, pp. 249–76. New York: Oxford University Press.

Petitti DB, Amster A (1998) Measuring the quality of health care. In: Brownson RC, Petitti DB (eds), Applied Epidemiology: Theory to Practice, pp. 299–321. New York: Oxford University Press.

Prochaska JO, Norcross JC, Diclemente CC (1995) Changing for Good. New York: Avon Books.

Prochaska JO, Johnson S, Lee P (1998) The transtheoretical model of behavior change. In: Shumaker SA, Schron EB, Ockene JK, McBee WL (eds), The Handbook of Health Behavior Change, 2nd edn, pp. 59–84. New York: Springer Publishing.

Redelmeier DA, Tibshirani RJ (1997) Association between cellular–telephone calls and motor vehicle collisions. N Engl J Med 336:453–8.

Reinke WH (1991) Applicability of industrial sampling techniques to epidemiologic investigations. Am J Epidemiol 134:1222–32.

Rice DP, MacKenzie EJ, Jones AL, Kaufman SR, deLissovoy GV, Miller TR, Robertson LS, Salkever DS, Smith GS (1989) Cost of injury in the United States; a report to Congress. San Francisco, CA: Institute for Health Aging, University of California and Injury Prevention Center, The Johns Hopkins University.

Rivara FP, Calonge N, Thompson RS (1989) Population-based study of unintentional injury incidence and impact during childhood. Am J Public Health 79:990–4.

Rivara FP, Thompson DC, Thompson RS, Rogers LW, Alexander B, Felix D, Bergman AB (1994) The Seattle Children's Bicycle Helmet Campaign: changes in helmet use and head injury admissions. Pediatrics 93:567–9.

Rothman R, Greenland (1998) Case control studies In: Rothman K, Greenland S (eds), Modern Epidemiology, 2nd edn, pp. 93–114. Hagerstown, MD: Lippincott-Raven.

Runyan CW (1998) Using the Haddon Matrix: introducing the third dimension. Injury Prev 4:302–7.

Schulman J, Provenzano G, Wolters C, Mitchell K (1998) Preventable injuries, costs, and related deaths (PICARD). Contract No 200-92-0534, Task No 36. Sponsored by Centers for Disease Control and Prevention. Baltimore, MD: Battelle, Centers for Public Health Research and Evaluation.

Shahian DM, Williamson WA, Svensson LG, Restuccia JD, D'Agostino RS (1996) Applications of statistical quality control to cardiac surgery. Annals of Thoracic Surg 62:1351–9.

Skinner H, Botelho R (eds) (1999) Beyond Advice: Changing Behavior in Health Organizations. Thousand Oaks, CA: Sage Publications.

Stewart AL, Hays RD, Ware JE (1988) The MOS short-form general health survey. Med Care 26:724–35.

Thompson RS, Rivara FP, Thompson DC, Barlow WE, Sugg NK, Mairuo RD, Rubanowice DM (2000) A Group randomized trial to improve identification and management of domestic violence in primary care practice. Am J Prevent Med.

Thompson NJ, McClintock HO (1998) Demonstrating Your Program's Worth: A Primer on Evaluation for Programs to Prevent Unintentional Injury. Atlanta, GA: Centers for Disease Control and Prevention, National Center for Injury Prevention and Control.

Thompson RS (1996) What have HMOs learned about clinical prevention services? An examination of the experience at Group Health Cooperative of Puget Sound. Milbank Q 74:469–509.

Thompson RS, Rivara FP, Thompson DC (1989) A case-control study of the effectiveness of bicycle safety helmets. NEJM 302:1361–7

Thompson RS, Thompson DC, Rivara FP, Salazar AA (1993) Cost-effectiveness analysis of bicycle helmet subsidies in a define population. Pediatrics 91:902–7.

Thomson MA, Oxman AD, Davis DA, Haynes RB, Freemantle N, Harvey EL (1998a) Outreach visits to improve health professional practice and health care outcomes. (Cochrane Review). In: The Cochrane Library, Issue 2. Oxford: Update Software.

(1998b) Audit and feedback to improve health professional practice and health care outcomes. (Cochrane Review). In: The Cochrane Library, Issue 2. Oxford: Update Software.

(1998c) Audit and feedback to improve health professional practice and health care outcomes (Part II). (Cochrane Review). In: The Cochrane Library, Issue 2. Oxford: Update Software.

(1998d) Local opinion leaders to improve health professional practice and health care outcomes. (Cochrane Review). In: The Cochrane Library, Issue 2. Oxford: Update Software.

Velicer W, Bothelo R, Prochaska J, Skinner H (1999) Expert systems for motivating health behavior change. In: Skinner H, Botelho R (eds), Beyond Advice: Changing Behavior in Health Organizations, Chapter 16. Thousand Oaks, CA: Sage Publications.

Vernick JS, Li G, Ogaitis S, MacKenzie EJ, Baker SP, Gielen AC (1999) Effects of high school driver education on motor vehicle crashes, violations and licensure. Am J Prev Med 16(Suppl. 1):40–6.

Walsh JME, McPhee SJ (1992) A systems model of clinical preventive care: an analysis of factors influencing patient and physician. Health Educ Q 19:157–75.

Ware JE (1994) SF–36 Physican and Mental Health Summary Scales: A Users Manual. Boston, MA: The Health Institute, New England Medical Center.

(1995) The status of health assessment 1994. Annu Rev Public Health 16:327–54.

Willey C, Laforge R, Blais L, Pallonen U, Prochaska J, Botelho R (1996) Public health and the science of behavior change. Curr Issues Public Health 2:18–25.

Zucker DM, Lakatos E, Webber LS (1995) Statistical design of the Child and Adolescent Trial for Cardiovascular Health (CATCH): implications of cluster randomization. Controlled Clin Trials 16:96–118.

Zeger SL, Liang KY (1986) Longitudinal data analysis for discrete and continuous outcomes. Biometrics 42:121–30.

16

The Development of Clinical Decision Rules for Injury Care

Ian G. Stiell

Introduction

Reports of clinical decision rules are becoming increasingly common throughout the medical literature. Clinical decision rules (prediction rules) are designed to help physicians with diagnostic and therapeutic decisions at the bedside. We define a clinical decision rule as a decision-making tool, which is derived from original research (as opposed to a consensus-based clinical practice guideline) and incorporates three or more variables from the history, physical examination, or simple tests (Laupacis et al., 1997). These tools help clinicians cope with the uncertainty of medical decision making, predict prognosis, and improve efficiency in using resources, an important issue as health-care systems demand more cost-effective medical practice. A recently published example of a decision rule that helps emergency physicians cope with uncertainty is a guideline about which patients with community acquired pneumonia require hospitalization (Fine et al., 1997). A decision rule that predicts prognosis, would be a recent study to predict outcome in children after near drowning (Graf et al., 1995). A typical example of a decision rule to improve resource use efficiency are the Ottawa Ankle Rules for the use of radiography in acute ankle injuries (Stiell et al., 1992a, 1993, 1994, 1995a; McDonald, 1994; Wasson and Sox, 1996).

Methodologic standards for the development of clinical decision rules have been described, originally by Wasson and Feinstein and more recently by our own research group (Wasson et al., 1985; Feinstein, 1987; Laupacis et al., 1997; Stiell and Wells, 1999). We consider the following to be the six important stages in the development and testing of a fully mature decision rule (Table 16.1). First, is there a need for a decision rule? Has current practice been shown to be inefficient or highly variable? Second, was the rule derived according to rigorous methodologic standards? Third, has the rule been properly validated prospectively in a new patient group? Fourth, has the rule been successfully implemented into clinical practice and been shown to change behavior? Fifth, would use of the rule be cost-effective according to a formal health economic analysis? Finally, how will the rule be disseminated to ensure widespread adoption in the injury care community?

This chapter will provide injury researchers with a guide to the methodologic standards for developing high-quality clinical decision rules. It will also serve as a guide to help readers critically appraise the methodologic quality of a paper or

Table 16.1 Checklist of standards for the six stages in the development of a clinical decision rule

(1) Is there a need for the decision rule?

  (a) prevalence of the clinical condition
  (b) current use of the diagnostic test
  (c) variation in practice
  (d) attitudes of physicians
  (e) clinical accuracy of physicians

(2) Was the rule derived according to methodological standards?

  (a) definition of outcome
  (b) definition of predictor variables
  (c) reliability of predictor variables
  (d) selection of subjects
  (e) sample size
  (f) mathematical techniques
  (g) sensibility of the decision rule
  (h) accuracy

(3) Has the rule been prospectively validated and refined?

  (a) prospective validation
  (b) selection of subjects
  (c) application of the rule
  (d) outcomes
  (e) accuracy of the rule
  (f) reliability of the rule
  (g) physicians interpretation
  (h) refinement
  (i) potential impact

(4) Has the rule been successfully implemented into clinical practice?

  (a) clinical trial
  (b) impact on use
  (c) accuracy of the rule
  (d) acceptability

(5) Would use of the rule be cost-effective?

(6) How will the rule be disseminated and implemented?

papers describing a clinical decision rule. We will consider the six major stages in the development and testing of a new clinical decision rule and will discuss a number of standards within each stage. We will use examples from injury care and, in particular, examples from our own research on clinical decision rules for radiography in trauma.

Example of a Clinical Decision Rule

Our research group has derived (Stiell et al., 1992a), validated (Stiell et al., 1993), and implemented (Stiell et al., 1994, 1995a) the Ottawa Ankle Rules in a series of

Table 16.2 Classification performance of the Ottawa Ankle Rule in a prospective validation study

	Actual fracture	
	Yes	No
Ottawa Ankle Rule		
Yes	121	557
No	0	354

studies involving several thousand patients. This is an example of a clinical decision rule designed to help clinicians be much more selective in their use of radiography for acute ankle injuries in adults without jeopardizing patient care. The rule states that an ankle radiography series is only required for patients with any one of these criteria: (1) bone tenderness at the posterior edge or tip of the lateral malleolus; or (2) bone tenderness at the posterior edge or tip of the medial malleolus; or (3) inability to bear weight both immediately after the injury and for four steps in the emergency department.

In a subsequent prospective validation study (Stiell et al., 1993), the Ottawa Ankle Rule was performed as shown in Table 16.2.

Hence it could be determined that the rule classified fracture cases with a sensitivity of 100% (95% CI, 97–100%) and a specificity of 39% (95% CI, 36–42%). In a later "before–after" implementation trial, the rule was shown actually to reduce the use of radiography by 28% with no missed fractures and no increase in health-care utilization (Stiell et al., 1994). Finally, an economic evaluation demonstrated the potential for significant health-care savings with widespread implementation of the rule (Anis et al., 1995).

Is There a Need for the Decision Rule?

Researchers should ask themselves whether there really appears to be a need for a particular decision rule or whether the rule appears only to represent the analysis of a convenient set of data. Is there a demonstrated inefficiency or variation in current medical practice and does there appear to be the potential for improved efficiency through guidelines or a decision rule?

Prevalence of the Clinical Condition

Does the proposed decision rule deal with a commonly seen clinical problem? A rule for an uncommon clinical entity is unlikely to be easily adopted by physicians and is unlikely to contribute significantly to the overall efficiency of clinical practice. For example, because ankle injuries are one of the most common problems seen in U.S. emergency departments, one might expect a decision rule for radiography to have an impact on the management of hundreds of thousands of patients annually (McCaig, 1994; National Center for Health Statistics, 1994). We have estimated that $500 million is spent annually on ankle radiographs in North America and that even a modest reduction in the use of ankle radiography could lead to large health-care savings. On the other hand, because injuries to the mandible are not common, a decision rule for this problem is unlikely to have a significant impact.

Current Use of the Diagnostic Test

If the decision rule proposes to guide the ordering of a diagnostic test, are there data clearly demonstrating that current use of the test has a low yield for positive results? For example, we have previously shown that 87.2% of ankle and foot radiographs and 92.4% of knee radiographs ordered in emergency departments are negative for fracture (Stiell et al., 1992b, 1995c). While we have no exact data, we suspect that a majority of hip radiographs ordered are, in fact, positive for fracture and that, consequently, hip radiography would not be a productive area for a decision rule.

Variation in Practice

Is there significant variability in clinical practice among similar physicians or similar institutions? The low yield of a diagnostic test for positive results may not necessarily imply wastefulness, especially if the cost of a missed diagnosis is high. One would expect the yield of cervical spine radiography to be low in that emergency physicians naturally tend to be cautious when dealing with the possibility of a broken neck. Hence, our recent finding that 98.5% of cervical spine radiographs ordered in Canadian emergency departments are negative would not surprise many physicians. What does suggest a need for a decision rule, however, is our finding that use of cervical spine radiography varies twofold among equivalent busy hospitals and sixfold among attending staff physicians in these emergency departments (Stiell et al., 1997c). We have also demonstrated great variation in the use of computed tomography (CT) for patients with minor head injury (Stiell et al., 1997b).

Attitudes of Physicians

The need for a clinical decision rule is further supported if there is evidence that physicians believe that many of the diagnostic tests they order are unnecessary. For example, we demonstrated in studies involving more than 1700 patients that experienced attending physicians expected the likelihood of fracture to be 10% or less in 57.8% of ankle injury cases and 75.6% of knee injury cases (Stiell et al., 1995a). Despite ordering radiography for the vast majority of cases, these same physicians indicated that they would have been theoretically comfortable with no radiography for 45.9% of ankle injury patients and 55.5% of knee injury patients. In a mail survey, we gathered compelling evidence that Canadian emergency physicians strongly support the development of decision rules for cervical spine radiography as well as CT for minor head injury (Graham et al., 1998).

Clinical Accuracy of Physicians

There is little likelihood that a decision rule will ultimately be effective if physicians are unable to predict accurately a patient's outcome based on clinical findings alone. We were convinced of the potential for improved use of both ankle and knee radiography when we demonstrated that, based on history and physical examination alone, experienced emergency physicians could very accurately discriminate between fracture and nonfracture cases (Stiell et al., 1992a, 1995a).

Was the Rule Derived According to Methodological Standards?

Research methodology standards for the derivation of a clinical decision rule were first reviewed in 1985 in a landmark paper by Wasson et al. (1985). Feinstein (1987) later added to the literature of evidence-based patient assessment in his book Clinimetrics. More recently, our research group at the University of Ottawa Clinical Epidemiology Unit assessed clinical decision rule articles in four major medical journals and proposed modifications to Wasson's original methodologic standards (Laupacis et al., 1997; Stiell and Wells, 1999). In the following discussion, numbers in parentheses indicate the percentage of published studies meeting these criteria (in Journal of the American Medical Association, New England Journal of Medicine, British Medical Journal, and Annals of Internal Medicine).

Definition of Outcome

The outcome being identified by the clinical decision rule should be clinically important (100% of reviewed studies met this criterion) (Laupacis et al., 1997) and clearly defined (83%). Survival (e.g., death), radiological results (e.g., fracture), and laboratory results (e.g., elevated white blood cell count) are all biological outcomes which can be clearly defined as well as reproduced in other settings. While survival and fractures are clinically important outcomes, most physicians would not consider a laboratory marker such as white blood cell count to be any more than a weak surrogate outcome. A behavioral outcome such as admission to hospital may be dependent upon local factors and difficult to replicate, and as a result not be of high clinical relevance. Similarly, the term positive computed tomography in a head injury study cannot be considered clearly defined unless the investigators explicitly indicate that the outcome refers only to acute brain findings attributable to trauma rather than to chronic or soft tissue findings (Madden et al., 1995; Borczuk, 1995).

In order to avoid the danger of observation bias, the outcome measure should be assessed blindly (41%), that is, without knowledge of the status of the predictor variables. This standard is more important when evaluation of the outcome is soft or subject to interpretation, for example days off work, and less important for a hard outcome such as death.

Definition of Predictor Variables

Potential predictor variables for a decision rule should be clearly defined (59%) and ideally collected in a prospective standardized fashion. Investigators should ensure that the physicians in their study have been adequately trained to evaluate the patients and collect data according to well standardized assessment techniques. Clinical data tend to be most reliable when collected prospectively and recorded on a data collection form designed specifically for a decision rule study. Less satisfactory are data collected prospectively as part of a clinical trial and then subjected to a post-hoc secondary data analysis. Large administrative databases may also be used as a source of predictor and outcome variables but they frequently lack key clinical variables. Data collected from review of clinical records suffer from lack of precision and missing information and are generally unacceptable other than for assessing feasibility.

Again, to avoid observation bias, the assessment of predictor variables should be done without knowledge of the outcome (79%). Knowing, for example, that a patient has a knee fracture, might very well influence how a physician interprets and records his physical examination on a data form.

Reliability of Predictor Variables

Decision rules are highly dependent upon findings from the clinical examination, so unless these findings are reliable the resultant rule will not be dependable. Reliability refers to the consistency or reproducibility of the findings by the same clinician (intraobserver reliability) or by different clinicians (interobserver reliability) (Landis and Koch, 1977; Fleiss, 1981; Kramer and Feinstein, 1982). In assessing reliability, the coefficient used for agreement depends on the level of measurement, namely: the simple kappa for dichotomous or nominal data (Fleiss, 1981; Roberts and McNamee, 1998); the weighted kappa for ordinal data (Fleiss, 1981); and the intraclass correlation coefficient for interval data (Fleiss, 1986). Several papers have been published regarding the determination of sample size for reliability studies from the perspective both of the precision of estimation and of comparison of coefficients.

We believe that the reliability of the predictor variables (3%) should be explicitly assessed and that only those with good agreement beyond that expected by chance alone should be considered for a decision rule. For example, during the derivation of the Ottawa Ankle Rules we assessed 32 variables for interobserver agreement by having patients assessed independently by pairs of physicians (Stiell et al., 1992c). Twenty-three of these findings were discarded when they proved to have kappa values of less than 0.6.

Selection of Subjects

It is important for readers to be able to understand the generalizability of the findings of a decision rule study as well as its applicability to their own patients. Hence, the study subjects should be well described in terms of inclusion criteria, method of selection, clinical and demographic characteristics (79%), and the study setting (66%). Explicit inclusion criteria allow readers to understand clearly what types of patients are being studied and, therefore, to which patients the derived rule may be applicable. For example, the Ottawa Ankle Rules were developed only with patients aged 18 and older and should not be considered appropriate for pediatric cases. Similarly, if a decision rule for cervical spine radiography were derived in patients who were alert and stable then clinicians could not apply the rule to patients who were obtunded or unstable. Some studies fail to define specifically their study population and enroll cases chosen for a particular diagnostic test at the discretion of the treating physician. As different physicians may use different criteria for ordering tests, the reader of these studies has a difficult time deciding if the study patients were similar to his or her own.

Ideally, the method of patient selection is free of bias. Study subjects should encompass a wide clinical and demographic spectrum and be representative of all patients seen at the site with the designated condition. The investigators should report all pertinent characteristics of patients included in the study as well as of those eligible but not included. For example, a study of knee radiography, which systematically excluded more severely injured patients because the physicians were too busy to complete the data form, may result in a decision rule with limited applicability.

The study site should be described in sufficient detail to permit the reader to make a comparison with his own clinical setting. Was the study actually conducted in an emergency department, in a clinic or office setting, or among admitted patients? Was the hospital a primary, secondary, or tertiary care facility? Was this a teaching institution? What was the referral filter, that is, what proportion of patients were self-referred as opposed to being sent in by a physician? As an example, the status of patients seen in a neurology clinic for migraine might be expected to differ considerably from that of patients presenting to an emergency department with severe intractable migraine.

Sample Size

The authors should justify the number of subjects enrolled in the study. Of particular importance is that the sample size be appropriate for the type of multivariate analysis chosen. There may be problems with overfitting the data if there are too few outcome events per predictor variable. A commonly employed rule of thumb is that there should be at least 10 outcome events per independent variable in the prediction rule (Wasson et al., 1985; Peduzzi et al., 1996). Another important consideration in choosing the study sample size is the degree of precision in the confidence interval around the measure of accuracy, for example, the sensitivity of the rule. For example, a study to develop a prediction rule for rib fractures would require at least 40 subjects with positive X-rays if the rule encompassed four predictor variables. If all rib fractures were identified in such a study, the rule could be said to have a sensitivity of 1.0; however, the confidence interval around the sensitivity would be 0.91–1.0.

Mathematical Techniques

The mathematical techniques employed to derive a decision rule should be adequately described and justified (100%). Many techniques are available, from a simple 2×2 cross-tabulation of each predictor variable with the outcome to

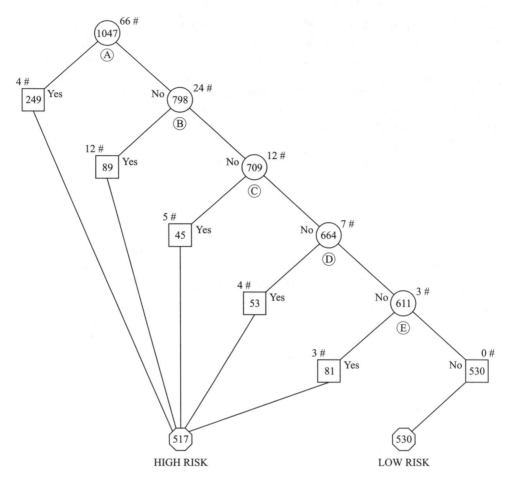

Figure 16.1 Example of Chi-square recursive partitioning analysis used to derive a clinical decision rule.

sophisticated multivariate analyses. While univariate analyses are easy to perform, they do not allow the exploration of the relationship of predictor variables with each other as well as with the outcome. To achieve this end, multivariate statistical approaches such as logistic regression and recursive partitioning are commonly used. The variables to be included in a multivariate analysis are usually screened by assessment of the univariate association with the outcome as well as an assessment of the reproducibility of the variable.

Chi-square recursive partitioning analysis progressively divides the patients into a sub-population that includes only patients with a particular outcome (Figure 16.1) (Friedman, 1977; Ciampi et al., 1986, 1988). This approach is quite appropriate when the objective of the study is to develop a decision rule with a very high sensitivity. Logistic regression analyses tend to lead to decision rules with higher overall accuracy (i.e., better overall classification of all cases), but in many situations it will not be possible to attain 100% sensitivity without unacceptably low specificity (Hosmer and Lemeshow, 1989; Heckerling et al., 1990).

Sensibility of the Decision Rule

Feinstein coined the term sensibility to describe whether a decision rule is clinically reasonable (97%), easy to use (41%), and provides a course of action (0%) (Feinstein, 1987). Assessment of sensibility depends on judgment rather than on statistical methods. Ideally, a decision rule would demonstrate content validity. This means that most clinicians would consider the items in the rule to be clinically sensible, that no obvious items are missing, that the method of grouping the individual variables is reasonable, and that the items seem appropriate for the purpose of the rule. Ease of use depends upon factors such as the length of time needed to apply the rule and simplicity of interpretation. In the emergency department, it is unlikely that physicians would embrace a rule that requires extensive calculations or use of a calculator. Similarly, a rule will not be useful if it depends upon laboratory results that are not available in a timely fashion.

We believe that decision rules are more likely to be used if they suggest a course of action rather than if they merely provide a probability of outcome. For example, a rule to predict the need for a cranial CT for nontrauma patients proposes a CT/no CT course of action rather than giving a percentage probability of abnormality on CT (Rothrock et al., 1997). In the case of the Ottawa Ankle Rules, clinicians are also advised whether to order radiography or not. We believe that merely giving the probability of fracture, for example, 2%, may lead to uncertainty in the clinician's decision to order a radiograph. An estimate of an outcome probability may, however, be useful for both the clinician and the patient in situations where the relative costs and benefits of a management option are less clear. Pauker and Kassirer (1980) have described the threshold approach to clinical decision making. A recently developed clinical model for deep vein thrombosis stratifies emergency department patients into low-, medium-, and high-probability groups (Wells et al., 1995, 1997, 1998).

Accuracy

Authors should make an effort to present the accuracy or classification performance (100%) based on the population from which the decision rule was derived. If the outcome is dichotomous (e.g., fracture or no fracture), then a 2 × 2 table should be presented along with calculations of sensitivity, specificity, negative predictive value, and positive predictive value, with the respective 95% confidence intervals (Diamond, 1989; Sackett et al., 1991). Sensitivity and specificity are characteristics of the decision rule itself and refer to the classification accuracy for patients with an abnormal outcome and a normal outcome, respectively. Negative and positive predictive values are greatly influenced by the prevalence of the outcome in the population being studied.

In many acute care scenarios high sensitivity, or the ability to rule out an outcome if the result is negative, is important. Alternately, a rule with a high specificity will rule in a condition or outcome if the result is positive. For conditions where the cost of missing the outcome is serious [e.g., myocardial infarction (Pozen et al., 1984; Goldman et al., 1988)] then a very high sensitivity is required. Unfortunately, a very high sensitivity tends to be associated with a decreased specificity and, consequently, overall decreased efficiency of the decision rule. For example, while the Ottawa Ankle Rules are designed to have a sensitivity of 100%, they have a relatively low specificity of 40%. Merely dropping the sensitivity to 96% would increase the specificity to 58% and greatly increase the potential for reducing radiography. However, we believe that many North American clinicians would be very uncomfortable using a rule with a sensitivity of only 96% (Feinstein, 1985; Long, 1985; Svenson, 1988).

The post-test probability of an outcome associated with the prediction of a decision rule can be calculated by the use of likelihood ratios (Koopman, 1984; Sox et al., 1988; Sackett et al., 1991). A likelihood ratio greater than 1.0 increases the probability of abnormality and a likelihood ratio less than 1.0 decreases it. Likelihood ratios are particularly useful for rules with more than two response categories. Receiver operator operating characteristic (ROC) curves result from the plotting of sensitivity versus 1-specificity using different cut points in the data (Hanley and McNeil, 1982). This technique allows a comparison of several rules and gives an overall estimate of accuracy, but is of limited clinical use because post-test probability can not be easily estimated (Choi, 1998).

Another important performance index of decision rules is an estimate of the potential impact of use. This estimation is usually overlooked and, while often optimistic, gives the reader a reasonable idea of the potential savings associated with implementation of the rule. For example, a rule for knee radiography would be of questionable value if it proved to be 100% sensitive for important fractures (which were normally never missed) but had such a low specificity that use of radiography would actually increase. Alternately, a decision rule for the use of abdominal CT in blunt trauma that led to increased use of CT might be valuable if subsequent laparotomy rates could be decreased.

Has the Rule been Prospectively Validated and Refined?

Unfortunately, many clinical decision rules are not prospectively assessed to determine, in a new patient population, their accuracy, reproducibility, acceptance to clinicians, or potential impact on practice. This validation process is very important because many statistically derived rules or guidelines fail to perform well when tested in a new population (Fischl et al., 1981; Centor et al., 1984; Rose et al., 1984). The reason for this poor performance may be statistical, that is, overfitting or instability in the original derived model (Charlson et al., 1987), or may be due to differences in prevalence of disease or differences in how the decision rule is applied (Poses et al., 1986; Wigton et al., 1986). The ideal characteristics of a validation study are described below.

Prospective Validation
    The clinical decision rule should be applied prospectively to a completely new patient population. Under ideal circumstances this would be performed in a new clinical setting by different clinicians from those involved in the derivation study.

Selection of Subjects

The patients should be chosen in an unbiased fashion and preferably in a complete population-based sample for that setting; for example, all eligible patients seen in a 12-month period in a particular emergency department. Patients who are not included in this validation phase need to be described so that their characteristics can be compared with those subjects who are included in the validation study. Readers should also be reassured that the patients included represent a wide spectrum of ages and severity for the clinical condition under question (see section on selection of subjects). For example, a study of minor head injury patients with Glasgow Coma Scale scores of 13–15 would best include cases with normal CT scans, those with minor abnormalities, and those with life-threatening hematomas.

Application of the Rule

Investigators conducting a validation study have an obligation to ensure that they fully understand how the decision rule is to be applied. If necessary, the investigator should discuss the accurate application of the decision rule with the original researcher and should be prepared to present accurately the decision rule to the study physicians. This must involve a brief but adequate training session (e.g., 15 minutes during a rounds presentation) and training tools such as posters, pocket cards, and audiovisual aids (Solomito et al., 1994; Pigman et al., 1994; Chande, 1995; McBride, 1997; Diercks et al., 1997). The literature includes clear examples where decision rules have faired suboptimally in validation studies where the treating physicians were not fully taught how to use the rule or were not in fact aware that they were assessing decision rules (Kerr et al., 1994; Lucchesi et al., 1995; Stiell et al., 1995b, 1996b). We believe that the purpose of validation studies is to assess rigorously the efficacy or accuracy of the rule itself. If the rule proves to be accurate, then subsequent implementation studies can serve to assess the effectiveness of the rule in the real world.

Outcomes

Ideally, all patients would be subjected to the gold or criterion standard to determine their true outcome compared with that predicted by the decision rule. For example, all patients undergoing a prospective validation of the Ottawa Ankle Rule underwent ankle radiography to determine the presence of fracture (Stiell et al., 1993). In many cases, however, the criterion standard is not normally applied to all potential patients. In this instance a suitable and reasonable proxy outcome may be substituted. For example, in the case of the Ottawa Knee Rule, knee radiography was not uniformly used for all knee injury patients in the study hospitals. Consequently, the investigators incorporated a proxy outcome for the 30% of patients who normally would not undergo radiography (Stiell et al., 1996a). In this instance, the proxy outcome included a structured telephone interview consisting of five explicit telephone questions (relating to pain, ability to walk, return to work, and need for medical care) applied by a registered nurse. Patients who could not satisfy all criteria were asked to return for an X-ray examination.

Accuracy of Rule

As described above, accuracy is best presented by a 2×2 table with calculation of classification performance in terms of sensitivity, specificity, negative predictive value, and positive predictive value, all with 95% confidence intervals. The sample size of a validation study primarily depends on the width of the confidence interval around the target sensitivity and the need to have an adequate number of outcomes to allow a satisfactory multivariate analysis in the refinement process.

Reliability of Rule

Rarely do investigators determine the interobserver agreement between physicians for assessing the actual rule itself. We believe that the reliability of interpretation of the decision rule (0%) should be explicitly measured in a validation study (e.g. radiography indicated – yes/no) (Stiell et al., 1993, 1996a). This is very important in that a rule which cannot be reliably assessed may lead to the misclassification of some patients and potentially to the misdiagnosis of serious outcomes.

Physicians' Interpretation

An important aspect of validation, which is often overlooked, is the ease with which clinicians can apply this rule. The investigator should make efforts to determine the interobserver agreement for interpreting the decision rule between pairs of physicians. Furthermore, the investigator should determine the accuracy with which the physicians interpret the decision rule as well as their comfort with its use (the latter may be determined by a simple survey question).

Refinement

A validation study provides a unique opportunity for the investigator to review the value of each of the component variables in the decision rule and possibly to improve upon the rule. Towards this end the investigator might well consider re-evaluating several variables that proved to be valuable but not essential in the original derivation study. By reassessing the reproducibility and accuracy of a limited number of variables it is quite possible that the study may lead to a more accurate rule or a simplified rule. In the case of the Ottawa Ankle Rule, the validation study led to a more streamlined ankle rule without the requirement for the age criterion. Furthermore, the refinement process led to a more accurate foot rule with slightly different criteria (Stiell et al., 1993). Once refined, of course, the rule must then be validated again in a new patient set.

Potential Impact

Having assessed the classification performance of the decision rule as well as the baseline ordering rate for the test in question, the investigator is now in a good position to estimate the potential impact of the decision rule. In other words, the investigator can now calculate the potential savings that might be realized if the decision rule were accurately and completely implemented into practice.

This determination is very important in predicting the potential usefulness of the rule as well as in determining the need or rationale for an implementation study.

Has the Rule been Successfully Implemented into Clinical Practice?

Very few clinical decision rules have been implemented and shown to alter clinical practice in what has been termed "the next painful step" for evaluating decision aids (Lee, 1990). A decision rule that has been shown to be valid and reliable still faces significant barriers to implementation in terms of both patient and physician acceptance (Long, 1985; Matthews, 1986; Svenson, 1988). Physicians dealing with acute injury are concerned about the medicolegal consequences of missing a diagnosis. Patients must place their trust in a physician whom they have never met before and whom they will not likely see again in follow-up. Hence, many physicians have the perception that their patients will only be satisfied with some form of diagnostic investigation (Feinstein, 1985). Consequently, widespread acceptance of a clinical decision rule must be preceded by an implementation study that clearly shows that clinical behavior can be altered.

Clinical Trial

Although the ideal implementation trial would be a randomized controlled trial, such a study is often not feasible when the intervention under study is a cognitive guideline that is learned by the individual physician. Randomizing by clinician is limited by the problem of contamination and randomizing by setting is limited by the inherent baseline practice variation among sites. Several implementation trials have adopted before–after comparisons, which also incorporate concurrent control groups from other hospitals (Stiell et al., 1994, 1997a). To enhance generalizability, an implementation trial should be conducted in as many different types of settings as possible and involve as many types of physician as possible (Stiell et al., 1995a; Auleley et al., 1997). The physicians must be carefully trained to interpret accurately and apply the decision rule and must have adequate reminders and cues so that they learn to apply the rule routinely. For example, we have employed pocket cards and posters as training tools, as well as memos and follow-up by study nurses, to encourage the accurate use of the Ottawa Ankle and Ottawa Knee Rules.

Impact on Use

The primary outcome measure of an implementation trial is generally the impact on use of the resource in question, for example, ordering of radiography. Follow-up of patients is important to ensure that those denied a procedure or test at the study hospital do not go elsewhere to obtain the same test. Ideally, physician practice would also be followed at a later date to assess the long-term effect of the decision rule (Verbeek et al., 1997).

Accuracy of the Rule

Careful follow-up is important to ensure that there are few missed diagnoses and that the sensitivity and specificity of the decision rule can be recalculated.

Acceptability

Physicians should be surveyed both formally as part of the study as well as informally to determine their comfort with applying the rule, as well as their impression regarding its ease of use. Finally, the patients should be surveyed to determine their attitudes to the process, and especially their satisfaction with care that may not include a diagnostic test.

Would Use of the Rule be Cost-effective?

If an implementation trial does, in fact, show that the decision rule alters clinical behavior, then a formal economic evaluation conducted by a health economist might be conducted (Anis et al., 1995; Nichol et al., 1997). The objective of such a study would be to clearly demonstrate the health-care savings that might be associated with widespread use of the decision rule. Economic assessment is concerned with choosing between alternative uses of resources. Resources are limited and choices must be made.

Three basic concepts are involved in any economic evaluation, namely: the type of analysis that is performed, the type of costs and benefits included, and the point of view from which the analysis is taken. There are three types of analysis: cost identification, cost-effectiveness and cost–benefit. The choice is determined by whether or not benefits are included in the analysis and the manner in which benefits are valued. Three types of costs and benefits can be considered, direct, indirect, and intangible. There are several points of view that can be taken including that of the patient, health-care provider, health-care payer, and society. An economic analysis must include reasonable assumptions regarding the accuracy and effectiveness of the rule as well as of the costs involved. Sensitivity analyses allow one to assess the robustness of the impact of the rule under a variety of conditions. More details on economic evaluations are presented in the chapter by Graham and Segui-Gomez (this volume).

How will the Rule be Disseminated and Implemented?

For a clinical guideline to have widespread impact on health-care delivery, there must be an active plan for dissemination and implementation. We are well aware that the simple passive diffusion of original study results (through publication in medical journals or presentation at scientific meetings) is unlikely to alter clinical practice significantly (Lee and Cooper, 1997; Greer, 1988). Strategies to ensure the dissemination and implementation of clinical research is currently the subject of intensive health services research (Anderson, 1993; Hayward and Laupacis, 1993; Greco and Eisenberg, 1993). Dissemination is a more active process which involves targeting modified information for a specific audience (Lomas, 1993, 1994).

Examples include secondary sources such as meta-analyses, reviews, practice guidelines, and consensus statements which are distributed by journal publication, the lay press, targeted mailings, or a campaign of visiting speakers. Implementation is the most active process and employs organizational and behavioral tools applied locally and persistently to overcome barriers to the use of the new information by practitioners.

Adoption of innovations (such as decision rules) is affected by a number of factors, including the attributes of the innovation itself, the characteristics of the physician, the practice setting, legal and financial issues, regulation, as well as patient factors (Basinski et al., 1992; Davis et al., 1995; Davis and Taylor-Vaisey, 1997). The attributes of the innovation which facilitate adoption are relative advantage (new practice is demonstrably superior to the old), compatibility (similar to prior experience or practice), complexity (ease of incorporation into practice), "trialability" (practitioner can "try it out"), and "observability" (can observe practice of other physicians) (Grilli and Lomas, 1994; Davis and Taylor-Vaisey, 1997).

Previous research has shown that some interventional strategies are much more effective than others in changing physician behavior (Davis et al., 1995; Oxman et al., 1995; Davis and Taylor-Vaisey, 1997). Relatively weak approaches are traditional lecture-based conferences and seminars and unsolicited, mailed information. More effective is audit and feedback, which is best when given concurrently rather than later, when directed at specific individuals, and when delivered by opinion leaders (respected local clinicians). The strongest implementation strategies are considered to be concurrent reminder systems (posters, pocket cards, sheets, computer-embedded prompts), academic detailing (face-to-face education in the physician's setting), and the use of multiple interventions concurrently (Anderson, 1993).

How should the impact of dissemination or implementation be assessed? Generally, studies evaluate either the process of care or patient outcome (Grimshaw and Russell, 1993). Examples of process of care evaluations might include rates of cervical spine radiography use, timely thrombolytic administration, or appropriate hospital admission for pneumonia. Analogous examples of important patient outcomes would be morbidity from missed cervical spine fractures, mortality from myocardial infarction, or morbidity and mortality from undertreated pneumonia. Ideally, investigators should discuss appropriate strategies for dissemination and implementation once their clinical decision rule has been proven to be valid and effective.

Conclusions

Very few clinical decision rules have been successfully derived, validated, and adopted into clinical practice. This is because development of an effective decision rule is a long, rigorous, and expensive process. Medicine has many clinical situations which would benefit from a decision rule and this provides many research opportunities. This chapter has outlined important methodologic issues for both the critical reader and the clinical researcher to consider.

References

Anderson G (1993) Implementing practice guidelines. Can Med Assoc J 148:753–5.

Anis AH, Stiell IG, Stewart DG, Laupacis A (1995) Cost-effectiveness analysis of the Ottawa ankle rules. Ann Emerg Med 26:422–8.

Auleley G-R, Ravaud P, Giraudeau B, Kerboull L, Nizard R, Massin P, Garreau de Loubresse C, Vallee C, Durieux P (1997) Implementation of the Ottawa Ankle Rules in France: a multicenter randomized controlled trial. JAMA 277:1935–9.

Basinski ASH, Naylor CD, Cohen MM, Ferris LE, Williams JI, Llewellyn-Thomas HA (1992) Standards, guidelines, and clinical policies. Can Med Assoc J 146:833–7.

Borczuk P (1995) Predictors of intracranial injury in patients with mild head trauma. Ann Emerg Med 25:731–6.

Centor RM, Yarbrough B, Wood JP (1984) Inability to predict relapse in acute asthma. N Engl J Med 310:577–80.

Chande VT (1995) Decision rules for roentgenography of children with acute ankle injuries. Arch Pediatr Adolesc Med 149:255–8.

Charlson ME, Ales KL, Simon R, MacKenzie CR (1987) Why predictive indexes perform less well in validation studies. Arch Intern Med 147:2155–61.

Choi BC (1998) Slopes of a receiver operating characteristic curve and likelihood ratios for a diagnostic test. J Clin Epidemiol 148:1127–32.

Ciampi A, Thiffault J, Nakache J-P, Asselain B (1986) Stratification by stepwise regression, correspondence analysis and recursive partition: a comparison of three methods of analysis for survival data with covariates. Comput Stat Data Anal 4:185–204.

Ciampi A, Hogg SA, McKinney S, Thiffault J (1988) RECPAM: a computer program for recursive partition and amalgamation for censored survival data and other situations frequently occurring in biostatistics I Methods and program features. Comput Methods Prog Biomed 26:239–56.

Davis DA, Taylor-Vaisey A (1997) A systematic review of theoretic concepts, practical experience and research evidence in the adoption of clinical practice guidelines. Can Med Assoc J 157:408–16.

Davis DA, Thomson MA, Oxman AD, Haynes RB (1995) A systematic review of the effect of continuing medical education strategies. JAMA 274:700–05.

Diamond GA (1989) Limited assurances. Am J Cardiol 63:99–100.

Diercks DB, Hall KN, Hamilton CA (1997) Validation of the Ottawa knee rules in an American urban teaching emergency department. Acad Emerg Med 4:408–9. (Abstract).

Feinstein AR (1985) The "chagrin factor" and qualitative decision analysis. Arch Intern Med 145:1257–9.

    (1987) Clinimetrics. New Haven: Yale University Press.

Fine MJ, Auble TE, Yealy DM, Hanusa BH, Singer DE, Coley CM, Marrie TJ, Kapoor WN (1997) A prediction rule to identify low-risk patients with community-acquired pneumonia. N Engl J Med 336:243–50.

Fischl MA, Pitchenik A, Gardner LB (1981) An index predicting relapse and need for hospitalization in patients with actue bronchial asthma. N Engl J Med 305:783–99.

Fleiss JL (1981) Statistical Methods for Rates and Proportions, 2nd edn. New York: John Wiley & Sons.

    (1986) The design and analysis of chemical experiments. In: Barnett V, Bradley RA, Hunter JS (eds), Reliability of Measurement, pp. 1–31. New York: John Wiley & Sons.

Friedman JH (1977) A recursive partitioning decision rule for nonparametric classification. IEEE Trans Comput 16:404–8.

Goldman L, Cook EF, Brand DA (1988) A computer protocol to predict myocardial infarction in emergency department patients with chest pain. N Engl J Med 318:797–803.

Graf WD, Cummings P, Quan L, Brutocao D (1995) Predicting outcome in pediatric submersion victims. Ann Emerg Med 26:312–19.

Graham ID, Stiell IG, Laupacis A, O'Connor AM, Wells GA (1998) Emergency physicians' attitudes toward the use of clinical decision rules for radiography. Acad Emerg Med 5:134–40.

Greco PJ, Eisenberg JM (1993) Changing physicians' practices. N Engl J Med 329:1271–4.

Greer AL (1988) The state of the art versus the state of the science: the diffusion of new medical technologies into practice. Int J Technol Assessment Health Care 4:5–26.

Grilli R, Lomas J (1994) Evaluating the message: the relationship between compliance rate and the subject of a practice guideline. Med Care 32:202–13.

Grimshaw JM, Russell IT (1993) Effect of clinical guidelines on medical practice: a systematic review of rigorous evaluations. Lancet 342:1317–22.

Hanley JA, McNeil BJ (1982) The meaning and use of the area under a receiver operating characteristic (ROC) curve. Radiology 143:29–36.

Hayward RSA, Laupacis A (1993) Initiating, conducting and maintaining guidelines development programs. Can Med Assoc J 148:507–12.

Heckerling PS, Tape TG, Wigston RS (1990) Clinical prediction rule for pulmonary infiltrates. Ann Intern Med 113:664–70.

Hosmer DW, Lemeshow S (1989) Applied Logistic Regression. New York: John Wiley.

Kerr L, Kelly AM, Grant J, Richards D, O'Donovan P, Basire K, Graham R (1994) Failed validation of a clinical decision rule for the use of radiography in acute ankle injury. NZ Med J 107:294–5.

Koopman PAR (1984) Confidence intervals for the ratio of two binomial proportions. Biometrics 40:513–17.

Kramer MS, Feinstein AR (1982) Clinical biostatistics: LIV The biostatistics of concordance. Clin Pharmacol Ther 29:111–23.

Landis JR, Koch GG (1977) The measurement of observer agreement for categorical data. Biometrics 33:159–74.

Laupacis A, Sekar N, Stiell IG (1997) Clinical prediction rules: a review and suggested modifications of methodological standards. JAMA 277:488–94.

Lee TH (1990) Evaluating decision aids: the next painful step. J Gen Intern Med 5:528–9.

Lee TH, Cooper HL (1997) Translating good advice into better practice. JAMA 278:2108–9.

Lomas J (1993) Diffusion, dissemination, and implementation: who should do what? Ann NY Acad Sci 703:226–35.

Lomas J (1994) Teaching old (and not so old) docs new tricks: effective ways to implement research findings. In: Dunn EV, Norton PG, Stewart M, Tudiver F, Bass MJ (eds), Disseminating Research/Changing Practice, pp. 1–18. CA: Sage Publications.

Long AE (1985) Radiographic decision-making by the emergency physician. Emerg Med Clin N Am 3:437–46.

Lucchesi GM, Jackson RE, Peacock WF, Cerasani C, Swor RA (1995) Sensitivity of the Ottawa Rules. Ann Emerg Med 26:1–5.

Madden C, Witzke DB, Sanders AB, Valente J, Fritz M (1995) High-yield selection criteria for cranial computed tomography after acute trauma. Acad Emerg Med 2:248–53.

Matthews MG (1986) Guidelines for selective radiological assessment of inversion ankle injuries. Br Med J 293:959.

McBride KL (1997) Validation of the Ottawa ankle rules: Experience at a community hospital. Can Fam Physician 43:459–65.

McCaig LF (1994) National Hospital Ambulatory Medical Care Survey: 1992 emergency department summary. Advance Data 245:1–12.

McDonald CJ (1994) Guidelines you can follow and can trust: an ideal and an example. JAMA 271:872–3.

National Center for Health Statistics (1994) National Hospital Ambulatory Medical Care Survey 1992. Hyattsville: National Center for Health Statistics.

Nichol G, Stiell IG, Wells GA, Cacciotti TF, McDowell I, Laupacis A (1997) Cost-benefit analysis of implementation of the Ottawa knee rule. Acad Emerg Med 4:433. (Abstract).

Oxman AD, Thomson MA, Davis DA, Haynes RB (1995) No magic bullets: a systematic review of 102 trials of interventions to improve professional practice. Can Med Assoc J 153:1423–31.

Pauker SG, Kassirer JP (1980) The threshold approach to clinical decision making. N Engl J Med 302:1109–17.

Peduzzi P, Concata J, Kemper E, Holford TR, Feinstein AR (1996) A simulation study of the number of events per variable in logistic regression analysis. J Clin Epidemiol 49:1373–9.

Pigman EC, Klug RK, Sanford S, Jolly BT (1994) Evaluation of the Ottawa clinical decision rules for the use of radiography in acute ankle and midfoot injuries in the emergency department: an independent site assessment. Ann Emerg Med 24:41–5.

Poses RM, Cebul RD, Collins M, Fager SS (1986) The importance of disease prevalence in transporting clinical prediction rules: the case of streptococcal pharyngitis. Ann Intern Med 105:586–91.

Pozen MW, D'Agostino RB, Selker HP, Sytkowski PA, Hood WB (1984) A predictive instrument to improve coronary-care-unit admission practices in acute ischemic heart disease: a prospective multicenter clinical trial. N Engl J Med 310:1273–8.

Roberts C, McNamee R (1998) A matrix of Kappa-type coefficients to assess the reliability of nominal scales. Stat Med 17:471–88.

Rose CC, Murphy JG, Schwartz JS (1984) Performance of an index predicting the response of patients with acute bronchial asthma to intensive emergency department treatment. N Engl J Med 310:573–7.

Rothrock SG, Buchanan C, Green SM, Bullard T, Falk JL, Langen M (1997) Cranial computed tomography in the emergency evaluation of adult patients without a recent history of head trauma: a prospective analysis. Acad Emerg Med 4:654–61.

Sackett DL, Haynes RB, Guyatt GH, Tugwell P (1991) Clinical Epidemiology: a basic science for clinical medicine, 2nd edn. Toronto: Little, Brown and Co.

Solomito AL, Singal BM, Radack M (1994) Ankle radiography in the emergency department: a prospective validation of Ottawa ankle rules. Acad Emerg Med 1:A64. (Abstract).

Sox HC, Blatt MA, Higgins MC, Marton KI (1988) Medical Decision Making. Boston: Butterworths.

Stiell IG, Greenberg GH, McKnight RD, Nair RC, McDowell I, Worthington JR (1992a) A study to develop clinical decision rules for the use of radiography in acute ankle injuries. Ann Emerg Med 21:384–90.

Stiell IG, McDowell I, Nair RC, Aeta H, Greenberg GH, McKnight RD, Ahuja J (1992b) Use of radiography in acute ankle injuries: physicians' attitudes and practice. Can Med Assoc J 147:1671–8.

Stiell IG, McKnight RD, Greenberg GH, Nair RC, McDowell I, Wallace GJ (1992c) Interobserver agreement in the examination of acute ankle injury patients. Am J Emerg Med 10:14–17.

Stiell IG, Greenberg GH, McKnight RD, Nair RC, McDowell I, Reardon M, Stewart JP, Maloney J (1993) Decision rules for the use of radiography in acute ankle injuries: refinement and prospective validation. JAMA 269:1127–32.

Stiell IG, McKnight RD, Greenberg GH, McDowell I, Nair RC, Wells GA, Johns C, Worthington JR (1994) Implementation of the Ottawa ankle rules. JAMA 271:827–32.

Stiell I, Wells G, Laupacis A, Brison R, Verbeek R, Vandemheen K, Naylor D, the MARS Group (1995a) A multicentre trial to introduce clinical decision rules for the use of radiography in acute ankle injuries. Br Med J 311:594–7.

Stiell IG, Greenberg GH, McKnight RD, Wells GA (1995b) Ottawa ankle rules for radiography of acute injuries. NZ Med J 108:11.

Stiell IG, Wells GA, McDowell I, Greenberg GH, McKnight RD, Cwinn AA, Quinn JV, Yeats A (1995c) Use of radiography in acute knee injuries: need for clinical decision rules. Acad Emerg Med 2:966–73.

Stiell IG, Greenberg GH, Wells GA, McDowell I, Cwinn AA, Smith NA, Cacciotti T, Sivilotti MLA (1996a) Prospective validation of a decision rule for the use of radiography in acute knee injuries. JAMA 275:611–15.

Stiell IG, Greenberg GH, McKnight RD, Wells GA (1996b) The "real" Ottawa ankle rules. Ann Emerg Med 27:103–4.

Stiell IG, Wells GA, Hoag RA, Sivilotti MLA, Cacciotti TF, Verbeek RP, Greenway KT, McDowell I, Cwinn AA, Greenberg GH, Nichol G, Michael JA (1997a) Implementation of the Ottawa knee rule for the use of radiography in acute knee injuries. JAMA 278:2075–8.

Stiell IG, Wells GA, Vandemheen K, Laupacis A, Brison R, Eisenhauer MA, Greenberg GH, MacPhail I, McKnight RD, Reardon M, Verbeek R, Worthington JR, Lesiuk H (1997b) Variation in ED use of computed tomography for patients with minor head injury. Ann Emerg Med 30:14–22.

(1997c) Variation in emergency department use of cervical spine radiography for alert, stable trauma patients. Can Med Assoc J 156:1537–44.

Stiell IG, Wells GA (1999) Methodological standards for the development of clinical decision rules in emergency medicine. Ann Emerg Med 33:437–47.

Svenson J (1988) Need for radiographs in the acutely injured ankle. Lancet i, 244–5.

Verbeek RP, Stiell IG, Hebert G, Sellens C (1997) Ankle radiograph utilization after learning a decision rule: a 12-month follow-up. Acad Emerg Med 4:776–9.

Wasson JH, Sox CH (1996) Clinical prediction rules: have they come of age? JAMA 275: 641–2.

Wasson JH, Sox HC, Neff RK, Goldman L (1985) Clinical prediction rules: application and methodological standards. N Engl J Med 313:793–9.

Wells PS, Anderson DR, Bormanis J, Guy F, Mitchell M, Gray L, Clement C, Robinson KS, Lewandowski B (1997) Value of assessment of pretest probability of deep-vein thrombosis in clinical management. Lancet 350:1795–8.

Wells PS, Anderson DR, Stiell IG, MacLeod B, Simms M, Lewandowski B (1998) The use of a clinical model to manage patients with suspected deep venous thrombosis. Acad Emerg Med 5:500. (Abstract).

Wells PS, Hirsh J, Anderson DR, Lensing AWA, Foster G, Kearon C, Weitz J, D'Ovidio R, Cogo A, Prandoni P, Girolami A, Ginsberg JS (1995) Accuracy of clinical assessment of deep-vein thrombosis Lancet 345:1326–30.

Wigton RS, Connor JL, Centor RM (1986) Transportability of a decision rule for the diagnosis of streptococcal pharyngitis. Arch Intern Med 146:81–3.

17

Trauma Performance Improvement

Ronald V. Maier and Michael Rhodes

Introduction

Professionals involved with trauma care, and medicine in general, are being asked to adopt new standards of accountability as a major societal responsibility. In addition to traditional accountability for the highest standards of care for each individual patient (trauma audit), there is an increasing need to demonstrate the efficacy and cost-effectiveness of medical practice in health systems and entire patient populations. This has led to the development of the field of performance improvement.

Performance improvement is the continuous evaluation of a system and the providers through structured review of the process of care as well as the outcomes. Performance improvement has evolved from previous quality assurance paradigms and represents a more scientific and evidence-based continuation of those standards. The goal of performance improvement is to ensure that trauma centers and trauma systems design processes to monitor, analyze, and improve performance systematically with the ultimate intent of improving patient outcomes. The primary focus has been shifted to the assessment of whole processes – not isolated individual components of care. A performance process may reside entirely within a department, but major processes will include several departments or disciplines. A process may be narrowly defined and formalized, or it may be fairly loose and informal. In order for performance improvement to occur, processes need to be (1) planned and designed, (2) monitored by means of ongoing data collection, (3) analyzed to determine process effectiveness, and (4) implemented with a commitment for sustained activity and improvement. Continuous monitoring, analysis, and sustained improvement are the key elements in ongoing performance improvement efforts (O'Leary, 1995).

This chapter will examine the current status of performance improvement methodology to assess the care of the injured patient. The development of performance improvement from preventable mortality studies, audit filters, assessment of complications, and institutional trauma registries is investigated. The current use of risk adjusted scoring and evidence-based medicine, and the need for better system-wide approaches and measures of quality of life outcomes is discussed.

History of Trauma Performance Improvement

Trauma performance improvement takes its roots from the surgical audit, which began in the nineteenth and earlier twentieth century as a system of counting procedures, complications and deaths (Wright, 1995). Codman, as a member of the American College of Surgeons at the beginning of the twentieth century, emphasized precise record keeping, including both physician and patient assessment of long-term outcome (Passaro and Organ, 1999). His plea for accountability was largely ignored for 50 years, until 1957, when the American College of Surgeons published a method of surgical audit based on chart abstraction of predetermined data designed to capture mostly quantitative measures (Myers and Slee, 1957). Simultaneously, Australian surgeons and anesthesiologists developed similar audit techniques, but added indications for surgical procedures (Smyth, 1959). A byproduct of these audit efforts was a lively interaction among staff members and a demand for intellectual honesty, which has come to be known as the Morbidity and Mortality conference. Several authors have further defined the purpose and conduct of these meetings, which have become an important element of surgical audit and performance improvement (Bosk, 1979; Campbell, 1988; Gordon, 1994). Traditionally, trauma care was part of the surgical audit process, and was frequently discussed at the surgical Morbidity and Mortality conference. Separate Morbidity and Mortality conferences for trauma patients now exist in many high volume trauma centers as part of the audit process.

A health-care industry-wide initiative known as quality assurance emerged a quarter century ago based on the Deming model of quality control in industry (Deming, 1982). These audits were characterized by retrospective chart review by nonphysicians searching for documentation of predetermined criteria, which were introduced to reflect acceptable quality in physician performance. Eventually recognition of the limitations of this bad apple approach led to the abandonment of this onerous process and endorsement of the concepts of total quality management and continuous quality improvement. These emphasized the process as well as the outcome of care, including the impact of the system (rather than the individual) on patient care. The ongoing evolution of this process has led to the concept of performance improvement (a term popularized by the Joint Commission for the Accreditation of Health Care Organizations), with the added goal of reducing unnecessary variation in trauma care (Joint Commission for Accreditation of Healthcare Organizations, 1998).

This evolution in performance improvement activities has included preventable death studies (Cales and Trunkey, 1985), interdisciplinary audits (Shackford et al., 1986), development of trauma-specific audit filters (Shackford et al., 1987a), requirements of structured and measurable quality improvement programs for trauma center recognition (Mitchell et al., 1994; Bazzoli et al., 1995), and a movement toward evidence-based performance improvement utilizing clinical pathways and protocols (American College of Surgeons Committee on Trauma, 1998; Cook, 1998). To date, although generally accepted as useful by trauma practitioners and researchers, there is unfortunately a dearth of data to support or refute the value of trauma performance improvement.

Preventable Mortality Studies

In the 1960s and 1970s, several studies expanded beyond the typical individual institutional audit of trauma deaths and utilized the concept of preventable mortality (i.e., the percentage of deaths retrospectively judged to have been preventable had optimal care been available), to examine multi-institutional or system level performance. These analyses were provided by panels of "experts" utilizing empiric assessments in the absence of evidence-based standards of care. Care was defined as unacceptable if the rate of preventable deaths in one locale was higher than that in similarly injured patients in another locale (West et al., 1979). Estimates vary, but some identified 20–40% of trauma deaths as preventable (Trunkey and Lewis, 1991). These studies relied on labor intensive reviews of charts by a panel of experts; assessments were based on empiric knowledge and experience. The outcome (death) was objective and easily measured. But, designation of a death as preventable was a much more subjective and often inaccurately determined endpoint (Mendeloff and Cayten, 1991; MacKenzie et al., 1992).

While lacking in quantitative precision, these studies provided a major stimulus for the improvement in the process of acute trauma care and an impetus for the development of modern trauma systems. A major study, in the early 1980s, from San Diego County reported that implementation of a regional trauma system reduced the proportion of preventable deaths from 13.6% to 2.7% of all trauma deaths (Shackford et al., 1986). This and other assessments of early trauma systems led to the development of a formal, multidisciplinary, trauma audit process for regional trauma systems (Shackford et al., 1987a). These new system-level approaches to trauma audit and audit filters served as a template for trauma care evaluation throughout the world (Shackford et al., 1987b). The Morbidity and Mortality conference, trauma audit, and audit filters have continued to evolve and are still the basis for most current trauma quality assurance and performance improvement programs, particularly in the United States.

Audit Filters

The concept of trauma audit filters to identify specific cases was based on the use of "ideal" criteria against which actual performance could be measured. These filters were intended to identify patients in whom care may have been suboptimal, and thus, should be further reviewed. In 1987, the American College of Surgeons Committee on Trauma first published 12 audit filters that were derived by expert opinion (American College of Surgeons, 1987). Most of the filters, sometimes referred to as critical indicators, were developed by consensus while some were backed by varying amounts of scientific evidence. Although each criterion or filter was designed to measure a standard or process that had an accompanying rationale, none are truly evidence-based (Table 17.1). For example, the audit filter,

Table 17.1 Trauma audit filters

- The absence of an ambulance report on the medical record for a patient transported by prehospital emergency medical service (EMS) personnel (system filter).
- A patient with a Glasgow Coma Scale score of < 14 who does not receive a computed tomographic scan of the head.
- A comatose trauma patient (Glasgow Coma Scale score of < 8) leaving the emergency department before a definitive airway (endotracheal tube or surgical airways) is established.
- Any patient sustaining a gunshot wound to the abdomen who is managed nonoperatively.
- Patients with abdominal injuries and hypotension (systolic blood pressure < 90 mm Hg) who do not undergo laparotomy within 1 hour of arrival in the emergency department; other patients undergoing laparotomy performed more than 4 hours after arrival in the emergency room.
- Patients with epidural or subdural brain hematoma receiving craniotomy more than 4 hours after arrival at emergency department, excluding those performed for intracranial pressure monitoring.
- Interval of > 8 hours between arrival and the initiation of debridement of an open tibial fracture, excluding a low velocity gunshot wound.
- Abdominal, thoracic, vascular, or cranial surgery performed > 24 hours after arrival.
- A trauma patient admitted to the hospital under the care of an admitting or attending physician who is not a surgeon.
- Nonfixation of femoral diaphyseal fracture in an adult trauma patient.
- Selected complications, monitored as either trends or sentinel events.
- All trauma deaths.

American College of Surgeons Committee on Trauma (1993). Resources for Optimal Care of the Injured Patient: 1993, Chicago, American College of Surgeons, pp. 79–80.

"subdural/epidural hematomas operated on after more than 4 hours," was based on a retrospective study which suggested that patients undergoing craniotomy within 4 hours had a better outcome than those undergoing craniotomy after 4 hours (Seelig et al., 1981). While it appeared reasonable to review all epidural/subdural hematomas that were operated on after 4 hours as an audit filter, subsequent studies have shown that management factors other than the timing of craniotomy have a greater influence on outcome (Wilberger et al., 1990; Schwartz et al., 1991).

The American College of Surgeons Committee on Trauma expanded the number of audit filters based on expert opinion to 22, in 1990 (American College of Surgeons, 1990). However, they subsequently, in 1993, recommended, based on further study, that only a limited number of filters be used very selectively in focused audits to avoid unrewarding costly reviews (American College of Surgeons, 1993). Several investigators have found that the yield, defined as opportunity for improvement, in mature trauma systems from audit filters was very low and the reviews costly to perform (Rhodes et al., 1990; Nayduch et al., 1994). In 1995, a study based on 21,000 patients in the Pennsylvania Trauma Registry found that 57% of the total cases were noncompliant (referred to as "fallouts" or "qualifiers") with regard to at least one filter, and that only nine of the 20 filters assessed, were found to identify patients who had a greater length of stay or increased mortality (Copes et al., 1995). A subsequent study from Los Angeles County examined five audit filters for nonfatal trauma and found that the yield was minimal (Cryer et al., 1996). A more recent study from Seattle, found that the patient care issues identified with audit filters did not predict an increased length of stay (O'Keefe et al., 1999).

The sensitivity, specificity, and accuracy of trauma audit filters has not been accurately estimated. The need for more rigorous testing and validation of audit filters has been recognized (Copes et al., 1995). In response, the American College of Surgeons Committee on Trauma, in their recent trauma resources document did not publish any trauma audit filters, but still recommend that selective utilization of filters in existing trauma registries or in hospital-wide performance improvement programs may have value (American College of Surgeons, 1998).

Although mortality and complications are frequently listed as audit filters, they should be considered separately in that the yield from tracking these markers of outcome has been much more fruitful.

Complications

Although not well quantified in the research literature, complications in trauma care have been demonstrated to affect outcomes as defined by cost, length of stay, and quality of life (Mattox, 1994; Maull et al., 1996; O'Keefe et al., 1997). The American College of Surgeons Committee on Trauma has defined and published a list of complications, which are commonly tracked by most trauma registries as well as hospital-wide performance improvement programs (Table 17.2) (American College of Surgeons, 1999). In a San Diego study reviewing 857 complications in 399 patients, only one-third were judged to be provider-related (defined as delays or errors in care) while two-thirds were disease-related (resulting from progression of a disease or sequelae of an injury), most of which were infectious in nature (Hoyt et al., 1992). In a prior San Diego County study, two-thirds of provider-related complications occurred in the resuscitative and operative phase of care while one-third were identified in the critical care phase (Davis et al., 1991). In a study designed to quantify the costs associated with the development of complications in injury victims, 32 complications defined by the American College of Surgeons Committee on Trauma were analyzed using a linear regression model (O'Keefe et al., 1997). Six complications were found to be important predictors of cost, including adult respiratory distress syndrome (ARDS), acute renal failure, sepsis, pneumonia, decubitus ulceration, and wound infection. The 1201 individuals with these complications had an observed average cost of $47,457 compared with a predicted average cost of $23,266, with mean excess costs ranging from $7,000 to $18,000 per complication.

It is important not to confuse pre-existing disease (co-morbidity) with complications. Cardiac disease, diabetes, liver disease, malignancy, chronic pulmonary disease, obesity, renal disease, neurologic disease, and hypertension have been shown to be outcome predictors independent of age and injury severity (Milzman et al., 1992). The effect of these co-morbidites must be recognized when analyzing complications. For example, one of the American College of Surgeons Committee on Trauma complications is jaundice as defined by serum bilirubin $> 2 \, mg/dL$.

Table 17.2 Trauma-related complications

- Acute respiratory distress syndrome
- Aspiration pneumonia
- Bacteremia
- Cardiac arrest
- Coagulopathy
- Compartment syndrome
- Deep vein thrombosis
- Disseminated fungal infection
- Dehiscence/evisceration
- Empyema
- Esophageal intubation
- Hypothermia
- Intraabdominal abscess
- Jaundice
- Failure of fracture fixation
- Mortality
- Myocardial infarction
- No response to resuscitation
- Pancreatitis
- Pneumonia
- Pneumothorax
- Skin breakdown
- Progression of original neurologic insult
- Pulmonary embolus
- Renal failure
- Sepsis-like syndrome
- Urinary tract infection
- Wound infection

American College of Surgeons Committee on Trauma (1998). Resources for Optimal Care of the Injured Patient: 1999, Chicago, American College of Surgeons, pp. 69–76.

However, if the patient had preinjury liver dysfunction with elevated bilirubin, this should not be considered a complication resulting from injury.

Tracking provider-related complications as part of performance improvement offers an opportunity to measure and improve the process and outcome of care. Tracking disease-related complication rates and pre-existing disease can help to provide strategies for prevention and resource allocation.

Institutional Registries

Timely collection and access to high-quality data remain major challenges in the implementation of performance improvement in most institutions and trauma systems. Institutional trauma registries generally have been used to provide an ongoing database of all or various subsets of trauma patients admitted to a given hospital. Variations in the definition of a "trauma patient" from institution to institution can greatly affect the comparability of data. The National Trauma Data Bank (NTDB) developed by the Committee on Trauma of the American College of

Table 17.3 Trauma patient definition (National Trauma Data Bank, NTDB)

- Any patient with ICD-9 CM discharge diagnosis 800.00–959.9
    Excluding 905–909 (late effects of injury)
    Excluding 910–924 (blisters, contusions, abrasions, and insect bites)
    Excluding 930–939 (foreign bodies)
- All injury-related deaths in emergency department

Surgeons has attempted to provide a national standard for the definition of trauma to ensure consistency of populations analyzed (Table 17.3) (American College of Surgeons, 1996). In addition, many institutions supplement the registry with simple data sets on all injured patients seen, including all emergency department visits, in an attempt to derive an institutional denominator to quantify their total service volume. Registries have become the primary source of performance improvement information, and, in turn, have been used for selected audit filters and focused performance improvement tracking (see chapter on case series and cross-sectional surveys).

Risk Adjusted Scoring

Once trauma data have been collected, they can be compared with other institutions as a method of assessing performance. Many states with formalized trauma systems require data submission on all trauma cases as a prerequisite for institutional designation as a trauma facility (Bazzoli et al., 1995). Trauma centers usually compare their mortality rate with that of a standard population; in the United States the usual standard has been the patient population in the Major Trauma Outcomes Study (MTOS). Data were provided voluntarily to MTOS over a 7 year period on approximately 160,000 trauma patients admitted to 140 US and Canadian hospitals (Champion et al., 1990). Recently, a national trauma registry sponsored by the American College of Surgeons, the NTDB has been developed to receive data from all existing trauma registries for the ultimate purpose of establishing national benchmarking (American College of Surgeons, 1996).

Originally, these databases were developed to serve as a benchmark for outcomes from individual institutions. As discussed in Jurkovich and O'Keefe (this volume) and Mock (this volume), the Trauma and Injury Severity Score (TRISS) methodology was developed as a weighted score to estimate the probability of survival (Ps) for a given individual based on the MTOS database (Champion et al., 1983; Boyd et al., 1987; Champion et al., 1989; Markle et al., 1992). Thus, individual patients can be identified as unexpected deaths or survivors for selective quality assurance review, Figure 17.1. In addition, TRISS-based probabilities of survival, can be used to compare the overall institutional death rate with the predicted death rate from the large national data set of seriously injured trauma patients or national norm, such as MTOS (Champion et al., 1990). In a longitudinal assessment of trauma deaths utilizing TRISS, one trauma center was able to demonstrate an increase of 13.4 more survivors than predicted per 100 seriously injured patients per

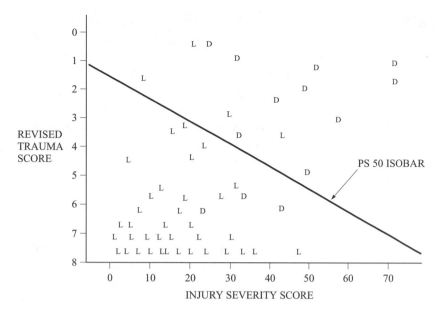

Figure 17.1 TRISS methodology.

year (Champion et al., 1992). In a Canadian study, which used TRISS methodology, designation of trauma centers led to a reduction in unexpected trauma deaths due to motor vehicle crashes from 8.8 to 3.6 per 100 patients treated following designation (Stewart et al., 1995).

To evaluate outcomes between trauma system versus trauma center implementation, risk stratified population-based registries have also been utilized. Mullins et al. (1994, 1996) in Oregon, used a statewide registry to analyze mortality outcomes in patients hospitalized for injuries before and after institution of a trauma system. The adjusted rate of mortality was reduced by one-third in level I trauma centers, while there was an overall decline in regional injury death rates. An additional study confirmed that improvement in mortality was due to trauma system development and not concurrent improvements of care by comparing trauma deaths in adjacent states with and without system implementation (Mullins et al., 1998).

Evidence-based Medicine (EBM) and Guidelines

EBM has been defined as a method of patient care, decision making and teaching that integrates high-quality research evidence with pathophysiologic reasoning, experience, and patient preference (Guyatt et al., 1995; Cook, 1998). EBM provides the scientific basis for guidelines from which institution specific pathways, protocols, or care plans can be developed (Rhodes, 1997). Clinical Decision Support Systems are rapidly evolving that will allow access to outcome data at the patient's bedside in an on-line fashion, facilitating the implementation of guidelines (Classen, 1998). Evidence-based guidelines should replace existing expert opinion-based audit filters and can be used to measure process and outcome as well as provide corrective action tools for both individual physicians and the system (Hoyt, 1997). Examples in the nontrauma surgical literature include a French study on the impact of clinical guidelines for breast and colon cancer which demonstrated that the percentage of evidence-based decisions significantly increased after implementation of the guidelines (Ray-Coquard et al., 1997). In another study, a prospective evaluation of a clinical guideline for upper gastrointestinal tract hemorrhage demonstrated a reduced length of stay for selected low-risk patients (Hay et al., 1997). In another recent study comparing two academic medical centers, development and implementation of a prophylactic ketoconazole practice guideline for intensive care unit patients at high risk for ARDS demonstrated increased use of ketoconazole and a lower rate of ARDS in the study hospital versus the control hospital (Sinuff et al., 1999).

Several trauma-related studies have suggested the utility of evidence-based guidelines for Performance Improvement. The international Cochrane Collaboration has taken a sophisticated approach to EBM by providing an electronic analytical database of the best available data from randomized clinical trials (Bero and Rennie, 1995). One such review of 26 randomized controlled trials of fluid resuscitation found no benefit from resuscitation with colloid solutions; colloids were associated with an increase in the mortality rate of 3.8% (Schierhout and Roberts, 1998). It should be feasible to measure compliance with the guidelines derived from EBM as a performance improvement tool (see Bunn et al., this volume).

The Eastern Association for the Surgery of Trauma has published guidelines on blunt cardiac injury, deep vein thrombosis prophylaxis, cervical spine clearance, and the management of colon injury (Pasquale and Fabian, 1998). Each of these guidelines present a level of recommendation based on the validity and the strength of the supporting data (Guyatt et al., 1995; Cook, 1998). The Brain Trauma Foundation has published evidence-based guidelines for severe head injury (Bullock et al., 1995). Although no study to date has prospectively demonstrated improved outcome with their use, these trauma guidelines have been adopted by many neurosurgeons and trauma surgeons worldwide. From these nationally derived evidence-based guidelines, trauma centers can develop institution-specific protocols and pathways, and compliance can be used as a measure of performance.

Process and Outcome Measures

The meaning and value of outcomes depend on the perspective from which they are viewed. The surgeon emphasizes quality of care. The patient anticipates a complete and rapid recovery. The administrator and payer review the cost of care. An overall goal is improving the value of trauma care. A useful method of viewing performance is through the value equation: (American College of Surgeons, 1999).

$$\text{Value} = \frac{\text{quality of process} + \text{quality of outcome}}{\text{cost}}$$

Value can be increased by improving the quality of the process or outcome or by decreasing cost. However, a modest increase in cost, which significantly improves quality can also add net value (see MacKenzie, this volume). This perspective can help prioritize performance improvement initiatives. Process measures are designed to examine the performance of the system as well as the practitioners. Therefore, the spectrum of performance evaluation can extend from measures of individual practitioner performance to institutional and system-wide variables. These categories of variables require defined criteria (expectations), which are determined from consensus, institutional guidelines, or ideally, evidence-based guidelines. Some variables will still require individualized peer review for determination. For most trauma centers, it is practical to monitor only selected criteria. Selection of variables to analyze will be dependent on the results of an in-depth institutional review of current patient care processes.

System Wide Performance Improvement

From the longstanding individualized and patient outcome driven audits in Morbidity and Mortality, to the experiences implementing, testing, and analyzing the effectiveness of trauma systems, trauma performance improvement can frequently set the tone for hospital-wide performance improvement processes. Assigning blame for poor outcomes is recognized as counterproductive and destructive to the performance improvement process. Most errors are system-level problems and should be addressed as such. Overall, broader-based performance improvement programs are most effective when integrated into both a hospital-wide and system-wide performance improvement plan.

It is likely that as medical informatics and hospital information systems improve, trauma performance improvement will become fully integrated into the hospital-wide or system-wide performance improvement processes. Stand-alone trauma registries, will become part of hospital information systems allowing for predetermined trauma-specific reports to be generated for local and national benchmarking. The expectations of the Joint Commission for the Accreditation of Healthcare Organizations as well as unique organizational needs will become integral to trauma performance improvement (O'Leary, 1995). Familiarity with the Joint Commission for the Accreditation of Healthcare Organizations performance improvement initiatives such as sentinel event reporting, accreditation watch, commendation, root cause analysis, and reporting tools will be essential for future institutional compliance with regulatory and societal expectations and cost-efficiency. However, the trauma Morbidity and Mortality conference/case audit, especially as it relates to peer review will likely continue to thrive as it has for years, as an established, culture appropriate qualitative tool.

Currently, most outcomes analyses have focused on the hospital phase of care. There is little information on outcomes derived from prehospital or postacute care rehabilitation phases of care. There are few prospective trials of effectiveness of prehospital trauma-related interventions. Even accepted standards, such as initiation of prehospital fluid resuscitation, have been recently challenged in a subset of patients with penetrating trauma to the torso (Bickell et al., 1994). In addition, morbidity, not merely mortality, must be tracked post discharge. Measurement of morbidity must include not only functional disability and loss of productivity, but also impact on quality of life, both short and long term (Dodds et al., 1993; MacKenzie, this volume).

Future

Several areas for future research are indicated. At this juncture, there are no compelling data to conclude that guidelines themselves have altered the traditional outcomes of mortality, complications, length of stay, cost, and quality of life. Equally apparent is the absence of research on the utility of guidelines, pathways, and protocols as Performance Improvement tools. It must be recognized that a substantial portion of trauma care will never be subjected to prospective, randomized controlled studies. Evaluating outcomes in trauma care requires development of appropriate, validated tools, for evaluating clinical effectiveness and patient outcomes (Dodds et al., 1993; MacKenzie, this volume). More reliable and valid measures of stratification: injury severity and case mix; and outcomes, sensitive to changes over time and differences in treatment are needed (Bonnie et al., 1999). To achieve these goals, improvements in population-based trauma data are necessary. A major requirement is improved linkage of data from prehospital to hospital to rehabilitation phases of care of the injured patient. The goal will be to identify the elements of the trauma care system responsible for reductions in Morbidity and Mortality and to identify problems to focus research and implement changes in clinical care.

References

American College of Surgeons (1987) Hospital and Prehospital Resources for Optimal Care of the Injured Patient: Appendices A through J, pp. 42–3. Chicago: American College of Surgeons.
   (1996) National Trauma Databank. Chicago: American College of Surgeons.
American College of Surgeons Committee on Trauma (1990) Resources for Optimal Care of the Injured Patient, pp. 67–76. Chicago: American College of Surgeons.
   (1993) Resources for Optimal Care of the Injured Patient: 1993, pp. 77–96. Chicago: American College of Surgeons.
   (1998) Resources for Optimal Care of the Injured Patient: 1999, pp. 69–76. Chicago: American College of Surgeons.
Bazzoli GJ, Madura KJ, Cooper GF, MacKenzie EJ, Maier RV (1995) Progress in the development of trauma systems in the United States Results of a national survey. JAMA 273(5):395–401.
Bero L, Rennie D (1995) The Cochrane Collaboration: preparing, maintaining, and disseminating systematic reviews of the effects of healthcare. JAMA 274:1935–8.
Bickell WH, Wall MJ, Pepe PE, Martin RR, Ginger VF, Allen MK, Mattox KL (1994) Immediate versus delayed fluid resuscitation for hypotensive patients with penetrating torso injuries. N Engl J Med 331(17):1105–9.
Bonnie RJ, Fulco CE, Liverman CT (1999) Trauma Care. In: Reducing the Burden of Injury Advancing Prevention and Treatment, pp. 138–77. Publication of the Committee on

Injury Prevention and Control, Division of Health Promotion and Disease Prevention, Institute of Medicine. Washington, DC: National Academy Press.

Bosk CL (1979) Forgive and Remember: Managing Medical Failure. Chicago: University of Chicago Press.

Boyd CR, Tolson MA, Copes WS (1987) Evaluating trauma care: the TRISS method Trauma Score and the Injury Severity Score. Journal of Trauma 27(4):370–8.

Bullock R, Chestnut RM, Clifton G et al. (1995) Guidelines for the Management of Severe Head Injury. The Brain Trauma Foundation. www.braintrauma.org/guideline.nsf

Cales RH, Trunkey DD (1985) Preventable trauma deaths: A review of trauma care systems development. JAMA 254:1059–63.

Campbell WB (1988) Surgical Morbidity and Mortality Meetings. Ann R Coll Surg Engl 70:363–5.

Champion HR, Sacco WJ, Hunt TK (1983) Trauma severity scoring to predict mortality. Wld J Surg 7:4–11.

Champion HR, Sacco WJ, Copes WS, Gann DS, Gennarelli TA , Flanagan ME (1989) A revision of the Trauma Score. J Trauma 29(5):623–9.

Champion HR, Copes WS, Sacco WJ, Lawnick NM, Keast SL, Bain LW, Flanagan ME, Frey CF (1990) The Major Trauma Outcome Study: establishing national norms for trauma care. J Trauma 30(11):1356–65.

Champion HR, Sacco WJ, Copes WS (1992) Improvement in outcome from trauma center care. Arch Surg 127(3):333–8.

Classen DC (1998) Clinical decisions support systems to improve clinical practice and quality of care. JAMA 280:1360–1.

Cook D (1998) Evidence-based critical care medicine: a potential tool for change. New Horizons 6:20–5.

Copes WS, Staz CF, Konvolinka CW, Sacco WJ (1995) American College of Surgeons audit filters: associations with patient outcome and resource utilization. J Trauma 38(3):432–8.

Cryer HG, Hiatt JR, Flemming AW, Gruen JP, Sterling J (1996) Continuous use of standard process audit filters has limited value in an established trauma system. J Trauma 41(3):389–95.

Davis JW, Hoyt DB, McArdle MS, Mackersie RC, Shackford SR, Eastman AB (1991) The significance of critical care errors in causing preventable death in trauma patients in a trauma system. J Trauma 31(6):813–19.

Deming WE (1982) Quality, Productivity and Competitive Position. Cambridge, MA: Massachusetts Institute of Technology, Center for Advanced Engineering Study.

Dodds TA, Martin DP, Stolov WC, Dey RA (1993) A validation of the functional independence measurement and its performance among rehabilitation inpatients. Arch Phys Med Rehab 74(5):531–6.

Gordon L (1994) Gordon's Guide to the Surgical Morbidity and Mortality Conference. Philadelphia: Hanley and Belfus.

Guyatt GH, Sackett DL, Sinclair JC, Hayward R, Cook DJ, Cook RJ (1995) Users' guides to the medial literature IX A method for grading health care recommendations. Evidence-Based Working Group. JAMA 274(22):1800–4.

Hay JA, Maldonado L, Weingarten SR, Ellrodt AG (1997) Prospective evaluation of a clinical guideline recommending hospital length of stay in upper gastrointestinal tract hemorrhage. JAMA 278(24):2151–6.

Hoyt DB (1997) Clinical practice guidelines. Am J Surg 173(1):35–6.

Hoyt DB, Hollingsworth-Fridlund P, Fortlage D, Davis JW, Mackersie RC (1992) An evaluation of provider-related and disease-related morbidity in a level I university trauma service: directions for quality improvement. J Trauma 33(4):586–601.

Joint Commission for the Accreditation of Healthcare Organizations (1998) Improving Organizational Performance. CAHM Update 3, pp. 1–36.

MacKenzie EJ, Steinwachs DM, Bone LR, Floccare DJ, Ramzy AI (1992) Inter-rater reliability of preventable death judgements. The Preventable Death Study Group. J Trauma 33(2):292–302.

Markle J, Cayten CG, Byrne DW, Moy F, Murphy JG (1992) Comparison between TRISS and ASCOT methods in controlling for injury severity. J Trauma 33(2):326–32.

Mattox KL (ed.) (1994) Complications of Trauma. New York: Churchill Livingstone

Maull KI, Rodriguez A, Wiles CE (eds) (1996) Complications in Trauma and Critical Care. Philadelphia: WB Saunders.

Mendeloff JM, Cayten CG (1991) Trauma systems and public policy. Annu Rev Public Health 12:401–24.

Milzman DP, Boulanger BR, Rodriguez A, Soderstrom CA, Mitchell KA, Magnant CM (1992) Pre-existing disease in trauma patients: A predictor of fate independent of age and ISS. J Trauma 32(2):236–44.

Mitchell FL, Thal ER, Wolferth CC (1994) American College of Surgeons Verification/ Consultation Program: analysis of unsuccessful verification reviews. J Trauma 37(4):557–562.

Mullins RJ, Veum-Stone J, Helfand M, Zimmer-Gembeck M, Hedges JR, Southard PA, Trunkey DD (1994) Outcome of hospitalized injured patients after institution of a trauma system in an urban area. JAMA 271(24):1919–24.

Mullins RJ, Veum-Stone J, Hedges JR, Zimmer-Gembeck MJ, Mann NC, Southard PA, Helfand M, Gaines JA, Trunkey DD (1996) Influence of a statewide trauma system on location of hospitalization and outcome of injured patients. J Trauma 40(4):536–45.

Mullins RJ, Mann NC, Hedges JR, Worrall W, Jurkovich GJ (1998) Preferential benefit of implementation of a statewide trauma system in one of two adjacent states. J Trauma 44(4):609–16.

Myers RS, Slee VN (1957) A new medical audit method. Bulletin of the American College of Surgeons 42:191–3.

Nayduch D, Moylan J, Snyder BL, Andrews L, Rutledge R, Cunningham P (1994) American College of Surgeons Trauma Quality Indicators: An analysis of outcome in a state wide trauma registry. J Trauma 37(4):565–75.

O'Keefe GE, Maier RV, Diehr P, Grossman D, Jurkovich GJ, Conrad D (1997) The complications of trauma and their associated costs in a level I trauma center. Arch Surg 132(8):920–4.

O'Keefe GE, Jurkovich GJ, Maier RV (1999) Defining excess resource utilization and identifying associated factors for trauma victims. J Trauma 46(3):473–8.

O'Leary MR (1995) Clinical performance data: a guide to interpretation. In: Joint Commission on Accreditation of Healthcare Organizations, pp. 65–96. Oakbrook Terrace, IL: The Commission.

Pasquale M, Fabian TC (1998) EAST Ad Hoc Committee on Practice Management Guideline Development Practice management guidelines for trauma from the Eastern Association for the Surgery of Trauma. J Trauma 44:941–57.

Passaro E, Organ CH (1999) Ernest A Codman: The Improper Bostonian. Bull Am Coll Surg 84(1):16–22.

Ray-Coquard I, Philip T, Lehmann M, Ferves B, Farsi F, Chauvin F (1997) Impact of clinical guidelines program for breast cancer in a French cancer center. JAMA 278(19):1591–5.

Rhodes M (1997) Clinical Practice Guidelines. Am J Surg 173:35–6.

Rhodes M, Sacco W, Smith S, Boorse D (1990) Cost effectiveness of trauma quality assurance audit filters. J Trauma 30(6):724–7.

Schierhout G, Roberts I (1998) Fluid resuscitation with colloid or crystalloid solutions in critically ill patients: a systematic review of randomized trials. Br Med J 316:961–4.

Schwartz ML, Sharkey PW, Anderson JA (1991) Quality assurance for patients with head injuries admitted to a regional trauma unit. J Trauma 31(7):962–7.

Seelig JM, Becker DP, Miller JD, Greenberg RP, Ward JD, Choi SC (1981) Traumatic acute subdural hematoma: Major mortality reduction in comatose patients treated within 4 hours. N Engl J Med 304(25):1511–18.

Shackford SR, Hollingsworth-Fridlund P, Cooper GF, Eastman AB (1986) The effect of regionalization upon the quality of trauma care as assessed by concurrent audit before and after institution of a trauma system: a preliminary report. J Trauma 26(9):812–20.

Shackford SR, Hollingsworth-Fridlund D, McArdle M, Eastman AB (1987a) Assuring quality in a trauma system–the Medical Audit Committee: composition, cost, and results. J Trauma 27(8):866–75.

Shackford SR, Mackersie RC, Hoyt DB, Baxt WG, Eastmen AB, Hammill FN, Knotts FB, Virgilio RW (1987b) Impact of trauma system on outcome of severely injured patients. Arch Surg 122(5):523–7.

Sinuff T, Cook DJ, Peterson JC, Fuller HD (1999) Development, implementation, and evaluation of a ketoconazole practice guideline for ARDS prophylaxis. J Crit Care 14(1):1–6.

Smyth JJ (1959) Surgical audits parts I and II. Med J Austr 46(1):313–19.

Stewart TC, Lane PL, Stefanits T (1995) An evaluation of patient outcomes before and after trauma center designation using Trauma and Injury Severity Score analysis. J Trauma 39(6):1036–40.

Trunkey D, Lewis FR (1991) Preventable mortality. In: Trunkey D, Lewis FR (eds), Current Therapy of Trauma, 3rd edn., pp. 3–4. Philadelphia: Decker.

West JG, Trunkey DD, Lim RC (1979) Systems of trauma care. A study of two counties. Arch Surg 114(4):455–60.

Wilberger JE, Harris M, Diamond DL (1990) Traumatic acute subdural hematoma: Morbidity and mortality related to timing of operative intervention. J Trauma 30(6):733–6.

Wright, JE (1995) The history of the surgical audit. J Quality Clin Practice 15:81–8.

18

Measuring Disability and Quality of Life Postinjury

Ellen J. MacKenzie

For every injury death there are approximately 18 nonfatal injuries resulting in hospitalization and 250 that are treated and released from emergency departments (Fingerhut and Warner, 1997). Although many of these nonfatal injuries are minor in nature and only result in 1 or 2 days of restricted activity, many others have far reaching consequences and are often significant enough to limit employment and recreation for the 40–50 years of life remaining for the typical patient. Productivity losses associated with nonfatal injuries alone have been shown to account for 40% of the total lifetime costs of injury (Rice et al., 1989; Miller et al., 1995). These considerations have challenged the field to find better ways to measure and monitor the impact of injuries in terms other than just lives saved. Measures of functional outcome, disability, and health-related quality of life are becoming increasingly important parameters in the evaluation of treatment and prevention strategies for reducing the burden of injury. In this chapter we begin with some definitions and an overall framework in which to discuss the epidemiology of injury outcome, proceed to a review of the most widely used measures of disability and health-related quality of life, and conclude with a discussion of the challenges ahead as we more broadly apply these measures in injury research and evaluation.

Defining Disability and Quality of Life: A Framework

A useful framework for distinguishing among different types of injury outcomes was first described by Nagi (1976) and more recently elucidated in two Institute of Medicine Reports, Disability in America (IOM, 1991) and Enabling America (IOM, 1997) (Figure 18.1). Nagi defined four related concepts of pathology, impairment, functional limitation, and disability. In the injury context, pathology refers to the cellular and tissue changes that describe the injury resulting from an acute exposure to physical agents. Impairment is defined as the discrete loss or abnormality of mental, physiological, or biochemical function, and reflects limitation in function at the organ or body system level. Examples of injury-related impairments include measures of reduced range of motion and strength following leg injuries and signs and symptoms consistent with cranial nerve damage following traumatic brain injury. The most direct way that impairments impact the individual is through the functional limitations they cause, including both physical limitations (e.g., difficulty walking, climbing stairs, stooping/bending) and neuropsychologic

Transitional Factors

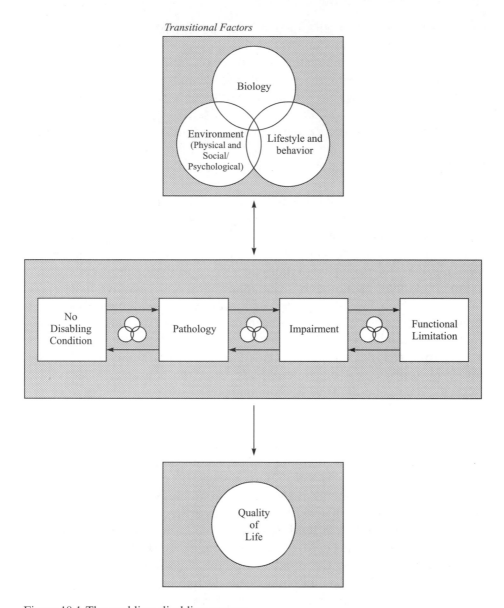

Figure 18.1 The enabling–disabling process.

limitations (e.g., ability to think, reason and problem solve). Functional limitations define function at the level of the individual independent of the physical and social environment and are most appropriately assessed using performance tests that measure the capacity of an individual to perform specific tasks within a controlled environment (e.g., self-selected walking speed, hand function tests, intelligence tests). As such, functional limitations are still expressions of limitations from the clinician's perspective and may bear little resemblance to what an individual can and does do in everyday life. Disability, on the other hand, is defined as difficulty performing activities or roles expected of an individual within the context of his or her environment, including self-care and independent living, major role activity, recreation, and social interaction. By definition, disability is a relational concept as it is a function of the interaction of the person (and his or her capacity to perform certain tasks) with the physical, social, and economic environment. Disability is typically measured from the consumer's perspective, using standardized questionnaires.

In revisiting Nagi's framework, the IOM added quality of life as a fifth element to reflect the relationship of impairment, functional limitations and disability to the individual's overall level of well-being and satisfaction with life. As the broadest definition of quality of life encompasses aspects of well-being that are not directly related to health, such as standard of living, quality of housing, and job satisfaction, the term health-related quality of life (HRQOL) is often used to focus attention on those aspects more directly related to health (Ware, 1995a). Measures of HRQOL (also referred to as general health status measures) traditionally extend beyond those of disability to encompass the consumer's perspective of his or her everyday function across multiple domains including physical and cognitive functioning, social roles, emotional well-being, energy and vitality, social interactions, and self-perceived health status. They also differ from measures of disability in that they often incorporate a qualitative judgment regarding the relative importance to the individual (or society) of various aspects of function and disability. By definition, HRQOL measures assess outcomes strictly from the consumer's perspective, through the use of standardized questionnaires.

It should be noted that other frameworks exist for defining and studying outcomes following illness and injury. Most notable is the International Classification of Impairments, Disability and Handicaps (ICIDH) (WHO, 1980) and its pending revision (ICIDH-2), which is currently being beta tested (WHO, 1997). The Nagi/IOM and ICIDH frameworks do not differ as much in their conceptual underpinnings as they do in terminology and emphasis. Much confusion about these alternative frameworks has arisen, however, because both the original ICIDH and Nagi/IOM models use the term disability but do so to describe different concepts (IOM, 1991). The original ICIDH also included the term handicap to describe the disadvantage for a person (resulting from an impairment or disability) that limits or prevents the fulfillment of a socially defined role. The term, handicap, has fallen into disuse in the United States, however, due in part to its negative connotation. The proposed revision of the ICIDH discards the use of both handicap and disability and replaces them with the more neutral concepts of activity and participation. This revision may well change the fundamental way in which we talk about and classify outcomes. Its further development should be monitored and its usefulness to the study of injury outcomes evaluated.

The remainder of this chapter will focus on a selected review of consumer reported measures of disability and HRQOL (as defined in the Nagi/IOM framework) that are relevant to the study of injury outcomes. The emphasis on these measures as opposed to those of impairment or functional limitations reflects the growing recognition that the consumer's perspective of his or her health and well-being is central to the development and evaluation of cost-effective programs and policy (Relman, 1988; Gold et al., 1996). In focusing our discussion on consumer-oriented measures of outcome, however, we in are in not advocating their use as a substitute for clinical measures of impairment and functional limitations. Rather, they should be used as complementary measures that tap into broader aspects of outcomes most relevant to the individual and to society as a whole. Indeed, only by examining the relationships between impairments, functional limitations, disability, and HRQOL (and the factors that influence these relationships) will we be able to identify appropriate opportunities for intervention.

Disability and Health-related Quality of Life Measures: A Review

Table 18.1 lists selected measures of disability and HRQOL that have been used in injury outcomes research; Table 18.2 summarizes the domains of functioning they cover. Examples are described below to give the reader a general understanding of the different types of available measures.

Instrumental Activities of Daily Living

Early measures of functional status and disability focused on documenting limitations in activities of daily living (or ADL) (Moskowitz, 1957; Katz et al., 1963; Mahoney and Barthel, 1965). These measures were initially developed for assessing function among the elderly and chronically ill and summarize the individual's degree of independence in self-care activities. Stimulated in part by the movement towards community based living for the elderly, these early ADL scales were later extended to include a broader set of activities (e.g., getting around the neighborhood, shopping, cooking, and managing money) that better reflect the more applied activities that community-based living necessitates (McDowell and Newell, 1996). These extended ADL measures are typically referred to as instrumental activities of daily living, or IADL measures.

The Functional Independence Measure (FIM)

One example of an IADL disability measure widely used today in assessing function among severely injured patients is the FIM. The FIM was developed by Granger and Hamilton (1993) for the purpose of monitoring patient progress and outcomes of inpatient rehabilitation; it is now the principal measure of outcome included in the Uniform Data System for Medical Rehabilitation (UDS) (Hamilton et al., 1987). The FIM consists of 18 items summarizing level of independence in six areas: self-care, sphincter control, transfer mobility, ambulation, communication, and social cognition. Although FIM scores are typically based on direct observation and evaluation by a nurse or therapist, a structured questionnaire has been developed that can be used to derive FIM scores based on self-reports. The questionnaire can be administered in person as well as over the phone. FIM scores based on direct observation versus patient interview may be quite different, however. The results of any study using the FIM must be interpreted in light

Table 18.1 Examples of disability and HRQOL measures for use in injury research

Measure	Abbreviation	Selected reference(s)	Number of Items/Questions	Scoring options[a]	Time to Administer (minutes)
Functional Independence Measure	FIM	Granger et al. (1993) Linacre et al. (1994)	18[b]	SS, SI	20–25
Sickness Impact Profile	SIP	Bergner et al. (1981) De Bruin et al. (1992)	136	P, SS, SI	20–25
Musculoskeletal Function Assessment Questionnaire[c]	MFA	Martin et al. (1996) Martin et al. (1997)	101	P, SI	15–20
Burn Specific Health Scale	BSFS	Munster et al. (1987) Munster et al. (1996)	80	P, SI	15–20
Medical Outcomes 36-Item Short Form Health Survey[d]	SF-36	Ware and Sherbourne (1992) McHorney et al. (1993)	36	P, SS	5–10
Child Health Questionnaire[e]	CHQ	Landgraf and Abetz (1996)	50	P, SS	10–15
Quality of Well Being Scale	QWB	Kaplan and Bush (1982)	107	SI	15–20
European Quality of Life Scale	EuroQol	EuroQol Group (1990) Brazier et al. (1993) Elvik (1995)	15	SI	5–10
Health Utilities Index Mark III	HUI:3	Feeney et al. (1995)	45[f]	SI	5–10
Functional Capacity Index	FCI	MacKenzie et al. (1996)	64[f]	P, SI	10–15

[a] P = profile; SS = summary scores; SI = single index.

[b] The FIM questionnaire consists of a structured series of probes designed to assist the interviewer in assessing respondent's level of independence in each of 18 activities.

[c] A short form of the MFA has been developed that consists of 46 items and takes 10–15 minutes to complete.

[d] A short form of the SF-36 has been developed that consists of 12 items and takes less than 5 minutes to complete.

[e] A short form of the CHQ has been developed that consists of 28 items and takes 5–10 minutes to complete.

[f] Includes screening questions used to identify persons with no limitations.

Table 18.2 Domains covered by selected disability and HRQOL measures

DOMAINS	SIP	MFA	BSHS	SF-36	CHQ-50	QWB	EuroQol	HUI:3	FCI	FIM
Physical activity	✓	✓	✓	✓	✓	✓			✓	✓
Ambulation/mobility	✓	✓	✓	✓	✓	✓	✓	✓	✓	✓
Hand/fine motor function	✓	✓	✓						✓	✓
Self-care	✓	✓	✓	✓	✓		✓	✓	✓	✓
Sensory function	✓					✓[a]		✓	✓	
Communication/speech	✓					✓[a]		✓	✓	✓
Cognitive function	✓	✓				✓[a]		✓	✓	✓
Role function	✓	✓	✓	✓	✓	✓	✓[b]			
Social function	✓	✓	✓	✓	✓	✓				✓
Family functioning			✓		✓					
Emotional well-being/distress	✓	✓	✓	✓	✓	✓[a]	✓	✓		
General behavior	✓	✓	✓		✓					
Self-esteem		✓				✓[a]				
Sleep/rest	✓	✓				✓[a]				
Energy/fatigue		✓	✓	✓	✓					
Leisure/recreational activities	✓	✓	✓							
Sexual function	✓	✓	✓			✓[a]			✓	
Symptoms/health problems										
General health perceptions	✓		✓	✓	✓	✓[a]	✓			
Bodily pain	✓		✓	✓	✓		✓	✓		

[a] These domains are covered by one to two items included as part of the QWB symptom checklist.
[b] Role function in the EuroQol is broadly defined to include both major role and other usual activities (work, study, housework, family or leisure activities).

of the approach used to obtain the scores, and caution should be exercised in combining the two approaches within the context of a single study.

Both an overall score as well as two subscores reflecting physical and cognitive functioning, respectively, can be derived (Granger et al., 1993; Heinemann et al., 1993; Linacre et al., 1994). The FIM was carefully designed with appropriate attention paid to issues of reliability and validity (Davidoff et al., 1990; Hamilton et al., 1991; Dodds et al., 1993; Stineman et al., 1996). It has now been applied in measuring outcomes following spinal cord injury, brain injury, and severe orthopedic trauma (e.g., see DiScala et al., 1992; Hetherington et al., 1995; Brenneman et al., 1997; Heinemann et al., 1997; Corrigan et al., 1998). A pediatric version of the FIM, the Wee FIM, has been developed for application to children (McCabe et al., 1990). Also, in response to criticism that the FIM is not sensitive to deficits specific to brain injury, the Functional Assessment Measure (FAM) was developed as an adjunct to the FIM and includes 12 items related to motor, cognitive, and psychological aspects of everyday functioning (Hall et al., 1993, 1994).

While the FIM is widely advocated as a measure of injury outcome, it is important to emphasize that like other ADL and IADL measures, it is not sensitive to variations in outcome at the higher end of functioning that would be more typical of many orthopedic injuries and mild to moderate brain injuries. In addition, the FIM does not incorporate broader issues of disability and quality of life such as role activity, psychological well-being, and general health perceptions. As a brief measure of physical disability, however, it remains a useful measure of rehabilitation outcomes, and should be considered for inclusion in studies of severe brain injuries, spinal cord injury, and multiple trauma.

Health-related Quality of Life

As described above, HRQOL scales go beyond measures of ADL and IADL and tap into several domains of function including not only physical and cognitive function, but role functioning, social functioning, mental health, vitality, and general health perceptions. Several measures have been proposed in the literature (McDowell and Newell, 1996). They vary widely in purpose, content, output, and mode of administration. Most are generic, developed to cut across different populations and clinical conditions, whereas others have been developed for application to specific diseases or treatments. Although some controversy still exists regarding the relative benefits of generic versus condition specific measures, most agree that the use of generic measures is important as they facilitate comparisons across different conditions and injuries, populations, investigations, and interventions (Ware, 1995a). Generic measures are particularly useful when measuring outcome from multiple trauma as multiple body systems are involved with consequences that affect multiple aspects of function. Disease-specific measures, however, are often more sensitive to small but clinically relevant differences in outcome that may be important in judging the relative effectiveness of specific treatments. They are also useful in identifying important concerns of patients that may be peculiar to specific conditions but may not be adequately reflected in a generic measure (Patrick and Deyo, 1989). Although the choice of measures will depend on the purpose of the investigation as well as practical constraints of the application, the use of a generic measure supplemented with a disease-specific instrument is often advocated to derive the benefits of each (Patrick and Deyo, 1989; Guyatt et al., 1996).

HRQOL measures are generally characterized as either (1) psychometric measures or health status profiles, or (2) preference-based or utility measures (Ware, 1995a). Psychometric measures describe the health status of a person across a comprehensive set of domains, yielding separate scores for each domain and one or more summary scores that provide measures of physical versus psychosocial health. A preference-based measure, on the other hand, provides a single summary score typically ranging from zero (representing death) to 1 (optimal health). These scores reflect the preferences of patients or consumers for different health profiles and are derived using decision theory and economic principles (Bennett and Torrance, 1996). Unlike health profiles, preference principles-based measures combine death and quality of life into a single metric and can be used together with survival data in calculating quality adjusted life years (QALYs). As discussed in Graham and Segui-Gomez (this volume), QALYs provide the foundation for cost-utility analyses that are particularly useful when evaluating tradeoffs in costs and effectiveness in terms readily interpretable by policy makers. They are less useful, however, for understanding specific dimensions of injury outcomes and are often of limited value in assessing the impact of particular treatments over time. Examples of both psychometric and preference-based measures are provided in the next sections and summarized in Table 18.1.

The Sickness Impact Profile (SIP)

The SIP (Bergner et al., 1981) was developed as a performance-based measure of the impact of illness and consists of 136 statements about limitations in 12 categories: sleep and rest, emotional behavior, body care and movement, eating, home management, mobility, social interaction, ambulation, alertness behavior, communication, recreation, and work. Respondents endorse statements that describe them on a given day and that are related to their health. Scores are computed for the overall instrument, for each of the 12 categories listed above and for two major dimensions of health (physical and psychosocial). Scores are calculated using a set of standard weights that reflect the relative severity of each limitation in the context of everyday living. The SIP has been tested extensively for its reliability and validity and is often used as a gold standard against which other instruments are compared (DeBruin et al., 1992). It is one of the most comprehensive measures of health status, tapping into most dimensions of health with considerable depth. It is also sensitive to a broad range of levels of dysfunction. It takes 20–25 minutes to administer, however, making it impractical for many applications. Shorter versions of the SIP have been proposed for specific applications, but have not been widely validated (Sullivan et al., 1993; Gerety et al., 1994; Post et al., 1996). The SIP can be self-administered or administered by an interviewer. It has been translated into several languages which has facilitated its use

Table 18.3 Mean SIP scores: pre-injury vs. 6 months vs. 12 months post-injury for 329 lower extremity fracture patients

	Mean SIP scores		
	Pre-injury	6 Months	12 Months
Overall	2.5	9.5[a]	6.8[a,b]
Physical Health	1.3	8.2[a]	5.5[a,b]
Ambulation	1.1	16.1[a]	9.9[a,b]
Mobility	2.4	6.0[a]	3.5[a,b]
Body care and movement	0.9	5.7[a]	4.3[a,b]
Psychosocial health	2.5	6.8[a]	5.5[a,b]
Social interaction	3.0	8.2[a]	5.9[a,b]
Alertness behavior	3.0	6.0[a]	5.2[a]
Emotional behavior	2.1	9.6[a]	8.9[a]
Communication	1.4	1.9	1.8
Independent categories			
Sleep and rest	5.1	12.8[a]	10.0[a,b]
Eating	1.2	1.2	1.3
Work	8.8	32.3[a]	21.0[a,b]
Home management	2.6	14.5[a]	99.3[a,b]
Recreation	4.2	17.6[a]	13.0[a,b]

[a] $p < 0.05$, compared with preinjury baseline.
[b] $p < 0.05$, compared with 6-month score.
Adapted from Jurkovich et al. (1995).

world-wide. An adaptation of the SIP for use in the United Kingdom was developed and renamed the Functional Limitations Profile (FLP) (Patrick et al., 1985).

The SIP has been used in several studies describing the outcomes of spinal cord injury, head injury, burns and orthopedic trauma (e.g., Patterson et al., 1987; Siosteen et al., 1990; Dikmen et al., 1995; Gruen et al., 1995; Beaton et al., 1997; Corrigan, 1998; Faergemann et al., 1998; Fleming et al., 1998; Richmond et al., 1998). Jurkovich et al. (1995), for instance, used the SIP to examine outcomes following blunt, lower extremity trauma and found it to discriminate among patients with multiple versus single fractures, severe versus moderately severe fractures, and high energy versus low energy fracture patterns. Higher SIP scores were also associated with the presence versus absence of a mild head injury in addition to the leg injury (patients with moderate–severe head injuries were excluded from the study). SIP scores decreased significantly between 6 and 12 months postinjury, although 12-month scores were still significantly higher than typically found in a general population of similar age and gender (Table 18.3). The authors found the SIP to be useful in documenting the multiple effects of extremity trauma across a wide range of daily activities including ambulation, sleep, psychosocial health, home management, work, and recreation.

Temkin and colleagues (1988, 1989) proposed modifications to the SIP in an attempt to make it more sensitive to outcomes specific to head injury. Modifications consisted of adding items, deleting nonapplicable items, and reweighting areas of function. Interestingly, they found little improvement in discrimination or responsiveness and concluded that the SIP in its original form could be used as a valid measure of outcome following head trauma.

The Medical Outcomes 36-Item Short Form Health Survey (SF-36)

The SF-36 was designed as a generic indicator of health status for use in large population-based studies. Derived from a set of more detailed measures developed for use in Rand's Health Insurance Experiment (Lohr et al., 1986) and the Medical Outcomes Study (Stewart et al., 1989), the SF-36 consists of 35 items that are scaled to measure eight health concepts: physical functioning, role limitations due to physical health problems, bodily pain, general health perceptions, vitality, social functioning, role limitations due to emotional problems, and general mental health (Ware et al., 1992; McHorney et al., 1993). An additional question asks respondents to describe changes in health status during a 1-year period but is not used to score any of the eight scales. When using the SF-36 to examine outcomes postinjury some modification to questions asking about change in status or abilities is recommended to ascertain changes from before the injury (as opposed to over the last year or past 4 weeks). Two summary scores can be derived that measure physical and mental health, respectively (Ware et al., 1995b). The SF-36 can be self-administered or administered by an interviewer and takes only 5–10 minutes to complete. Because the SF-36 is relatively short in length, it can be readily incorporated as part of a telephone interview. In 1996, the developers published a 12-item version of the SF-36 (Ware et al., 1996). Although validation studies have shown a high correlation of the SF-12 with the SF-36, each subscore of the SF-12 is measured with less precision. The SF-12 is largely advocated for use in population monitoring of health status.

A British-English version of the SF-36 has been developed (Brazier et al., 1992) and the instrument has also been adapted for use in several other languages (Ware et al., 1998). Norms for the general U.S. and British populations (by specific age and gender groups) are available as are norms for persons with varying medical conditions (Ware et al., 1993). The SF-36 was developed with exquisite attention paid to issues of reliability and validity. As will be true with any abbreviated measure, however, the SF-36 is somewhat more limited in scope when compared with some of the more detailed instruments. Of particular concern with regards to the application of the SF-36 in trauma outcomes research is the lack of items specifically relating to cognitive function. The SF-36 does not appear to discriminate well among major trauma patients with and without head injury. However, by supplementing the SF-36 with three or four items asking about limitations in attention, problem solving, and memory, one can derive a subscore specific to cognitive function, that when used in combination with the standard eight subscores of the SF-36, provides a health profile more relevant to head injury.

The use of the SF-36 in outcomes research is now widespread across a variety of conditions and populations (Shiely et al., 1996). However, fewer published examples of its application to injury are available (e.g., Kopjar, 1996; Beaton et al., 1997; Martin et al., 1997; Corrigan et al., 1998). A study by McCarthy and colleagues on

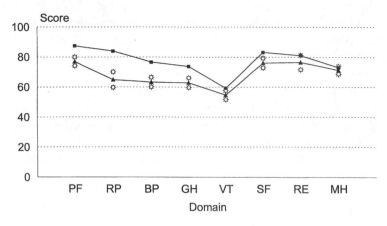

Figure 18.2 SF-36 health profile following orthopedic trauma women, ages 18–45.

pelvic fractures among young women illustrates how the SF-36 can be used in examining outcomes postinjury and also points to limitations of generic measures when focusing on specific types of injury (McCarthy et al., 1995; Copeland et al., 1997). A group of 123 women with pelvic ring fractures were retrospectively identified and compared with a similar group of 110 women who sustained a lower extremity fracture (matched on age, year of injury, and injury severity). Compared with age and gender appropriate population norms, both groups of women scored significantly worse (lower scores) on all dimensions of the SF-36 except mental health (Figure 18.2). There was no significant difference between the fracture groups, however, suggesting that outcomes from major pelvic fractures were no worse than those associated with lower extremity fractures. Of particular interest in examining outcomes from pelvic fracture, however, is the impact on genitourinary and sexual function. As the SF-36 does not include items related to either of these problem areas, the SF-36 was supplemented with questions related to urinary and bowel complaints as well as sexual function. Results showed that after adjusting for demographics and co-morbidities, women with moderate to severe pelvic fracture were significantly more likely than women with mild pelvic fractures or extremity fractures to have urinary problems and gynecologic pain during sexual activity. This result would not have been evident if the SF-36 alone were used as a measure of outcome.

The Child Health Questionnaire (CHQ)

Until recently, there were few generic HRQOL measures applicable to measuring outcomes from trauma in children. Examples include: the Rand Health Insurance Experiment Child Health Scale (Eisen et al., 1979); the Functional Status II-R (Stein and Jessop, 1990); the Child Health and Illness Profile (Starfield et al., 1995); and the Child Disability Scale (Gofin and Adler, 1997). Landgraf and Abetz (1996) review these and other measures and point to their inadequacies, especially in assessing outcomes of young children. Their Child Health Questionnaire (CHQ) was subsequently introduced to address some of these inadequacies (Landgraf et al., 1996). It was originally constructed to measure the well-being of children and adolescents 5 years and older; a version of the CHQ applicable to toddlers is currently under development. The CHQ assesses health across 14 domains: physical functioning, role/social function – physical problems, role/social function – emotional problems, role /social function – behavioral problems, bodily pain, general behavior, mental health, self-esteem, general health perceptions, change in health, parental impact-time, parental impact-emotional, family limitation in activities, and family cohesion. Twelve of these 14 domains (excluding family limitations and family cohesion) can be combined into two summary measures of physical and psychosocial health status.

Although relatively new, the CHQ was developed using sound principles of measurement science and holds great promise as an effective tool for assessing outcome from childhood injury. It is one of the more comprehensive generic health status measures available, tapping into several domains of functioning with considerable depth. For this reason it is likely to be sensitive to differences in outcomes across a broad range of types and severities of injury. Four different versions of the instrument exist consisting of 28, 50, 87, and 98 items, respectively; all versions tap into the same 14 domains but with varying depth. The CHQ can be self-administered or interviewer administered and both parent and child versions exist for children ages 10 and older. Normative data are available for both the 50- and 28-item versions. One potential deficiency of the CHQ for application in studies of outcome from injury is the lack of attention paid to the assessment of cognitive function; only one CHQ question taps into this important domain. As discussed above in relation to the SF-36, however, this deficiency could be addressed by supplementing the CHQ with a short battery of questions specifically designed to measure the important aspects of cognitive functioning in children.

The Quality of Well-Being (QWB)

The QWB is a preference-based measure of health that combines patient-reported symptoms and disability into a single index that provides an expression of well-being that ranges from 0 for death to 1 for asymptomatic full functioning (Kaplan and Bush, 1982). QWB scores are derived from a structured interview consisting of two parts. The first part assesses the level of performance across three domains of function: mobility, physical activity, and social activity. The second part of the interview asks about the presence of 27 different symptoms or problem complexes. Respondents are asked about their symptoms and level of function over the past 6 days; final scores are produced by weighting the responses averaged across the 6 days. Weights were empirically derived and reflect societal judgments about the relative importance of symptoms and levels of function and their impact on overall quality of well-being. The QWB interview takes 15–20 minutes to administer and in its current form is not well suited to self-administration (Anderson et al., 1988). A self-administered version of the QWB is currently under development, however, which should enhance the applicability of the QWB in outcomes research and evaluation. Limited norms for the general population exist for the QWB (Erickson et al., 1989).

Table 18.4 Mean QWB scores (and SD) for major trauma patients[a] at discharge and follow-up

	N	Mean QWB (SD)
Hospital discharge	1048	0.40 (0.04)
6 months post injury	826	0.63 (0.12)
12 months post injury	805	0.67 (0.14)
18 months post injury	712	0.68 (0.13)

[a] Adult admissions excluding patients with Glasgow Coma Scale (GCS) less than 12. Source: Holbrook et al. (1999).

A distinguishing feature of the QWB is its inclusion of symptoms, even if those symptoms do not impact on function. As such, the QWB is particularly sensitive to minor deviations from complete asymptomatic well-being. An additional concern regarding the QWB as a global health related quality of life measure is its emphasis on physical health. While one of the symptom and problem complexes relates to "spells of feeling upset, being depressed, or of crying" the QWB is generally viewed as under-representing the domain of mental health (McDowell and Newell, 1996). Also of some concern is the extent to which the QWB addresses cognitive functioning. As with mental health, cognitive function is reflected by only one symptom complex: "trouble learning, remembering or thinking clearly." This particular symptom, however, is assigned a relatively high weight and may be sensitive to the impact of significant head trauma; to our knowledge the QWB has not been widely tested for its applicability to head injury.

Holbrook and colleagues (1998, 1999) used the QWB to examine outcomes following multiple trauma not involving significant head injury (i.e., Glasgow Coma Scale (GCS) score on admission less than 12) (Table 18.4). While significant improvements (increase in scores) were noted in mean QWB scores between hospital discharge and 6 months follow-up, scores at 6 months were low and remained low at both 12 and 18 months. At 18 months, only 20% of the study cohort were assigned QWB scores typical of a general population. These low scores did not translate into major disability as reflected by limitations in IADL. Exactly what the scores do represent in terms of outcome, however, is not entirely clear as no domain specific subscores are reported for the QWB. Thus, compared to the detailed information provided by the SIP (Table 18.2) or the SF-36 (Figure 18.2) the QWB provides little information that would be helpful in identifying opportunities for intervention.

While not as widespread in its use as the SIP or SF-36, the QWB represents a potentially powerful outcome measure especially for examining the impact of an intervention in terms of QALYs. Because the QWB is a preference-based measure that incorporates the consequences of both fatal and nonfatal injuries into one metric, it can be used in cost–utility analyses (Chapter 19). It does, however, take 15–20 minutes to administer making it impractical for large-scale studies. Other preference-based measures such as the European Quality of Life Scale (EuroQol Group, 1990; Brazier et al., 1993; Elvik, 1995), the Health Utilities Index Mark III

(Feeny et al., 1995) and the Functional Capacity Index (MacKenzie et al., 1996) may be more practical, although none has been widely validated. It should be noted that the FCI was developed specifically for measuring outcomes postinjury; its scope, however, is limited to physical and cognitive functioning. Recent work has also suggested that a preference-based metric can be derived from the SF-36 health profile (Brazier et al., 1998). This work is particularly exciting and its development should be closely monitored.

Challenges and Future Directions

As increasing attention is focused on the prevention and treatment of nonfatal injuries and their consequences, the broader use of disability and HRQOL measures becomes imperative. Significant advances have been made over the past two decades in defining the components of a valid and reliable measure and in using these measures for monitoring health outcomes, evaluating specific treatments and health care policy, and, more directly in clinical practice (Ellwood, 1988; Epstein, 1990). Their application presents many challenges, however, some of which are inherent to the field of outcomes research, while others are specific to the study of injury.

Critical to the study of outcome following multiple trauma is the use of a measure that is sensitive to decrements in function across multiple body systems. Instruments like the SIP appear to meet the criteria of a measure that taps into multiple domains with considerable depth. However, the SIP takes 20–25 minutes to administer and is therefore impractical for many applications. The SF-36, used in conjunction with a small number of items that measure cognitive function, holds promise as a brief measure of HRQOL relevant to the multiple trauma patient. An underlying challenge of outcomes research, in general, is the need for measures that are both practical and sensitive enough to identify important differences in outcomes.

Measuring outcomes from head injury poses significant challenges. In addition to choosing a measure sensitive to decrements in cognitive function, one is faced with difficult decisions regarding the use and interpretation of proxy respondents. Only a handful of studies have examined the relationship of proxy respondents to self-reports and these have typically focused on ADL and IADL limitations among the elderly (e.g., DeBruin, 1992; Rodgers and Miller, 1997). The work that has been done suggests that proxy reports tend to identify more limitations than perceived by the individual him or herself. Whether these differences represent over reporting on the part of the proxy or under reporting by the individual him or herself is not clear. More work is needed to investigate the appropriate role of proxy respondents in trauma outcomes research, especially when impaired cognition is a factor.

In trauma, there are typically no before measures which one can use to assess recovery in relation to pre-injury status. Recollections of activity limitation before the injury are often used as baseline measures. When assessed as soon after the injury as possible this approach may be reasonable, especially for measuring changes in physical function and role function; its validity when measuring psychosocial and cognitive function is less certain. The use of proxy assessments of pre-injury status has been advocated by some, although their use is highly debatable given our lack of understanding of the relationship of proxy to self-reports. For children, school records and assessments of pre-injury function by teachers are often used; this approach can be expensive, however, and not practical for large surveys and population-based studies. Given the lack of pre-injury measures and the uncertain validity of the approaches mentioned above, the use of appropriately defined comparison groups is often particularly important to the study of trauma outcomes and their relationship to treatment. In addition, the use of disability and HRQOL measures for which age and gender specific population norms exist is encouraged. Population norms provide some benchmark against which to compare postinjury outcomes.

Even with well developed measures of outcome that have been extensively evaluated for their reliability, validity and responsiveness, determining the impact of different interventions is difficult. This is true because some of the largest observed differentials in disability and HRQOL outcomes are related to a host of personal, social, and environmental factors that interact to influence access to postacute care services and the overall course of recovery (Yelin et al., 1980; Wilson and Cleary, 1995). While several studies have documented the important role that severity of illness, age, and co-morbidities play in determining outcome, few have looked beyond this narrow set of predictors in developing appropriate models for explaining variations in HRQOL. The few studies that have used a broader framework have documented that several characteristics of the individual and their environment are important in determining the trajectory of recovery, including: level of education, amount and source of income, the availability of social support, motivation, and health habits, including drinking behavior (e.g., Rimel et al., 1981; DeVivo et al., 1987; MacKenzie et al., 1987; Dikmen et al., 1995; Holbrook et al., 1999). When examining vocational outcomes, the physical demands of the pre-injury job and the work setting, together with type and amount of disability compensation, also influence the extent and rate of return to work (MacKenzie et al., 1998). For the purpose of identifying effective interventions that mediate the impact of injury on quality of life, it will be important to understand how these multiple factors interact to influence the transitions among the different levels or complexities of function that were described earlier in this chapter, that is impairments, functional limitations, and disability. Only by doing so will we better understand how and when to intervene.

References

Anderson JP, Bush JW, Berry CC (1988) Internal consistency analysis: a method for studying the accuracy of function assessment for health outcome and quality of life evaluation. J Clin Epidemiol 41:127–37.

Beaton DE, Bombardier C, Hogg-Johnson S (1997) Choose your tool: a comparison of the psychometric properties of five generic health status instruments in workers with soft tissue injuries. Qual Life Res 3:50–6.

Bennett KJ, Torrance GW (1996) Measuring health state preferences and utilities: rating scale, time trade-off, and standard gamble techniques. In: Spilker B (ed), Quality of Life and Pharmacoeconomics in Clinical Trials. Philadelphia, PA: Lippincott-Raven Publishers.

Bergner M, Bobbitt RA, Carter WB et al. (1981) The SIP: Development and final revision of a health status measure. Med Care 19:787.

Brazier J, Harper R, Jones NMB et al. (1992) Validating the SF-36 Health Survey questionnaire: new outcome measure for primary care. Br Med J 305:160–4.

Brazier J, Jones N, Kind P (1993) Testing the validity of the Euroqol and comparing it with the SF-36 Health Survey questionnaire. Qual Life Res 2:169–80.

Brazier J, Usherwood T, Harper R, Thomas K (1998) Deriving a preference-based single index from the UK SF-36 Health Survey. J Clin Epidemiol 51:1115–28.

Brenneman FD, Katyal D, Boulanger BR et al. (1997) Long-term outcomes in open pelvic fractures. J Trauma 42:773–7.

Copeland CE, Bosse MJ, McCarthy ML et al. (1997) Effect of trauma and pelvic fracture on female genitourinary, sexual, and reproductive function. J Orthoped Trauma 11:73–81.

Corrigan JD, Smith-Knapp K, Granger CV (1997) Validity of the functional independence measure for persons with traumatic brain injury. Arch Phys Med Rehabil 78:828–34.

(1998) Outcomes in the first 5 years after traumatic brain injury. Arch Phys Med Rehabil 79:298–305.

Davidoff GN, Roth EJ, Haughton JS et al. (1990) Cognitive dysfunction in spinal cord injury patients: sensitivity of the Functional Independence Measure subscales vs neuropsycholic assessment. Arch Phys Med Rehabil 71:326–9.

DeBruin AF, De Witte LP, Stevens F et al. (1992) Sickness Impact Profile: the state of the art of a generic functional status measure. Soc Sci Med 35:1003–14.

DeVivo MJ, Rutt RD, Stover SL, Fine PR (1987) Employment after spinal cord injury. Arch Phys Med Rehabil 68: 494–8.

Dikmen SS, Ross BL, Machamer JE, Temkin NR (1995) One year psychosocial outcome in head injury. J Int Neuropsychol Soc 1:67–77.

DiScala C, Grant CC, Brooke MM et al. (1992) Functional outcome in children with traumatic brain injury: agreement between clinical judgement and the Functional Independence Measure. Am J Phys Med Rehabil 71:145–8.

Dodds TA, Martin DP, Stolov WC et al. (1993) A validation of the Functional Independence Measurement and its performance among rehabilitation inpatients. Arch Phys Med Rehabil 74:531–6.

Eisen M, Ware JE, Donald C (1979) Measuring components of children's health status. Med Care 17:901–21.

Ellwood P (1988) Outcomes management: A technology of patient experience. N Engl J Med 318:1549–56.

Elvik R (1995) The validity of using health state indexes in measuring the consequences of traffic injury for public health. Soc Sci Med. 40: 1385–98.

Epstein AM (1990) Sounding Board: The outcome movement; Will it get us where we want to go? N Engl J Med 3223:266–70.

Erickson P, Kendall EA, Anderson JP et al. (1989) Using composite health status measures to assess the nation's health. Med Care 27:S66–76.

EuroQol Group (1990) EuroQol: a new facility for the measurement of health-related quality of life. Health Policy 16:199–208.

Faergemann C, Frandsen PA, Rock ND (1998) Residual impairment after lower extremity fracture. J Trauma 45:123–6.

Feeny D, Furlong W, Boyle M, Torrance GW (1995) Multi-attribute health status classification systems: the Health Utilities Index. PharmacoEconomics 7:490–502.

Fingerhut LA, Warner M (1997) Injury Chartbook. Health, United States, 1996–1997. Hyattsville, MD: National Center for Health Statistics.

Fleming JM, Strong J, Ashton R (1998) Cluster analysis of self-awareness levels in adults with traumatic brain injury and relationship to outcome. J Head Trauma Rehab 13:39–51.

Gerety MB, Cornell JE, Mulrow CD et al. (1994) The Sickness Impact Profile for Nursing Homes (SIP-NH). J Gerontol 49:M2–8.

Gofin R, Adler B (1997) A seven item scale for the assessment of disabilities after child and adolescent injuries. Injury Prev 3:120–3.

Gold MR, Siegel JE, Russell LB, Weinstein MC (1996) Cost-Effectiveness in Health and Medicine. Oxford: Oxford University Press.

Granger CV, Hamilton, BB, Linacre JM et al. (1993) Performance profiles of the Functional Independence Measure. Am J Phys Med Rehabil 72:84–9.

Gruen GS, Leit ME, Gruen RJ et al. (1995) Functional outcome of patients with unstable pelvic ring fractures stabilized with open reduction and internal fixation. J Trauma 39:838–44.

Guyatt GH, Jaeschke R, Feeny DH, Patrick DL (1996) Measurements in clinical trials: choosing the right approach. In: Spilker B (ed), Quality of Life and Pharmacoeconomics in Clinical Trials. Philadelphia, PA: Lippincott-Raven Publishers.

Hall KM, Johnston W (1994) Outcomes evaluation in TBI rehabilitation. Part II: Measuring tools for a National Data System. Arch Phys Med Rehabil 75: SC75–18.

Hall KM, Hamilton BB, Gordan WA, Zasler ND (1993) Characteristics and comparisons of functional assessment indices: Disability Rating Scale, Functional Independence Measure, and Functional Assessment Measure. J Head Trauma. 8:60–74.

Hamilton BB, Granger CV, Sherwin FS et al. (1987) A uniform national data system for medical rehabilitation. In: Fuhrer MJ (ed), Rehabilitation Outcomes: Analysis and Measurement. Baltimore, MD: Paula H. Brookes.

Hamilton BB, Laughlin JA, Granger CV et al. (1991) Interrater agreement of the seven level Functional Independence Measure (FIM). Arch Phys Med Rehabil 72:790.

Heinemann AW, Linacre JM, Wright BD et al. (1993) Relationships between impairment and physical disability as measured by the Functional Independence Measure. Arch Phys Med Rehabil 74:566–73.

Heinemann AW, Kirk P, Hastie BA et al. (1997) Relationships between disability measures and nursing effort during rehabilitation for patients with traumatic brain injury and spinal cord injury. Arch Phys Med Rehabil 78:143–9.

Hetherington H, Earlam RJ, Kirk CJ (1995) The disability status of injured patients measured by the Functional Independence Measure (FIM) and their use of rehabilitation services. Injury 26:97–101.

Holbrook TL, Anderson JP, Sieber WJ et al. (1998) Outcome after major trauma: Discharge and 6 month follow-up results from the Trauma Recovery Project. J Trauma 45:315–24.

(1999) Outcome after major trauma: Twelve and eighteen month follow-up results from the Trauma Recovery Project. J Trauma 46:765–71.

Institute of Medicine (1991) In: Pope AM, Tarlov AR (eds), Disability in America: A National Agenda for Prevention. Washington, DC: National Academy Press.

(1997) In: Brandt EN, Pope AM (eds), Enabling America: Assessing the Role of Rehabilitation Science and Engineering. Washington, DC: National Academy Press.

Jurkovich GJ, Mock C, MacKenzie EJ et al. (1995) The Sickness Impact Profile as a tool to evaluate functional outcome in trauma patients. J Trauma 39:625–31.

Kaplan RM, Bush JW (1982) Health-related quality of life measurement for evaluation research and policy analysis. Health Psychol 1:61–80.

Katz S, Ford AB, Moskowitz RW et al. (1963) Studies of illness in the aged. The Index of ADL: a standardized measure of biological and psychosocial function. JAMA 185:914–19.

Kopjar B (1996) The SF-36 Health Survey: A valid measure of changes in health status after injury. Injury Prev 2:135–9.

Landgraf JM, Abetz LN, Ware JE (1996) The CHQ User's Manual, 1st edn. Boston, MA: The Health Institute, New England Medical Center.

Landgraf JM, Abetz LN (1996) Measuring health outcomes in pediatric populations: Issues in psychometrics and application. In: Spilker B (ed), Quality of Life and Pharmacoeconomics in Clinical Trials. Philadelphia, PA: Lippincott-Raven Publishers.

Linacre JM, Heinemann AW, Wright BD et al. (1994) The structure and stability of the Functional Independence Measure. Arch Phys Med Rehabil 75:127–32.

Lohr KN, Brook RH, Kamberg CJ et al. (1986) Use of Medical care in the Rand Health Insurance Experiment: diagnosis and service specific analyses in a randomized controlled trial. Med Care 24 (Suppl):S1–87.

MacKenzie EJ, Shapiro S, Smith RT et al. (1987) Factors influencing return to work following hospitalization for traumatic injury. Am J Public Health 77:329–34.

MacKenzie EJ, Dainiano AM, Miller T, Luchter S (1996) The development of the Functional Capacity Index. J Trauma 41:799–807.

Mackenzie EJ, Morris JA, Jurkovich GJ et al. (1998) Return to work following injury: the role of economic, social, and job-related factors. Am J Public Health 88:1630–7.

Mahoney Fl, Barthel DW (1965) Functional evaluation: The Barthel Index. Md State Med J 14:61–5.

Martin DP, Engelberg R, Agel J et al. (1996) Development of a musculoskeletal extremity health status instrument: the Musculoskeletal Function Assessment instrument. J Orthop Res l4:113–81.

Martin DP, Engelberg R, Agel J, Swiontkowski M (1997) Comparison of the Musculoskeletal Function Assessment Questionnaire with the Short Form-36, the Western Ontario, McMaster Universities Osteoarthritis Index, and the Sickness Impact Profile Health Status Measures. J Bone Joint Surg 70A:1323–35.

McCabe MA, Granger CV (1990) Content validity of a pediatric Functional Independence Measure. Appl Nurs Res 3:120–2.

McCarthy ML, MacKenzie EJ, Bosse MJ et al. (1995) Functional status following orthopedic trauma in young women. J Trauma 39:828–37.

McDowell I, Newell C (1996) Measuring Health. New York: Oxford University Press.

McHorney CA, Ware JE Jr, Raczek AE (1993) The MOS 36-item Short Form Health Survey (SF-36): II. Psychometric and clinical tests of validity in measuring physical and mental health constructs. Med Care 31:247–63.

Miller TR, Pindus NM, Douglass JB, Rossman SB (1995) Databook on Nonfatal Injury: Incidence, Costs and Consequences. Washington, DC: Urban Institute Press.

Moskowitz E, McCann CB (1957) Classification of disability in the chronically ill and aging. J Chronic Dis 5:342–6.

Munster AM, Fauerbach JA, Lawrence J (1996) Development and utilization of a psychometric instrument for measuring quality of life in burn patients, 1976 to 1996. Acta Chirurgiae Plasticae 38:128–31.

Munster AM, Horowitz GL, Tudahl LA (1987) The Abbreviated Burn–Specific Health Scale. J Trauma 27:425–8.

Nagi S (1976) An epidemiology of disability among adults in the United States. Milbank Mem Fund Q. 54:439–68.

Patrick DL, Sittampalam Y, Somerville SM et al. (1985) A cross-cultural comparison of health status values. Am J Public Health 75:1402–7.

Patrick DL, Deyo (1989) Generic and disease specific measures in assessing health status and quality of life. Med Care 27:S217–32.

Patterson DR, Questad KA, Boltwood MD et al. (1987) Patient self-reports three months after sustaining a major burn. J Burn Care Rehabil 8:274–9.

Post MW, deBruin A deWitte L, Schrijvers A (1996) The SIP68: a measure of health-related functional status in rehabilitation medicine. Arch Phys Med Rehabil 77:440–5.

Relman AS (1988) Assessment and accountability: The third revolution in health care. N Engl J Med 319:1220–2.

Rice DP, MacKenzie EJ, Associates (1989) The Cost of Injury in the United States. San Francisco, CA: Institute for Health and Aging, University of California and the Injury Prevention Center, Johns Hopkins University.

Rothman ML, Hedrick SC, Bulcroft KA et al. (1991) The validity of proxy-generated scores as measures of patient health status. Med Care 29:115–24.

Read JL, Quinn RJ, Hoefer MA (1987) Measuring overall health: an evaluation of three important approaches. J Chronic Dis 40 (Suppl 1):S7–21.

Richmond TS, Kauder D, Schwab CW (1998) A prospective study of predictors of disability at 3 months after non-central nervous system trauma. J Trauma 44:635–42.

Rimel RW, Giordani B, Barth et al. (1981) Disability caused by minor head injury. Neurosurgery 9:221–8.

Rodgers W, Miller B (1997) A comparative analysis of ADL questions in surveys of older people. J Gerontol 52B:21–36.

Shiely J-C, Bayliss MS, Keller SD, Tsai C, Ware JE (1996) SF-36 Health Survey Annotated Bibliography, 1st edn (1988–95). Boston, MA: The Health Institute, New England Medical Center.

Siosteen A, Lundqvist C, Blomstrand C et al. (1990) The quality of life of three functional spinal cord injury subgroups in a Swedish community. Paraplegia 28:476.

Starfield B, Reiley A, Green B et al. (1995) The adolescent child health and illness profile: a population-based measure of health. Med Care 33:553–66.

Stein REK, Jessop DJ (1990) Functional status II(R): a measure of child health status. Med Care 28:1041–55.

Stewart AL, Greenfield S, Hays RD et al. (1989) Functional status and well-being of patients with chronic conditions. JAMA 262:907–13.

Stineman MG, Shea JA, Jette A et al. (1996) The Functional Independence Measure: Tests of scaling assumptions, structure, and reliability across 20 diverse impairment categories. Arch Phys Med Rehabil 77:1101–8.

Sullivan M, Ahlmen M, Bjelle A et al. (1993) Health status assessment in rheumatoid arthritis. II. Evaluation of a modified Shorter Sickness Impact Profile. J Rheumatol 20:1500–7.

Temkin N, McLean A Jr, Dilunen S et al. (1988) Development and evaluation of modifications to the Sickness Impact Profile for head injury. J Clin Epidemiol 41:47–57.

Temkin NR, Dikmen S, Macrame J et al. (1989) General versus disease-specific measures: further work on the Sickness Impact Profile for head injury. Med Care 27 (Suppl):S44–53.

Ware JE (1995a) The status of health assessment in 1994. Annu Rev Public Health 16:327–54.

Ware JE, Sherbourne CD (1992) The MOS 36-item Short-Form Health Survey (SF-36) I. Conceptual framework and item selection. Med Care 30:473–83.

Ware JE Jr, Snow KK, Kosinki M et al. (1993) SF-36 Health Survey: manual and interpretation guide. Boston, MA: The Health Institute, New England Medical Center.

Ware JE, Kosinski M, Keller SD (1994) SF-36 physical and mental health summary scores: a user's manual. Boston, MA: The Health Institute, New England Medical Center.

(1996) A 12 item Short Form Health Survey: Construction of scales and preliminary tests of relability and validity. Med Care 3:220–33.

Ware JE, Kosinski M, Bayliss MS et al. (1995b) Comparisons of methods for the scoring and statistical analysis of the SF-36 health profile and summary measures: Summary of results from the Medical Outcomes Study. Med Care 33:AS264–79.

Ware JE, Gandek B, Kosinski M et al. (1998) The equivalence of SF-36 summary health scores estimated using standard and country-specific algorithms in 10 countries: results from the International Quality of Life Assessment Project. J Clin Epidemiol 51:1167–70.

Weinstein MC, Stason WB (1977) Foundations of cost-effectiveness analysis for health and medical practices. N Engl J Med 296:716–21.

Wilson IB, Cleary PD (1995) Linking clinical variables with health related quality of life: A conceptual model of patient outcomes. JAMA 273:59–65.

World Health Organization (WHO) (1980) The International Classification of Impairments, Disabilities and Handicaps. A Manual Relating to the Consequences of Disease. Geneva: WHO.

World Health Organization (WHO) (1997) The International Classification of Impairments, Activities and Participation. A Manual of Dimensions of Disablement and Functioning. Beta-1 Draft for Field Trials. Geneva: WHO.

Yelin E, Nevitt M, Epstein W (1980) Towards an epidemiology of work disability. Milbank Mem Fund Q Health Soc 58:386–415.

19

Economic Evaluation of Injury Control

John D. Graham and Maria Segui-Gomez

Purposes of Economic Evaluation

As the problem of injury garners increasing attention in the public and private sectors of the economy, the amount of resources dedicated to the prevention, treatment, and rehabilitation of injuries can be expected to grow. These resources are the scarce labor and capital that could be applied to other productive uses in the economy (e.g., better housing or education) if they were not allocated to the field of injury control. Even if we restrict the allocation issue to the injury control field (e.g., prevention vs. treatment, unintentional vs. intentional injuries, injuries to adults vs. injuries to children, and technological vs. behavioral interventions), resource-allocation decisions regarding which interventions to implement still need to be made. Currently, these types of decisions are often made informally or implicitly, without analytical consideration of what would be in the best interests of society.

Effectiveness is one of the few objective criteria applied in the selection of recommended best practices (US Preventive Task Force, 1996). Efficiency, that is the relationship between the effectiveness of an intervention and the resources needed to implement it, is more rarely used as a selection criterion.

The purpose of economic evaluation is to assist decision makers in allocating resources efficiently by taking into account the costs and effects (or consequences) of an intervention compared with the status quo or the most-likely alternative to the intervention. Efficiency considerations become even more necessary as the number of effective interventions continues to grow, exceeding the resources available to implement all of them. On occasion, nonefficiency considerations, such as fairness or equity, may induce informed departures from efficient resource allocation. Thus, economic evaluation offers information, insight, and guidance; it is not an algorithm that replaces the need for human judgment and ethical considerations in resource allocation (Drummond et al., 1997).

Types of Economic Evaluation

Economic evaluation consists of a set of three techniques (Drummond et al., 1997). The choice among them depends on the type of consequences produced by the interventions being compared (Table 19.1).

Table 19.1 Types of economic evaluation

Type of analysis	Units used to measure cost	Units used to measure consequences	The interventions being compared produce:
Cost minimization	Money (e.g., US dollars)	None	identical consequence(s) (in type and quantity)
Cost effectiveness	Money (e.g., US dollars)	Natural units (e.g., lives saved, life-years gained, number of injuries averted)	same type of consequence(s), but produced in different amount
		Non-natural units[a] (e.g., quality-adjusted life years)	identical or not identical consequences
Cost benefit	Money (e.g., US dollars)	Money (e.g., US dollars)	identical or not identical consequences

Note: [a]historically referred to as cost utility analysis.
Adapted from: Drummond et al., 1997.

When the interventions under comparison lead to identical consequences, both in type and in quantity, only costs deserve attention and cost-minimization techniques are used to evaluate which of the interventions is more economical. When the interventions under evaluation produce different types of outcomes and/or in different amounts, cost-minimization techniques become insufficient and the consequences need to be compared using either natural, non-natural, or monetary units.

When non-monetary outcomes are used to measure effectiveness, the techniques are either cost-effectiveness or cost-utility analysis. The result of the analysis is presented as the ratio between the net resources consumed by the intervention (expressed as costs) and the net effectiveness accrued by the intervention. This ratio indicates how many resources (e.g., dollars) are expended to gain one unit of outcome. The term cost-effectiveness analysis (CEA) has been used, historically, when the outcomes are described in one or several of the available natural units (e.g., lives saved, injuries averted, hospital days prevented, days of work saved, potential years of life saved). This diversity of effectiveness measures limits the use of this technique. It is impossible to compare cost-effectiveness ratios of alternative interventions when different units have been employed in their evaluation. In injury prevention, this becomes particularly limiting if one tries to compare the fatal and nonfatal injury prevention benefits of different interventions. For example, if the effectiveness of safety belts is measured by the number of lives saved while air bag effectiveness is measured by the number of head injuries prevented (both nonfatal and fatal), then it is not feasible to compare the cost-effectiveness of the two restraint systems.

Cost-utility is the name traditionally given to CEA in which the consequences of the intervention are described in non-natural, preference-weighted units, such as utility values. Some experts prefer these "utility-based" measures because they are based on the preferences of citizens who are at risk of injury and who might benefit from (and bear the cost of) the intervention programs. The word "utility" refers to an approach to measuring citizen well-being that was developed by decision theorists, economists, and psychologists and that is the basis for measures such as the quality-adjusted life years (QALYs) or the disability-adjusted life years (DALYs). These measures are increasingly used in decision problems involving clinical and preventive interventions where the subjective preferences of patients are critical to the choice of optimal therapy (Weinstein and Stason, 1977; Torrance, 1986; Gold et al., 1996) or to quantify the burden of disease and injury in a population (Murray and Lopez, 1996). In the field of injury control, the Functional Capacity Index (MacKenzie et al., 1996) is an example of this type of measure (see Mackenzie, this volume).

Despite the conceptual distinction between natural and non-natural (i.e., pre-ference-based) units, any economic evaluation involving non-monetary outcomes is often termed CEA, regardless of whether natural or non-natural units have been used to describe the outcomes (Gold et al., 1996). In this chapter, we will use the term CEA in this broader sense.

CEA is particularly well designed to help identify the most efficient mix of interventions, where efficiency implies achieving the maximum amount of effec-tiveness with the resources available. When several cost-effectiveness ratios are presented together, this is often referred to as a "league table," because it resembles the rank ordering of sports teams by wins and losses.

Cost–benefit analysis (CBA) is the technique used when the consequences are measured in monetary terms. In CBA one subtracts the benefits that the inter-vention produces from the amount of resources required to implement the inter-vention (that is, the net cost of implementing the intervention). From the perspective of economic theory, CBA is the best-grounded technique (Pauly, 1995; Johannesson, 1996; Kenkel, 1997) and it allows for comparison of all types of interventions (e.g., within the injury field, across other health care-related fields, and across other fields such as education or housing). Despite this strength, CBA has had only limited influence in the health sector because of its requirement that an explicit monetary loss be assigned to premature death and health impair-ments. Many citizens, scientists, and policy makers consider this practice to be unscientific and/or unethical. For example, it has been noted that whether a health-related intervention is "worth its cost" is not an economic issue but "a moral and ethical issue" (Petitti, 1994). Consequently, CEA – in the broader definition of the term, has emerged as the dominant economic-evaluation technique in the evalua-tion of health-related interventions (Johannesson and Jonsson, 1991; Gold et al., 1996).

State-of-the-art Methods

An economic evaluation is typically performed from the societal perspective, which means that all costs and benefits of an intervention are counted, regardless of who in society is affected. It is also feasible to conduct evaluations from narrower perspectives, such as the accounting perspective of a managed care organization or the budgetary perspective of the Medicare program. Analyses undertaken from these targeted perspectives can be useful to specific decision makers but will not provide the overall insight that is provided by an evaluation undertaken from the societal perspective. It is important for any economic evaluator to state explicitly the perspective that is being taken.

The problem definition in economic evaluation goes beyond the choice of perspective. It entails specification of the particular morbidity, mortality, or disability outcomes that are of concern as well as the specific target population (e.g., age, gender, and geographic location) for analysis. The same intervention (e.g., seat belts) may offer fewer benefits for some target populations (e.g., rear-seat car occupants) than others (e.g., car drivers) because the baseline levels of injury risk vary enormously by target population and/or the effectiveness of the intervention is different (e.g., seat belt effectiveness on drivers vs. children).

Comparison of decision alternatives is essential to any evaluation. The costs and benefits of a particular intervention (e.g., an automobile air bag system) are not defined unless the comparator to the chosen intervention is defined (e.g., a manual lap/shoulder belt system). The same intervention may appear attractive or unattractive depending upon the comparator that is chosen. Thus, air bags may look like a better investment when applied to a vehicle with few safety features than when applied to a vehicle that already has numerous safety features. When evaluating a new technology or program, the standard practice in economic evaluation is to select the status quo (or current technology, treatment, or program) as the comparator.

The choice of comparator is a concept closely related to that of incremental analysis. An incremental analysis of alternatives needs to be conducted any time the economic evaluation compares more than two interventions that are not mutually exclusive. Suppose three alternatives are being considered to address fire-related injuries: no action, installation of smoke detectors, and installation of sprinkler systems. It may be the case that smoke detectors and sprinkler systems are each a good economic investment compared with no action. Yet that does not mean that it makes sense to purchase both systems. An incremental analysis needs to be undertaken that quantifies the extra (or additional or incremental) net cost and net benefit of doing both systems compared with doing only one system. The technical literature in economic evaluation has devised some fairly rigorous guidelines for how such incremental comparisons should be performed in order to achieve efficient investment strategies (Weinstein, 1995). It has been shown that a decision-making algorithm based on incremental CEA can be used to achieve the maximum amount of overall effectiveness with the resources available (Sloan, 1995; Weinstein, 1995; Gold et al., 1996).

The temporal issues that are important in an economic evaluation are the lifetime of the program or technology and the "analytic time horizon." Explicit assumptions must be made because these times typically differ. The useful life of a bicycle helmet may be 5 or 10 years. Yet an analysis of the benefits and costs of using bicycle helmets may require a much longer time horizon as, for example, the economic and quality-of-life impacts of head injuries may extend for the entire life of people who are injured in bicycle crashes.

When measuring the net cost of the intervention (the cost of the intervention minus the savings from the intervention), the governing principle will be one of opportunity cost. All resources used by the intervention (including the long run costs associated with the intervention and its effects) should be included. Resources that will be consumed regardless of adoption of the intervention should be excluded from the analysis. Market prices are (most frequently) used as they are presumed to reflect the marginal opportunity costs of labor and material resources. When market prices are neither available nor valid, shadow prices can be devised and used. Constant dollars are used when aggregating price information across time (removing any effects of general price inflation). In CEA, the net cost of the intervention becomes the numerator of the ratio; this numerator should not include productivity impacts (i.e., loss of capability of working) of the intervention to avoid double counting (Gold et al., 1996). In contrast, in CBA, productivity impacts of the intervention should be included and wages are used as a surrogate measure for the value of time for those in the labor force.

Sensitivity analyses of key inputs to the economic evaluation (e.g., the discount rate, effectiveness estimates, utility values) should be conducted to determine the degree of uncertainty in the results (i.e., uncertainty analysis). Additionally, information on any qualitative issues associated with an intervention that cannot be included in the analysis but may be of concern to policy makers (e.g., a target population with a disproportionate number of low-income or minority citizens which would bring into consideration equity arguments) should be presented. These issues are sometimes called intangible considerations (Mishan, 1994) and should be explicitly stated.

There are multiple textbooks that cover the technical aspects associated with the use of these techniques (Petitti, 1994; Johannesson, 1996; Drummond et al., 1997). Although most of these books have been written with a more generic application to health issues, there is no barrier to their application in the injury field. In 1994, the U.S. Department of Health and Human Services appointed an Expert Panel that recommended that analysts use standard practices when conducting CEA of public health and clinical interventions and proposed such standards (Gold et al., 1996). These standard practices cover how costs are defined and measured, how effectiveness is defined and quantified, why and how future costs and effectiveness are discounted to present value, and how cost-effectiveness ratios are computed and reported. (Table 19.2 summarizes these recommendations.) Adherence to these recommended practices can be expected to bring more rigor and consistency to economic evaluations. In the example that follows in this chapter, we follow fairly closely these standard practices.

Review of Injury-control Economic Evaluations

Only in rare occasions do injury prevention interventions lead to identical consequences; thus, cost-minimization analysis is seldom used. Indeed, we are not

Table 19.2 Summary of the steps required to perform a cost-effectiveness analysis

(1) Identify problem and promising intervention to evaluate.
(2) Identify alternative (or set of alternatives) against which to compare the intervention, including any incremental comparisons.
(3) Identify baseline data for the population of interest: mortality, morbidity, disability.
(4) Identify (incremental) effectiveness estimate(s): mortality, morbidity, disability.
(5) Identify (incremental) gross costs and savings costs.
(6) Control for inflation (if necessary) by computing constant dollars by using the Consumer Price Index.
(7) Discount future costs and savings at the same real discount rate.
(8) Compute the (incremental) number of fatalities, morbidity, and disability averted.
(9) Compute the discounted (incremental) number of years of life gained (by averting the fatalities).
(10) Compute the discounted (incremental) quality-adjusted life years gained (by averting morbidity and disability).
(11) Compute the discounted (incremental) total quality-adjusted years of life by adding the discounted (incremental) years of life gained and the discounted (incremental) quality-adjusted years gained.
(12) Compute the (incremental) costs of implementing the intervention.
(13) Compute the (incremental) savings in resource costs.
(14) Compute the net costs by subtracting the (incremental) savings in resource costs from the (incremental) costs of implementing the intervention.
(15) Compute the discounted (incremental) net costs.
(16) Compute the cost-effectiveness ratio by dividing the discounted (incremental) net cost by the discounted (incremental) total quality-adjusted years of life gained.
(17) Perform sensitivity analysis of important inputs such as effectiveness, discount rate, intervention cost, and utility values.

Adapted from: Gold et al., 1996.

aware of any peer-reviewed publication using this technique to evaluate an injury prevention intervention.

There is a burgeoning literature on economic evaluation (usually CEA) of interventions aimed at preventing or treating chronic and infectious diseases (Elixhauser, 1993). Yet, the literature on injury prevention is quite limited and is restricted primarily to the regulatory impact analyses of proposed rules issued by U.S. federal agencies such as the National Highway Traffic Safety Administration, Federal Aviation Administration, Consumer Product Safety Commission, and the Occupational Safety and Health Administration, and that are required by the Office of Management and Budget (OMB).

In a systematic review by Segui-Gomez et al. (in press) 54 studies were identified that reported information on the cost and effectiveness of 128 injury control interventions. Besides the fact that the use of the terminology (CEA, CBA) was very frequently inconsistent and/or inappropriate, the survey uncovered a similar problem that has emerged in the reviews of other economic evaluations of public health and medicine: inconsistent and poor analytical practices. In one-third of the reviewed papers, it was impossible to know what the viewpoint of the analysis was (i.e., whether societal, governmental, or other). Many different types and

Table 19.3 A league table of selected injury control interventions (1995 US$)

Intervention evaluated	Comparator	Target population	$ per LY	$ per QALY
Lap/shoulder belt (50% use)	No restraint	Drivers or front-right occupants (passenger vehicles)	< 0	< 0
Compulsory helmet use	Voluntary helmet use	Motorcyclist	< 0	< 0
Daytime running lights	Nighttime lights only	All motorvehicle occupants	< 0	< 0
Frontal air bags	Manual lap/shoulder belt (50% use)	Drivers (passenger cars)	24,000	96,000
Strengthened side door beams	Status quo	All occupants (light trucks)	53,000	160,000
Frontal air bags	Manual lap/shoulder belt (50% use)	Front-right occupant (passenger cars)	61,000	213,000
55 m.p.h speed limit	65 m.p.h. speed limit	Rural interstate travelers	82,000	220,000
Lap-only belts (9% use)	No restraint	Rear-center seat occupants	830,000	1,300,000
Lap/shoulder belts (9% use)	No restraint	Rear-center seat occupants	2,400,000	6,000,000

LY, Life-Year saved; QALY, Quality-Adjusted Life-Year saved.
Adapted from: Graham et al., 1998.

combinations of monetary cost savings and gross costs were identified, making any rigorous comparison of interventions impossible. The analytic treatment of the morbidity-reduction effects of the interventions was not comprehensive, and was far less detailed than the treatment of mortality-reduction effects, which emphasizes the need for valid outcome measures that encompass mortality and morbidity effects. There was substantial variation in discounting practices. Uncertainties (e.g., about effectiveness or costs) were either not quantified, or were addressed in a rudimentary manner (with sensitivity analysis of one or two parameters at a time), or were not addressed at all. Despite all these limitations, some of these analyses are particularly insightful illustrations of economic evaluation (Muler, 1980; Arnould and Gabrowski, 1981; Loeb and Gilad, 1982; Petak and Atkisson, 1982; Rodgers, 1985; Eastern Research Group, 1987). Other examples of more recent economic evaluations are Levy and Miller (1995) and Miller and Lestina (1997).

The first peer-reviewed CEA published using the Expert Panel recommendation was an evaluation of the incremental costs and benefits of driver- and passenger-side air bags compared to safety belts (Graham et al., 1997). The cost per year of life saved (LY) and quality-adjusted life years (QALY) saved from this evaluation are summarized in a league table (Table 19.3) together with other selected motor vehicle-related injury prevention interventions re-evaluated using the panel's recommendations (Graham et al., 1998).

The limited number of economic evaluations of injury prevention interventions reflects a variety of factors such as a lack of definitive information on the effectiveness of interventions and a lack of information on the costs of treating injuries – costs that might be averted if effective interventions were implemented. Furthermore, there has been a lack of methodology to combine mortality and nonfatal impairment information into a unified effectiveness scale. The cost-effectiveness evaluations reviewed reflect the lack of common methodology that would allow for comparison of their results.

An Illustrative Example

Imagine a society that is considering whether to mandate driver-side air bags in all new motor vehicles produced in the near future (10 million per year). If air bags are not mandated, it is assumed that the driver's fatality rate will be 125 cases per million vehicles per year. For each fatality, additional 15 severe, yet nonfatal, and 150 minor injuries are expected in the absence of air bags. We assume that this baseline rate of fatality and injury is spread evenly over a 10-year vehicle life (i.e., we follow 10 million vehicles for 10 years). We will use a 3% annual discount rate. We assume further that each fatality is associated with a loss of 23 discounted life years of full quality and that each significant and minor injury are associated with the loss of five and 0.01 discounted QALYs, respectively. In our example, these air bag systems are 10% effective in preventing fatal and significant nonfatal injuries, but increase the rate of minor nonfatal injuries by 50%.

We assume also that the driver air bag system costs $250 per vehicle and that the total lifetime injury-related treatment costs, discounted to present value, are $10,000 per fatality, $60,000 per significant injury, and $5000 per minor injury. The question then is, will there be any net resource savings to society due to the installation of these air bags? (The numbers presented next are rounded for simplicity purposes.)

The total gross discounted savings will equal $11 million for the fatality prevention ($10,000 \times 125 \times 0.10 \times 10$ years) – (with discounting) plus $990 million for the significant injury prevention ($60,000 \times 1875 \times 0.10 \times 10$ years), or a total gross savings of $1001 million. Yet the driver air bag will cause numerous minor injuries (9375 per year for 10 years) that will cost a total of $412 million to treat. Overall, the net costs of mandating the air bags will be $2.5 billion ($250 per air bag system $\times$ 10 million vehicles) minus the net savings in treatment costs ($589 million), or about $1.91 billion.

Although the driver air bag will not produce a net savings in resources in the economy (i.e., it is not a "cost saving" intervention), it may still be a reasonable investment in length and quality of life (Russell, 1986). The annual number of discounted life years saved will be 2875 (125×23), or a total of 24,848 for the 10 years of protection after discounting (i.e., 2875 + (2875 × 0.97) + (2875 × 0.94) + ⋯ + (2875 × 0.77)). The impact on nonfatal injuries includes a reduction in significant nonfatal injuries (1250 × 15 × 0.10 × 5), or 9375 QALYs saved per year of air bag protection, or a total of 82,406 QALYs saved over 10 years. A deduction must be made for the QALYs lost from minor injuries (1250 × 150 × 0.5 × 0.01 = 938 per year), which amount to a total loss of 8241 QALYs from air bag-induced minor injuries over 10 years. Overall, the total effectiveness of the driver air bag is 99,013 QALYs saved. It is worth noting here the distinction between the discounted life-years gained by preventing a fatality and the discounted QALYs lived after preventing the long-term consequences of a nonfatal injury.

The net cost-effectiveness ratio for the driver air bag (compared with the safety forecast with no air bag) is equal to the net resource costs ($1.91 billion) divided by the net number of QALYs saved (99,013), or about $19,290 per QALY saved ($19,000 when rounded). Interestingly, this hypothetical calculation is a close approximation to the finding of the recent cost-effectiveness evaluation of driver air bag systems in the United States referred to before (Graham et al., 1997).

Is $19,000 per QALY saved a large or small ratio? There is no correct answer to this question. One can only compare the ratio with the ratios for other interventions. For example, many well-accepted procedures in the prevention and treatment of heart disease and cancer have cost-effectiveness ratios in the range from $50,000 to $150,000 per QALY saved (calculated using the same procedures) (Table 19.3) (Tengs et al., 1995; Graham et al., 1998). Some economists, based on surveys and studies of the implicit preferences of consumers and workers, have estimated that the implicit value of a QALY saved is as high as $400,000 (Viscusi, 1993). Yet it may be preferable to treat a cost-effectiveness ratio as information that decision makers should consider in conjunction with other legal, political, and ethical information about the proposed air bag mandate.

Challenges Ahead

An economic evaluation is only as good as the input values that one uses for the analysis. Fortunately, scientific progress in recent years has made it possible to apply economic evaluation techniques to a variety of injury control interventions. Despite this encouraging progress, much work is needed in (1) better defining the effectiveness of interventions; (2) characterizing the costs of injuries; (3) describing alternative and more comprehensive outcome measures; (4) promoting standardization of the methodology; and (5) encouraging the training of researchers in this area.

First, more rigorous research needs to be conducted to evaluate the effectiveness of injury prevention interventions. Although relatively few injury control interventions have been evaluated through randomized clinical trials (for both ethical and practical reasons), a number of other methods (e.g., case–control, case crossover, time-series studies) can be (and are being) properly used in effectiveness research. Several chapters of this book contain references to this issue (see chapters 7–13, and 15).

Second, although a variety of investigators have made important contributions to our understanding of the costs of injuries, both the costs of treating injuries (from the emergency department to long-term care) and the productivity losses, consensus on the methods used to compute these costs needs to be achieved. To date, most of the research on the cost of injuries has been done in the context of motor vehicle injuries. Faigin (1975) produced the first major categories and estimates of motor vehicle-related injury costs. These costs have been updated regularly by the National Highway Traffic Safety Administration (Blincoe and Luchter, 1983; Blincoe and Faigin, 1992; Blincoe, 1996) and refined including long-term consequences and separating types and severity of injury (Smart and Sanders, 1976; Hartunian et al., 1981; MacKenzie et al., 1988a, b).

Rice and MacKenzie (1989) published the first comprehensive cost-of-injury study, including costs of injuries by age and sex, with breakdowns into six major cause categories: motor vehicle crashes, falls, firearms, fires/burns, poisonings, and near drowning. More recently, Miller (1993; Miller et al., 1995) provided the first U.S. cost information for nonfatal injury by body region, body part, and nature of injury (e.g., fracture, laceration). There is also a growing literature on the "pain and suffering" costs of injuries based on the willingness-to-pay method (Jones-Lee, 1985, 1995; Viscusi, 1993). These costs, while relevant to CBA, are not relevant to CEA (Gold et al., 1996), where the effectiveness measure (if a utility-based type of measure) is adjusted for impacts on personal well-being, such as pain and suffering.

Third, various utility-based scales and elicitation procedures have been developed that can be employed to combine information on mortality, morbidity, and sequelae into a single numerical index (Kaplan et al., 1976; Kaplan, 1982; Kind et al., 1982; Torrance, 1986). For example, using the time-tradeoff technique (one of the elicitation methods available), one might ask a citizen to decide how many years of life with good health are equivalent in value to 30 years confined to a wheelchair. If the citizen responded 15, then each year in a wheelchair would be assigned a utility value of 0.5 on a scale from 0 to 1.0, where 0 represents death (or the worst health state) and 1.0 represents good health. Thus, if all citizens in a community shared this opinion, a community intervention that saved 1000 life years and averted 500 wheelchair years would, using the utility scale, be said to save a total of 1250 (undiscounted) QALYs. These utility-based scales, while inherently subjective and a source of some controversy, are now frequently used in CEA of public health and medicine (Neumann et al., 1997)

The effort to combine information on mortality, morbidity and impairment due to injuries was initiated by Hirsch et al. (1983), while Carston and O'Day (1986) laid the groundwork for linking the Abbreviated Injury Scale (AAAM, 1990) values and measures of impairment (disutility). Luchter (1987), Miller et al. (1989), and Guria (1993) stimulated interest in the development of utility-based approaches to the valuation of nonfatal traffic injuries. Miller et al. (1995) published the first set of estimates of utility losses attributable to nonfatal injuries, taking into account previous research on limitations in physical capability due to injury, functional capacity losses (impairment), and disability at work and at home.

MacKenzie et al. (1996) through the development of the Functional Capacity Index (FCI) has advanced this work.

The FCI was conceptualized for application to patients of all ages but the initial application was only performed on middle-aged adults living in the United States who sustained only one injury and whose functional limitations lasted at least 1 year. Several projects are now underway to clinically validate the scale, refine the utility values, expand the scale to include pediatric and geriatric injuries, integrate multiple injuries, and encompass injuries with consequences that last less than 1 year. Future work should also explore the applicability of these U.S.-based utility values to other societies. Although more work on FCI is certainly appropriate, it is apparent that, compared with other utility-based scores used in the literature, the FCI is a relatively sophisticated and well-developed measure (Neumann et al., 1997).

Finally, methodologic consensus in the application of economic evaluation techniques is being widely promoted and encouraged (Gold et al., 1996; Drummond et al., 1997).

Given these recent scientific developments, the next years are an appropriate time for more researchers to seek proper training in the basic tenets of decision theory and economic evaluation, and to conduct economic evaluations of injury prevention interventions using comparable methods, good quality data, and valid assumptions. Without good-quality information on effectiveness and costs, it is difficult to make a convincing economic case in favor (or in opposition) to any specific injury prevention intervention.

References

Arnould RJ, Gabrowski H (1981) Auto safety regulation: an analysis of market failure. Bell J Econ 12:27–48.

Association for the Advancement of Automotive Medicine (1990) The Abbreviated Injury Scale. Des Plaines, IL:AAAM.

Blincoe LJ (1996) Plans and Policy. The Economic Cost of Motor Vehicle Crashes, 1994. DOT HS# 808 425. Washington, DC: National Highway Traffic Safety Administration.

Blincoe LJ, Faigin BM (1992) The Economic Cost of Motor Vehicle Crashes 1990. DOT HS# 807 876. Washington, DC: National Highway Traffic Safety Administration.

Blincoe LJ, Luchter S (1983) The Economic Cost of Motor Vehicle Accidents. DOT HS# 806 342. Washington, DC: National Highway Traffic Safety Administration.

Carston O, O'Day J (1986) Relationship of Accident Type to Occupant Injuries UMTRI 14–24.

Drummond, MF, O'Brien B, Stoddart GL, Torrance GW (1997) Methods for the Economic Evaluation of Health Care Programmes, 2nd edn. Oxford: Oxford University Press.

Eastern Research Group (1987) Economic Impact Analysis of the Proposed Revision of OSHA Subpart P Standard 1926. 650–652 Governing Trenching and Excavation Work. Arlington, MA: Eastern Research Group.

Elixhauser A, Luce BR, Taylor WR, Reblando J (1993) Health care CBA/CEA: An update on the growth and composition of the literature. Med Care 31:JS1–11.

Faigin B (1975) The Societal Costs of Motor Vehicle Accidents. Washington, DC: National Highway Traffic Safety Administration.

Gold MR, Siegel JE, Russell LB, Weinstein MC (1996) Cost-effectiveness in Health and Medicine. Oxford: Oxford University Press.

Graham JD, Thompson K, Goldie SJ, Segui-Gomez M, Weinstein MC (1997) The cost-effectiveness of airbags by seating position. JAMA 278:1418–25. Reply in (1998) JAMA 279:506–7.

Graham JD, Corso P, Morris J, Segui-Gomez M, Weinstein MC (1998) Evaluating the cost-effectiveness of clinical and public health measures. Annu Rev Public Health 19:125–52.

Guria JC (1993) The expected loss of life quality from traffic injuries requiring hospitalization. Accid Anal Prev 25:765–72.

Hartunian N, Smart C, Thompson M. (1981) The Incidence and Economic Costs of Major Health Impairments. Lexington, MA: Lexington Books.

Hirsch A, Eppinger R, Shame T, Nguyen R, Levine R, Machenzie J, Marks, M, Ommaya A (1983) Impairment scaling from the Abbreviated Injury Scale. DOT HS# 806 648. Washington, DC: National Highway Traffic Safety Administration.

Johannesson M (1996) Theory and Methods of Economic Evaluation of Health Care. Boston, MA: Kluwer Academic Publishers.

Johannesson M, Jonsson B (1991) Economic evaluation in health care: Is there a role for cost-benefit analysis? Health Policy 17:1–23.

Jones-Lee M, Hammerton M, Philips P (1985) The value of safety: results of a national survey. Econ J 95:49–72.

Jones-Lee M, Loomes G, Philips P (1995) Valuing the prevention of non-fatal road injuries: contingent valuation versus standard gambles. Oxford Econ Papers 47:676–95.

Kaplan RM, Bush JW, Berry CC (1976) Health status: Types of validity for an index of well being. Health Serv Res 10:478–507.

Kaplan RM (1982) Human preference measurement for health decisions and the evaluation of long-term care. In: Kane RL, Kane RA (eds), Values and Long-term Care Lexington, pp. 157–88. MA: Lexington Books.

Kind P, Rosser R, Williams A (1982) Valuation of quality-of-life: Some psychometric Evidence. In: Jones-Lee MW (ed.), The Values of Life and Safety, pp. 159–70. New York: North-Holland Publishing.

Kenkel (1997) On valuing morbidity, cost-effectiveness analysis and being rude. J Health Econ 16:749–57.

Levy DT, Miller TR (1995) A cost benefit analysis of enforcement efforts to reduce serving intoxicated patrons. J Stud Alcohol 56:240–7.

Loeb PD, Gilad B (1984) The efficacy and cost-effectiveness of vehicle inspection: a state-specific analysis using time series data. J Transport Econ Policy 18:145–64.

Luchter S (1987) The Use of Impairment for Establishing Accident Injury Research Priorities. SAE Paper Number 87-1078. Warrenton, PA: Society of Automotive Engineers.

MacKenzie E, Shapiro S, Siegel J (1988a). The economic impact of vehicular trauma: One-year treatment related expenditures. JAMA 260:3290–7.

MacKenzie E, Siegel J, Shapiro S, Moody M, Smith R. (1988b) Functional recovery and medical costs of trauma: An analysis by type and severity of injury. J Trauma 28:281–97.

MacKenzie EJ, Damiano AM, Miller T, Luchter S (1996) The development of the Functional Capacity Index. J Trauma 41:799–807.

Miller TR, Calhoun CC, Arthur WB (1989) Utility-adjusted Impairment Years: A Low-cost Approach to Morbidity Evaluation: Estimating and Valuing Morbidity in the Policy Context. Proceedings of the Association of Environmental and Resource Economists Workshop, Washington, DC.

Miller TR, Pindus NM, Douglass JB (1993) Medically related motor vehicle injury costs by body region and severity. J Trauma 34:270–5.

Miller TR, Pindus NM, Douglass JB, Rossman SB (1995) Databook on Nonfatal Injury: Incidence, Costs, and Consequences. Washington, DC: The Urban Institute Press.

Miller TR, Lestina D (1997) The costs of poisoning in the US and the savings from poison control centers: a benefit-cost analysis. Ann Emerg Med 29:239–45.

Mishan EJ (1994) Cost-Benefit Analysis, 4th edn. New York: Routledge.

Muler A (1980) Evaluation of the costs and benefits of motorcycle helmet laws. Am J Public Health 70:586–92.

Murray JL, Lopez AD (1996) The Global Burden of Disease: A comprehensive assessment of mortality and disability from diseases, injuries, and risk factors in 1990 and project to 2020. Cambridge, MA: Harvard University Press.

Neumann PJ, Zinner DE, Wright JC (1997) Are methods for calculating QALYs in cost-effectiveness analyses improving? Med Dec Making 17:402–8.

Pauly M (1995) Valuing health care benefits in monetary terms. In: Sloan FA (ed.), Valuing Health Care: Costs, Benefits, and Effectiveness of Pharmaceuticals and Other Medical Technologies, pp. 99–124. New York: Cambridge University Press.

Petak WJ, Atkisson AA (1982) Natural hazard mitigation costs and impacts. In: Natural Hazard Risk Assessment and Public Policy. New York: Springer-Verlag.

Petitti DB (1994) Meta-Analysis, Decision Analysis, and Cost-effectiveness Analysis: Methods of Quantitative Synthesis in Medicine. New York: Oxford University Press.

Rice DP, MacKenzie EJ (1989) Economic cost of injury. In: Red I (ed.) Cost of Injury in the United States: A Report to Congress. San Francisco, CA: Institute for Health & Aging, University of California and Injury Prevention Center, The Johns Hopkins University.

Rodgers GB (1985) Preliminary Economic Assessment of the Chain Saw Standard. Washington, DC: US Consumer Product Safety Commission, Division of Program Analysis, Directorate for Economic Analysis.

Russell LB (1986) Balancing cost and quality: methods of evaluation. Bull NY Acad Med 62:55–60.

Segui-Gomez M, Wright J, Graham J (In press) Economic evaluation of injury prevention interventions: The need for standardization. Accid Anal Prev.

Sloan FA (ed.) (1995). Valuing health care. Cost, Benefits and Effectiveness of Pharmaceuticals and Other Medical Technologies. New York: Press Syndicate of the University of Cambridge.

Smart C, Sanders CR (1976) The Costs of Motor Vehicle Related Spinal Cord Injuries. Report. Washington, DC: Insurance Institute for Highway Safety.

Tengs TO, Adams ME, Pliskin JS, Safran DG, Siegel JE, Weinstein MC, Graham JD (1995) Five hundred life-saving interventions and their cost-effectiveness. Risk Anal 15:369–90.

Torrance GW (1986) Measurement of health state utilities for economic appraisal: A review. J Health Econ 5:1–30.

US Preventive Task Force (1996) Guide to Clinical Preventive Services. Washington, DC: Department of Health and Human Services.

Viscusi W (1993) The value of risk to life and health. J Economic Literature 31:1912–46.

Weinstein MC, Stason WB (1977) Foundations of cost-effectiveness analysis for health and medical practices. N Eng J Med 296:716–21.

Weinstein MC (1995) From cost-effectiveness ratios to resource allocation: Where to draw the line? In: Sloan FA (ed.), Valuing Health Care: Cost, Benefits and Effectiveness of Pharmaceuticals and Other Medical Technologies, pp. 77–96. New York: Press Syndicate of the University of Cambridge.

20

Ethical Issues

Helen McGough and Marsha E. Wolf

Ethical Principles

Injury control research, like any other research involving the collection of information from or about human beings, is guided by ethical principles (International Guidelines for Ethical Review of Epidemiological Studies, 1991). These principles have evolved during the twentieth century beginning with the Nuremberg Code (US Government Printing Office, 1949) to the Helsinki Convention (World Medical Assembly, 1964, 1975) to the Belmont Report (National Commission for the Protection of Human Subjects of Biomedical and Behavioral Research, 1978) and including the International Conference on Harmonisation of Technical Requirements for Registration of Pharmaceuticals for Human Use (Baber, 1994). They include the principles of respect, beneficence, and justice.

The principle of respect, sometimes referred to as autonomy is the proposition that researchers should treat potential research subjects as autonomous and respect their choices. Individuals, for example, have the right to decide for themselves whether or not to become subjects of a human research experiment. The principle of respect also recognizes that some people may have limited autonomy because of developmental, chronic, or acute diminished capacity, and that they are entitled to special protections when they are asked to take part in research activities.

The principle of beneficence requires that the potential benefits to society of a research activity must outweigh the foreseeable risks to those who would be subjects of that research. Researchers are obligated by this principle to conduct their research so as to minimize the possible harm to subjects that may result and to maximize the potential benefits to individual subjects and to society.

The principle of justice requires researchers to select subjects equitably, so that all affected groups are represented in the subject population, and so that no one group of subjects is inappropriately or exclusively burdened with the risks of research. This principle protects subjects who may be vulnerable to coercion because of educational, social, or economic disadvantage, or who are members of a population of convenience from potential exploitation.

The process of informed consent is fundamental to the recognition and implementation of these principles. Robert J. Levine, in his classic text on the ethics of clinical research points out that research consent must be informative, comprehensible (presented in language understandable to the subject), voluntary (given without coercion), and be given by a person who is legally competent to do so (Levine, 1981).

Applying the Principles to Injury Control Research

While these principles and the concept of informed consent apply to all research involving human subjects, implementing them in the design of injury control research may be a particular challenge for several reasons. First, we think of these principles as applicable, for the most part, to research that tests experimental treatments of diseases. This kind of research typically involves subjects who are sick or injured and uses traditional clinical research methodologies such as randomization and placebo controls. Second, clinical research is often conducted in traditional health-care settings where there is direct interaction between the researchers and subjects. Injury control research, however, may involve healthy control subjects as well as injured cases. It may use research methodologies such as random digit dialing, snowball recruitment, and linkage of data sets (see chapters by Mueller; Runyan and Bowling; and Grossman and Rhodes, this volume). It may be conducted in non-clinical settings and may involve no interaction between the researchers and the subjects. Third, when injury research is conducted in the clinical setting, it may involve human subjects whose competence to provide informed consent is compromised, requiring non-traditional consent procedures such as proxy consent or waived consent.

Another challenge is evaluating the risks peculiar to injury control research. While most clinical research involves relatively predictable and ideally remediable risks, injury control research often results in risks of harm to privacy and confidentiality – harms that are less predictable and often irremediable. The researcher's tasks are to evaluate both the probability of these risks as well as their magnitude, to minimize both to the fullest extent possible, and to insure that the potential benefits of the research to individual subjects and society outweigh the risks to individual subjects.

Three topics emerge as particularly important ethical considerations in injury control research: the protection of vulnerable subjects, variations on the informed consent process, and maintaining the confidentiality of research data. We will examine each of these topics in the context of injury control research and provide examples of the ethical issues involved in each.

Protection of Subjects

Because of the nature of injury research, potential research participants of interest often include vulnerable populations who are victims of trauma and violence. The types of vulnerable populations in injury research include: victims of intimate partner violence, cognitively impaired subjects, critically injured trauma patients, minors, incarcerated persons or ones involved in illegal activities, and non-English or non-native speakers. In conducting research with these vulnerable populations, injury researchers need to ensure adequate protection and make ethical decisions and study policies that consider the legal/moral, safety, psychoemotional, and social aspects of the vulnerable potential participant. The following sections will describe some of the ethical risks and what researchers can do to minimize them. We have chosen to discuss the research involving victims of intimate partner violence in greater detail because of the wide range of issues involved, some of which are applicable to other vulnerable groups.

Victims of Intimate Partner Violence

Protection of victims of intimate partner violence presents several ethical challenges to the injury researcher (Chalk and King, 1998). One aspect of planning a study on intimate partner violence is to develop and implement detailed study protocols regarding subject recruitment, data collection, data storage, subject reimbursement, and emergency procedures that address the important issues of safety and confidentiality and help minimize risk to the research participant and study staff. For example, with subject recruitment, study materials are not mailed to potential subjects without verifying in advance if it is a safe mailing address regardless of whether the subject is currently involved with the abusive partner or not. Safety measures for the study may include features that help ensure office location and phone numbers are not easily traced or obtained by a potentially violent partner of a participant. In addition, safety and confidentiality issues must be balanced while keeping the participant informed even though this balance may come in conflict. For example, emergency protocols which may necessitate breaching confidentiality are developed if the staff become concerned about the immediate safety of a participant. At the onset of the study, the participant is informed these measures may be implemented if necessary. For example, at the start of a telephone interview a study participant is told that if the interviewer becomes concerned about the safety of the participant (i.e., hearing shouting or a struggle) or the phone is disconnected and the interviewer cannot reach the participant after calling back immediately, then the study staff will break confidentiality for the safety of the participant and call the police. The confidential nature of the study is important not only for safety reasons, but also for social reasons. For example, the name used for the study in official mail or telephone correspondence should be general and not identifiable as a domestic violence study. This protects the participant not only from the abuser, but also protects confidentiality and privacy from co-workers, neighbors, or others.

Victims of intimate partner violence are also vulnerable because of their psychological–emotional state. The desire to achieve a high response rate for scientific validity is balanced with the respect for the potential participant to make an independent choice to participate without undue pressure or coercion. The interview may be emotionally distressing to a victim. As part of the informed consent the participant is informed in advance about the content and nature of the questions to be asked as well as the right to stop the interview at any time. In anticipation of possible emotional distress, the opportunity to provide the participant with resources or a referral if the need arises are included in the study protocol.

Although there is the risk of emotional distress, some subjects may actually find participation a positive and empowering act (Hutchinson et al., 1994).

Cognitively Impaired or Critically Injured Patients

Cognitively impaired injury research subjects may include head injured or critically injured patients whose impairment may be acute (short-term) or chronic (long-term). Injury researchers determine whether the potential subject is competent to consent to the research study (US President's Commission for the Study of Ethical Problems in Medicine and Biomedical and Behavioral Research, 1983; Drane, 1985; Bonnie, 1997). If the patient is not competent, the investigator needs to address the legal issue of who can provide informed consent for the subject (US Department of Health and Human Services, 1992). In addition, researchers must be sensitive to and respect the psychological–emotional state of the subjects and their family members in timing the contact with families for recruitment of their relatives into a study. Proxy consent and waiver of consent for research in emergency settings are discussed in a later section of this chapter. With cognitively impaired subjects, researchers also need to clarify their role with regard to local reporting obligations of specified medical conditions to driver's license agencies and inform subjects or their legally authorized representatives of these requirements.

Minors

Research involving children who are minors involves additional ethical considerations and regulations as set forth in the National Commission Report (National Commission for the Protection of Human Subjects of Biomedical and Behavioral Research, 1977). Inclusion of minors in studies often involves obtaining permission (not consent) from their parents or legal guardians as minors typically cannot give legal consent (Leikin, 1996). However, the principle of respect is applied to minors by providing them with the choice of assent, the affirmative agreement to participate in a study. The determination of whether to offer minors the opportunity for assent is based on the combination of age, psychological state, and maturity to make an informed decision. Adolescents are not addressed separately in regulations on minors. Mammel and Kaplan (1995) reported a broad range of practices in the United States concerning parental consent and minor assent for adolescents. A waiver of parental permission may be allowed if the major risk of harm from the study results from contact with the parents, as for example, in studies of child abuse and homelessness (English, 1991). Depending on the nature and content of the study and the age and developmental stage of the children, the most appropriate or reliable sources of information for the study may be the children and/or the parent (Kim and Spivey, 1994; Zinner, 1995; Silkand et al., 1997). No matter which family member is the source, the data collected are confidential and cannot be shared with others, including other members of the family without the source's permission. Suspected cases of child abuse may require breach of confidentiality and reporting to proper authorities according to the law as discussed in a later section on reporting obligations.

Incarcerated Persons

Injury patients are sometimes incarcerated because of activities such as use of illegal drugs, assault, or driving while intoxicated. The federal regulations protecting human research subjects include special protections for prisoners (US Department of Health and Human Services, 1992). An incarcerated person is a vulnerable research subject with regard to the principle of respect and autonomy to choose. Research involving prisoners needs to meet certain requirements and an advocate or representative for incarcerated subjects needs to be present when the study undergoes ethical review.

Persons Involved in Possibly Illegal Activities

Injury research subjects may have been involved in illegal activities (such as use of illegal drugs or assault) at the time they were injured. In addition, past illegal activities may be revealed during the study data collection. The data these subjects provide as part of the study are considered confidential unless the activity (such as child or elder abuse) is one that must, by law, be reported. The related moral issue is discussed in a subsequent section on Reporting Obligations.

Non-native Speaking Subjects

Immigrants or non-native speaking persons may be at high-risk for some kinds of injuries because of membership in high risk occupational groups or lack of information or access to injury interventions such as bicycle helmets or smoke detectors. Thus as a corollary of the principle of justice, efforts are necessary to include non-native speaking subjects as part of a representative sample of subjects for studies on some injury topics. However, the injury researcher has the obligation not to make an undue burden to these subjects and an obligation to make the consent and interview comprehensive by using a trained translator for verbal or written translation. Respect for privacy and cultural sensitivity are needed in choosing appropriate interpreters. For example, it is usually inappropriate to use a family member or friend of the subject as an interpreter if the information to be conveyed is private. For research conducted outside of the cultural realm in which the researcher is at home, careful training in neutrality and confidentiality must be provided to local research assistants who will have contact with subjects.

Informed Consent

Written Consent

Obtaining and maintaining the consent of research subjects is a continuous process. The process must include elements that assure the subject is informed about the purpose, procedures, risks, and potential benefits of the research. Customarily, it begins with a signed and dated agreement between a researcher and research subject – the consent form – written in language that is understandable to the subject. The process continues with regular discussions between the researchers and subjects to make sure that the latter continue to be informed about the research and its risks and continue to be willing to participate. The consent form is valuable for both the researcher and the research subject. For the former, it is evidence of when and by whom consent was obtained from the subject. For the subjects, the consent form serves not only this evidentiary function, but is also a relatively permanent reminder about what they agreed to do, and whom to contact when they have questions or in the case of a research-related adverse event. Although written informed consent is the gold standard, other kinds of consent are permissible under certain circumstances.

Implied or Veto Consent

In many kinds of injury control research written informed consent is not practicable, possible, or necessary. For example, suppose data will be collected through a mailed questionnaire. If appropriate measures have been taken to reduce the risks of invasion of privacy and breach of confidentiality and the activity does not include the collection of personally identifiable information, implied consent may be appropriate. This technique involves including the necessary elements of informed consent in a cover letter or introductory paragraph, including the reminder that participation is voluntary. A returned questionnaire implies that the subject consented to take part in the study. Veto consent offers potential subjects the opportunity to withdraw from the study after the data have been collected. Re-contacting nonresponders may be possible if the initial contact material includes both an explanation of plans to re-contact (If we don't hear from you by the end of two weeks we will send you another copy of this questionnaire), and an opportunity to decline further invitations (If you don't want us to contact you again, please leave a message at our toll-free number).

Researchers who wish to work with minor subjects are required to obtain parental permission before doing so. When the risks of the research to the child and family are minimal, parental permission may also be implied. For example, when a nonsensitive survey of adolescents is administered in a school setting, the researcher may send a letter to the parents explaining the study and asking only for a response from those parents who do not want their children to participate in the study. Such arrangements will require, of course, approval from the local ethics review committee.

Oral Consent

Suppose that data will be collected through telephone interviews. Again, assuming the risks of the study qualify as minimal, oral consent may be perfectly reasonable. Researchers who use an oral consent procedure are obligated to convey the elements of consent orally to the subject and to document in their records how and when the consent was given. The ethical principle of respect is upheld through use of a consent mechanism that assures that subjects are informed and have the right to decline to participate.

With both oral and written consent, one of the most important goals is using language that is understandable to the target population. Meeting this goal may require that the researcher employ professional translators or interpreters, and drafters who are familiar with the subjects' culture or subculture. Understanding the nuances of oral and written language is crucial to the success of truly informed consent.

Proxy or Surrogate Consent

Most government regulations allow researchers to obtain consent either from the subject or the subject's legally authorized representative (US Department of Health and Human Services, 1992). Proxy consent would be appropriate in a variety of research circumstances. Examples include: research on trauma in which the subject is not conscious at the time of data collection, and research involving decisionally impaired subject populations. Unless local jurisdiction or policy prohibits this arrangement, researchers may enroll subjects who are not competent to provide informed consent because of acute, developmental, or chronic conditions, if a legally authorized representative (LAR) is available and gives permission. Local jurisdiction will provide a list, in descending order, of people (usually related to the subject) eligible to provide proxy consent. Usually, researchers do not need to ask a court to declare who shall be the LAR. Consenting requirements for the LAR are the same as for the actual subject, although in cases of acute conditions, researchers should bear in mind that the LAR may be under considerable stress and may be, in fact, unable to act as a proxy decision-maker. While human subjects protection regulations do not usually address this issue, researchers should be aware that there are different bases on which proxy decisions are made. The proxy decision-makers may determine what is in the best interests of the subject, or may make the decision on the basis of what they believe the subject would have wanted (Gutheil and Applebaum, 1983). The differences are especially important when the incompetent subject is expected to regain competence during or after the research activity. In that case, the subjects themselves must give consent for continued participation in the study.

Waiver of Consent

Suppose, however, that the research is based on data from public or nonpublic sources of information about individuals or groups. The question is, how can the researcher collect (and even link) information about people without their explicit consent and still uphold the ethical principle of respect? The U.S. regulations protecting human research subjects (US Department of Health and Human Services, 1992) allow the research ethics review committee [Institutional Review Board (IRB)] to waive some or even all the elements of informed consent under certain circumstances. First, the research activity must pose no more than minimal risk to the subjects. Minimal risk is defined as "the probability and magnitude of harm or discomfort anticipated in the research are not greater in and of themselves than those ordinarily encountered in daily life or during the performance of routine physical or psychological examinations or tests" (US Department of Health and Human Services, 1992). Second, the researcher should be able to demonstrate that the research could not practically be done without the waiver. This qualification is intimately tied to the risk–benefit evaluation of the research project. The issues of the feasibility, cost, and time required to obtain informed consent must be balanced against the risks of invasion of privacy and breach of confidentiality. Third, the waiver must not adversely affect the rights and welfare of subjects. The usual interpretation of this qualification is that the data could not be used to deny rights or benefits to which the subjects would be otherwise entitled. Health services research on benefits programs whose results may be used to eliminate such programs poses ethical concerns, and might disqualify such a project from using a waiver of consent. Fourth, the researcher should, where appropriate, provide information to subjects after their participation (US Government Printing Office, 1993). The difficulty here is determining when postparticipation information to subjects is appropriate, how this information should be delivered, and what to do if subjects express concern over having been included as a research subject without a priori consent. If the IRB is able to determine that the research meets these qualifications and that the benefits of the activity outweigh the risks, a waiver of consent may be in order. Consideration must also be given when requesting a waiver of consent, however, to local, state, or other governmental regulations, which may supersede the authority of an IRB to waive consent.

Emergency Medicine Waiver

In 1996, the U.S. regulations were changed to allow IRBs to grant consent waivers to researchers conducting research in emergency settings that poses more than minimal risk to subjects. The additional conditions the researchers must satisfy before the waiver is allowed include: consultation with and public disclosure to the communities in which the research will be conducted and from which the subjects will be drawn about plans for the study and its risks and benefits; public disclosure of the results of the study after completion; establishment of an independent data monitoring committee for the study; and procedures in place to inform each subject, or the subjects' legally authorized representative of the subjects' inclusion in the study, of the details of the study, of the information contained in the consent form, and that either may decide to discontinue participation at any time. Researchers requesting a waiver of informed consent for studies involving an investigational drug or device must obtain a unique investigational new drug application (IND) or investigational drug exemption (IDE) from the U.S. Food and Drug Administration (FDA) even if an IND or IDE for the intervention already exists.

Confidentiality of Data

The ethical issue of respect also comes in to play with regard to confidentiality and sharing of data. Research data may be obtained by a variety of methods, whether primary or secondary data, and from public and nonpublic sources. However, obtaining and linking injury research data can present ethical challenges for maintaining confidential and secure data as discussed in the following sections.

Public Information

The use of public information (e.g., information from telephone books, the publicly available portions of birth records, death records, driver registration, voter registration, U.S. Census data, and Centers for Disease Control data) is not considered to be subject to the U.S. regulations protecting human research subjects (US Department of Health and Human Services, 1992). While this implies that consent is not required, it is important to remember that even uses of public information may result in risks of harms or wrongs to individuals and to communities. Publication of data comparing the dropout rates from high school between two ethnically distinct neighborhoods may lead to stigmatization of the ethnic groups, decisions not to locate new businesses in those neighborhoods, and decreased ability of the neighborhood governing body to obtain loans. The moral burden lies on the researcher to anticipate these problems and to minimize the risk of their occurrence.

Nonpublic Information

Nonpublic information includes data from medical records, records of psychiatric, drug, and alcohol treatment, school records, police records, the nonpublic portions of birth and death certificates, or any other individually identifiable information that a person can reasonably expect to be treated confidentially. The ethical issue is how to balance the need to protect individuals' privacy with the need to conduct research to protect the public health. Much records-based injury prevention research could not be conducted if the researchers were required to obtain informed consent from each of the individuals whose records are part of the database. The resolution of this dilemma lies in the careful analysis of the risk-benefit ratio posed by each research project by the ethics review committee. The evaluation of risks of harms and wrongs hinges largely on the steps that the researcher plans to take to minimize the possibility of invasion of privacy, breach of confidentiality, and potential misuse of the published data.

Sharing Data

There are several ethical issues associated with sharing study information. One problem encountered is when the researcher obtains data from other databases (public or nonpublic) to link with study data. Is it ethical for a researcher to reveal the subjects' identities in order to retrieve data about them from another source of data (e.g., criminal history data from courts or emergency room visits for the study population of police-identified domestic violence victims)? Revealing identifiers to an agency unconnected with the research may constitute both an invasion of privacy and a breach of confidentiality. If consent was obtained for the collection of data for one particular purpose, is it ethical to share those data with a colleague who wishes to link them with another source of information or use them for a different purpose? The answer for both questions depends largely on the conditions under which the data were collected, whether or not the data are identifiable, an evaluation of the risks posed by the proposed new use of the data, and the experience of the agencies involved in dealing with confidential data. The utility of the data may be inversely related to the level of protections available to the subject. Sharing identifiable, sensitive data poses the highest level of risk to the subjects; aggregate data with no identifiers poses the least risk. An additional issue is use of the researcher's already collected and linked data for a different research purpose than the original one. This secondary use of data is allowable if adequate protections are made for maintaining confidentiality of the data and necessary steps are taken for obtaining approval from the human subjects review board or the proper authority for this secondary, but new research purpose.

Protections

Fortunately, there are several avenues available to researchers to minimize these risks. The most effective way to protect against breach of confidentiality is to strip the data of all identifiers or links to identifiers as soon as possible after the data have been collected and linked. If it is necessary to retain identifiers (e.g., in longitudinal studies), the use of encryption and coding methodologies, which have become quite sophisticated over the past two decades, is recommended. It is important to recognize that identifiers include not only items like subject's name, hospital number, Social Security number, insurance claim number, telephone number, or address, but some compilations of demographic information may also serve as inadvertent identifiers. Deductive disclosure may result when unique information (ethnicity, age, gender, occupation, education, birth order, and so forth) is revealed during a study. Making sure that enough cases are represented in one cell (e.g., by aggregating age) may minimize this risk. Other standard operating procedures (such as keeping hard copy and computerized data in secured locations, conducting interviews in private, using letterhead and telephone scripts that do not immediately reveal the purpose of the study until a bona fide subject has been identified, compensating subjects with cash or checks made out to cash) can also minimize the chances that individuals will be harmed or wronged by their participation.

Government agencies may issue confidentiality protections for research data in the form of protective statues, confidentiality agreements, or certificates of confidentiality. For example, the specific federal government agencies may issue Certificates of Confidentiality to researchers collecting sensitive individually identifiable data, regardless of the source of the funding for the research (NIH Office of Extramural Research, 1998). These agreements are designed to protect the researcher from revealing individually identifiable data in response to a subpoena or court order. The certificates and agreements, however, are only as strong as the willingness and the ability of the researcher and the researcher's institution to enforce them.

Reporting Obligations

A common concern in injury control research is the apparent conflict between the moral obligation to protect data from disclosure and the legal obligation to report to governmental agencies information about subjects such as harm to self or others and abuse of children or elders. While a certificate of confidentiality may provide the researcher with legal protections against releasing such information to the appropriate authority, researchers also have the moral obligation to protect their subjects from harming themselves, from harming others, or from being harmed by others. The resolution of this conflict lies in discussing the protections available to protect identifiable information from disclosure and the moral obligation to report dangerous or illegal behavior with subjects before they decide whether or not to take part in the research project. Researchers may object to this discussion, fearing that subjects may be more likely to refuse to take part in the study if they know that information they reveal about themselves and others may be reported to governmental authorities. On the other hand, this discussion not only upholds the principle of respect, but may also buttress the rapport that researchers try to develop with subjects by establishing an open and honest communication from the beginning.

It is incumbent upon the researcher conducting injury control studies to emphasize the confidential nature of the study to the participant as well as reveal the obligation to report harmful behavior. For example, in most jurisdictions, the law requires reporting cases of suspected abuse of children or developmentally disabled or vulnerable adults or harm to self or others to the proper authorities. After notifying the authorities, the researcher may want to give courtesy notification to the study participant. Although the proper authorities may have been contacted and the legal requirement met by the researcher, if the first agency does not seem responsive (e.g., a child protection agency), then the researcher may also want to contact another proper authority such as the police. Additionally, clarification of these reporting obligations and the challenging related ethical issues may need to be explored in a supportive manner with the study staff involved in the implementation of these procedures.

Conclusions

Communication is key to the ethical conduct of injury control research – communication with the research subjects first and foremost, but also with the ethical review committee, the study sponsor, and those peripherally involved in the research – law enforcement agencies, manufacturers, employers, insurance companies, and other stakeholders. The highest quality research will emerge from an open dialogue about the research and an agreement among all parties that, although there are inevitable risks, the research is worth conducting. Our discussion of the ethical challenges should not be seen as limiting injury control research, but as assisting the researcher in dealing with these issues.

Additional Resources

The National Institutes of Health Office of Extramural Research maintains a web site at http://www.nih.gov/grants/oprr/library_human.htm which has many useful materials on this topic including regulations, guidelines, sample documents, and some of the references cited in this chapter.

References

Baber N (1994) International Conference on Harmonisation of Technical Requirements for Registration of Pharmaceuticals for Human Use (ICH). Br J Pharmacol 37(5):401–4.
Bonnie RJ (1997) Research With Cognitively Impaired Subjects: Unfinished Business in the Regulation of Human Research. Arch Gen Psychiatry 54(2):105–11.
Chalk R, King PA (eds), (1998) Violence In Families: Assessing Prevention and Treatment Programs. Washington, DC: National Academy Press.
Drane J (1985) The many faces of competency. Hastings Center Report 15:17–21.
English A (1991) Runaway and street youth at risk for HIV infection: legal and ethical issues in access to care. J Adolesc Health 12(7):504–10.
Gutheil TG, Applebaum PS (1983) Substituted judgment: best interests in disguise. Hastings Center Report 13(3):8–11.
Hutchinson SA, Wilson ME, Wilson HS (1994) Benefits of participating in research interviews. Image, J Nurs Scholarship 26(2):161–4.
International Guidelines for Ethical Review of Epidemiological Studies (1991) Law Med and Health Care 19(3–4):247–58.
Kim DT, Spivey WH (1994) A retrospective analysis of institutional review board and informed consent practices in EMS research. Ann Emerg Med 23(1):759–60.
Leikin S (1996) Ethical issues in epidemiologic research with children. In: Coughlin SS, Beauchamp TL (eds), Ethics and Epidemiology, pp. 197–218. New York: Oxford University Press.
Levine RJ (1981) Ethics and Regulation of Clinical Research, pp. 98–9. New Haven: Yale University Press.
Mammel KA, Kaplan DW (1995) Research consent by adolescent minors and institutional review boards. J Adolesc Health 17(5):323–30.
National Commission for the Protection of Human Subjects of Biomedical and Behavioral Research (1977) Research Involving Children: Report and Recommendations. DHEW Pub. No. (OS) 77-0004 (Appendix), and DHEW Pub. No. (OS) 77-0005. Washington, DC.
   (1978) The Belmont Report: Ethical Principles and Guidelines for the Protection of Human Subjects of Research. DHEW Pub. No. (OS) 78-0012. Washington, DC.
NIH Office of Extramural Research (1998) Certificate of confidentiality: privacy protection for research subjects. In: OPRR Human Subject Protections: Guidance Documents by Topic. Web Address: http://www/nih.gov/grants/oprr/humansubjects/guidance/certconpriv.htm
Silkand A, Schubiner H, Simpson PM (1997) Parent and adolescent perceived need for parental consent involving research with minors. Arch Pediatr Adolesc Med 151(6):603–7.
US Department of Health and Human Services (1992) Protection of human subjects: Title 45, Code of Federal Regulations, part 46, revised June 18, 1991. Bethesda, MD: Department of Health and Human Services, NIH, OPRR.
US Government Printing Office (1949) Trials of War Criminals before the Nuremberg Military Tribunals Under Control Council Law 10(2): pp. 181–2. Washington, DC.
   (1993) Protecting Human Research Subjects: Institutional Review Board Guidebook. Washington, DC.
US President's Commission for the Study of Ethical Problems in Medicine and Biomedical and Behavioral Research (1983) Making Health Care Decisions: The Ethical and Legal Implications of Informed Consent in the Patient–Practitioner Relationship. Washington, DC: US Government Printing Office.

World Medical Assembly (adopted and revised by) (1964 and 1975) World Medical Association Declaration of Helsinki: Recommendations Guiding Medical Doctors in Biomedical Research Involving Human Subjects. Helsinki, Finland: adopted by the 18th World Medical Assembly, and Tokyo, Japan: revised by the 29th World Medical Assembly.

Zinner SE (1995) The elusive goal of informed consent by adolescents. Theor Med 16(4):323–31.

Index